AF545200

123,90

50 12/87

oRg.

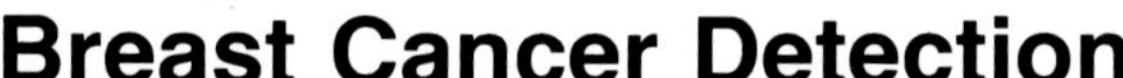

Breast Cancer Detection

Breast Cancer Detection

Mammography and Other Methods in Breast Imaging

Second Edition

Edited by

Lawrence W. Bassett, M.D.

Associate Professor of Radiological Sciences
UCLA School of Medicine and
Jonsson Comprehensive Cancer Center at UCLA
Director, The Iris Cantor Mammography Screening Clinic
Los Angeles, California

Richard H. Gold, M.D.

Professor of Radiological Sciences
UCLA School of Medicine and
Jonsson Comprehensive Cancer Center at UCLA
Los Angeles, California

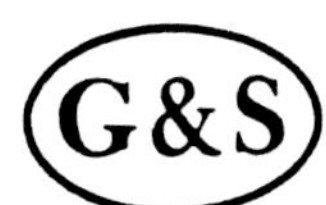

Grune & Stratton, Inc.
Harcourt Brace Jovanovich, Publishers
Orlando New York San Diego London
San Francisco Tokyo Sydney Toronto

Library of Congress Cataloging-in-Publication Data

Breast cancer detection.

Rev. ed. of: Mammography, thermography, and ultrasound in breast cancer detection. c1982.
Includes bibliographies and index.
1. Breast—Cancer—Diagnosis. 2. Diagnostic imaging. I. Bassett, Lawrence W. (Lawrence Wayne), 1942– II. Gold, Richard H. III. Mammography, thermography, and ultrasound in breast cancer detection. [DNLM: 1. Breast Neoplasms—diagnosis. 2. Mammography. 3. Thermography. 4. Ultrasonics—diagnostic use. WP 870 B825]
RC280.B8B678 1987 616.99′4490754 87-7580
ISBN 0-8089-1842-7

Grune & Stratton, Inc.
Orlando, Florida 32887

Distributed in the United Kingdom by
Grune & Stratton, Ltd.
24/28 Oval Road, London NW 1

Library of Congress Catalog Number
International Standard Book Number 0-8089-1842-7
Printed in the United States of America
87 88 89 90 10 9 8 7 6 5 4 3 2 1

This book
is dedicated to the memory of
Andrew H. Dowdy, M.D., D.Sc. (1904–1976),
father of mammography at UCLA, and
Stafford L. Warren, M.D. (1896–1981),
pioneer in mammography.

Contents

Acknowledgments

We are indebted to Wanda Batiste and Youlanda Mitchell, our chief mammography technologists. They personify the qualities needed in dedicated mammography technologists and were instrumental in collecting many of the cases presented in this book.

We are also very grateful to Mary Frazier, our secretary, for her invaluable assistance and dedication to the completion of this book.

Foreword

Cancer of the breast is the major health problem of women. Although new knowledge has led to a changing philosophy in its management, one factor remains of undisputed importance: early diagnosis. If the diagnosis is made while the cancer is still silent or occult, it may be treated by conservative surgical measures, with or without additive radio- or chemotherapy, with favorable short-term results. The long-term results of these measures are still to be determined.

In the routine examination of asymptomatic women and in screening programs, several diagnostic tools assume importance. Breast self-examination (BSE) is the simplest of these tools, but unfortunately only about 20 percent of women instructed in BSE perform it regularly. Physical examination by a professional has limitations in identifying early lesions; in the Breast Cancer Detection Demonstration Projects (BCDDP), only 6 percent of minimal cancers (less than 1 cm in diameter or in situ) were detected by physical examination alone. The remaining minimal cancers were identified either by mammography alone (57 percent) or by both mammography and physical examination (37 percent). This clearly illustrates the vital role of mammography in the early detection of breast cancer.

Mammography remains the most valuable technique of breast imaging. With a new generation of dedicated mammography equipment, the theoretical risk of radiation-induced cancers is now so low that it can hardly be considered of importance provided that high image quality is maintained. With ongoing improvements such as increased sensitivity of image receptors, more uniform and effective breast compression, and possibly digital mammography, the effectiveness of mammography as a diagnostic tool should be further improved.

Although ultrasonography is of particular value in differentiating cystic from solid lesions, it has not been effective in identifying cancers less than 1 cm in diameter. With further experience and advances in equipment, improvements may be forthcoming in both hand-held real-time ultrasonography and automated whole breast ultrasonography.

Thermography was proved not to be effective in breast cancer detection in the BCDDP, and was discontined after the second year of the five-year program. Transillumination light-scanning is of quesitonable value. Magnetic resonance imaging has yet to be established as a practical diagnostic tool for breast cancer detection. All of the aforementioned methods of imaging except x-ray mammography require further development and evaluation to determine their place in the diagnosis and screening of asymptomatic women.

The cost of breast imaging needs to be carefully considered. The benefit of decreased mortality derived from the annual screening of women age 50 and older by mammography and physical examination has been firmly established by the Health Insurance Plan (HIP) of Greater New York. The BCDDP data implies that mammography and physical examination are also of value in screening women age 40 to 49. However, high cost remains a major adverse factor in the widespread use of mammography for screening purposes.

The authors, in preparing this text on the state of the art of breast imaging, have fairly and accurately presented the relative merits and limitations of the imaging methods currently available. Most importantly, they have emphasized that mammography makes possible the early detection of breast cancer, offering the patient the most favorable prognosis and the highest quality of life.

Oliver H. Beahrs, M.D.

Preface

Since the appearance of the first edition of this textbook, the field of breast imaging has continued its remarkably rapid evolution. X-ray mammography has finally gained recognition as the single most successful technique for the detection of early, clinically occult breast cancer. Ultrasonography has undergone a realistic appraisal, leading to its current position as a practical adjunct to mammography and physical examination, useful for the determination of the cystic or solid nature of a mass, but not for breast cancer screening. Lightscanning and magnetic resonance imaging, two newer modalities that do not produce ionizing radiation, are still undergoing preliminary evaluation to determine their usefulness for breast cancer detection. Progress in breast thermography seems to have come to a standstill, the modality having been found to be generally ineffective in the detection of clinically occult cancer. Because thermography is still in use, although on the wane, we have again chosen to include it.

Part I of this new edition discusses breast imaging. Section 1 brings together all of the imaging techniques that are later to be discussed in detail, presenting the state of the art and possible future directions for each of them.

The principles of mammographic diagnosis are presented in Section 2. As in the first edition, we have placed major emphasis on the signs of early cancer. For this new edition, some mammographic illustrations have been added, some replaced with better examples, others enlarged, and still others augmented with histology in order to further elucidate the x-ray findings.

Section 3 highlights alternate methods of performing mammography. Experts in each technology discuss the advantages and limitations of their method.

In Section 4, convincing evidence is presented that screening mammography can consistently detect significant numbers of subclinical cancer and can reduce breast cancer mortality, and that these benefits far surpass any hypothetical risk.

Part II presents the technique, interpretation, advantages, and drawbacks of breast thermography, ultrasound, lightscanning, and magnetic resonance imaging by experts in these fields.

We hope that this new edition will again prove useful to diagnostic radiologists interested in breast cancer detection, especially those who are seeking guidance in mammographic interpretation and in the selection of breast imaging equipment.

Contributors

Franklin S. Alcorn, M.D.

Senior Attending in Diagnostic Radiology
Director of Mammography
Rush-Presbyterian St. Luke's Medical Center
Chicago, Illinois

Royal J. Bartrum, M.D.

Associate Professor of Radiology
Department of Radiology
Mary Hitchcok Hospital
Hanover, New Hampshire

Lawrence W. Bassett, M.D.

Associate Professor of Radiological Sciences
UCLA School of Medicine and
Jonsson Comprehensive Cancer Center at UCLA
Director, The Iris Cantor Mammography Screening Clinic
Los Angeles, California

Oliver H. Beahrs, M.D.

Professor of Surgery
Mayo Medical School and
Consultant in Surgery
Mayo Clinic
Rochester, Minnesota

Catherine Cole-Beuglet, M.D.

Professor in Residence
Department of Radiological Sciences
Department of Radiology
University of California Irvine Medical Center
Orange, California

Walter F. Coulson, M.D.

Professor of Pathology and
Chief, Division of Surgical Pathology
UCLA School of Medicine
Los Angeles, CA

Carl J. D'Orsi, M.D.

Professor of Radiology
Department of Radiology
University of Massachusetts Medical Center
Worcester, Massachusetts

Stephen A. Feig, M.D.

Professor of Radiology
Jefferson Medical College
Chief, Division of Mammography
Thomas Jefferson University Hospital
Philadelphia, Pennsylvania

Richard H. Gold, M.D.

Professor of Radiological Sciences
UCLA School of Medicine and
Jonsson Comprehensive Cancer Center at UCLA
Los Angeles, California

Robert V. P. Hutter, M.D.

Chairman, Department of Pathology
St. Barnabas Medical Center
Livingston, New Jersey

Joyce A. Janus, M.D.

Assistant Professor
Department of Diagnostic Radiology
University of Rochester School of Medicine and Dentistry
Rochester, New York

Lester Kalisher, M.D.

Clinical Director
Department of Radiology
Division of Diagnostic Radiology
St. Barnabas Medical Center
Livingston, New Jersey

Carolyn Kimme-Smith, Ph.D.

Adjunct Assistant Professor of Radiological Sciences
UCLA School of Medicine
Los Angles, CA

Wende W. Logan, M.D.

Breast Clinic of Rochester
Rochester, New York

John R. Milbrath, M.D.

Associate Clinical Professor of Radiology
Medical College of Wisconsin
Milwaukee, Wisconsin
Director, Breast Diagnostic Clinic
Milwaukee, Wisconsin

Myron M. Moskowitz, M.D.

Professor of Radiology
Department of Radiology
University Hospital Breast Consultation Center
Cincinnati, Ohio

Edward A. Sickles, M.D.

Associate Professor
Department of Radiology
University of California School of Medicine
San Francisco, California

Barbara Threatt, M.D.

Director, Comprehensive Breast Center
Ann Arbor, Michigan

PART I

X-ray Mammography

Section 1
Introduction to Breast Imaging: State of the Art and Future Directions

Richard H. Gold, M.D.
Lawrence W. Bassett, M.D.
Carolyn Kimme-Smith, Ph.D.

Breast cancer is not only the most frequent cancer in women, it is also the leading cause of their cancer deaths. Approximately 1 in every 10 American women will develop breast cancer. Regardless of the type of treatment employed, the prognosis ultimately depends on how early the disease is detected. Although the 5-year survival for cases with regional lymph node extension is only 59 percent, when the disease is localized to the breast, the 5-year survival is as high as 91 percent.[2] The smaller the cancer at detection, the greater the likelihood that it is localized to the breast.

X-RAY MAMMOGRAPHY

Mammography is the only proven method capable of detecting nonpalpable breast cancers. Some of these are carcinomas in situ or carcinomas "minimally" invasive and less than 5 mm in diameter—lesions that are associated with a 93 percent 20-year survival.[25]

Early detection, the key to successful management of breast cancer, is the fundamental objective of x-ray mammography. Early detection allows the application of therapeutic procedures that conserve the breast, and makes fear of mastectomy a thing of the past.

Historical Perspectives

In 1930, Stafford Warren reported the first performance of in vivo mammography (Fig. 1-1).[76] Thereafter, progress in mammography was impeded by the lack of a reproducible method for obtaining satisfactory images until 1960, when Robert Egan reported on a high-milliamperage/low-kilovoltage technique that yielded reproducible images on industrial film.[22] Remarkable advances since then have led to a striking improvement in image quality and a dramatic reduction in radiation dose.

The first modern x-ray unit dedicated to mammography was developed in the mid-1960s.[30] A molybdenum target, in place of tungsten, heightened contrast between water, fat, and calcific densities, while a built-in compression device diminished scattered radiation and motion artifacts and separated breast structures. In 1972, the introduction of a high-definition intensifying screen with a single-emulsion film, held in intimate contact by a vacuum, revolutionized mammography. It permitted rapid automatic processing and shorter exposures with diminished motion unsharpness, and greatly reduced surface exposure.[78]

Meanwhile, the introduction of xeromammography in 1972 provided an alternate imaging method that improved image quality by enhancing the edges of high-density structures, particularly calcifications.[46,80] Unfortunately, the aluminum filtration and negative mode processing that was required to reduce surface exposure to acceptable levels somewhat degraded the exquisite detail characterizing the images made with the original unfiltered positive-mode technique.[60]

State of the Art

Clinical investigations have failed to reveal a significant difference in accuracy between screen-film mammography performed with dedicated equipment and xeromammography.[50,67] However, although more than 90 percent of the mammographic examinations in the United States are currently performed with screen-film or xeromammographic image receptors,[37] not all mammograms are being performed with compression. Some screen-film mammographers are not utilizing x-ray equipment designed specifically for screen-film mam-

BREAST CANCER DETECTION
ISBN 0-8089-1842-7

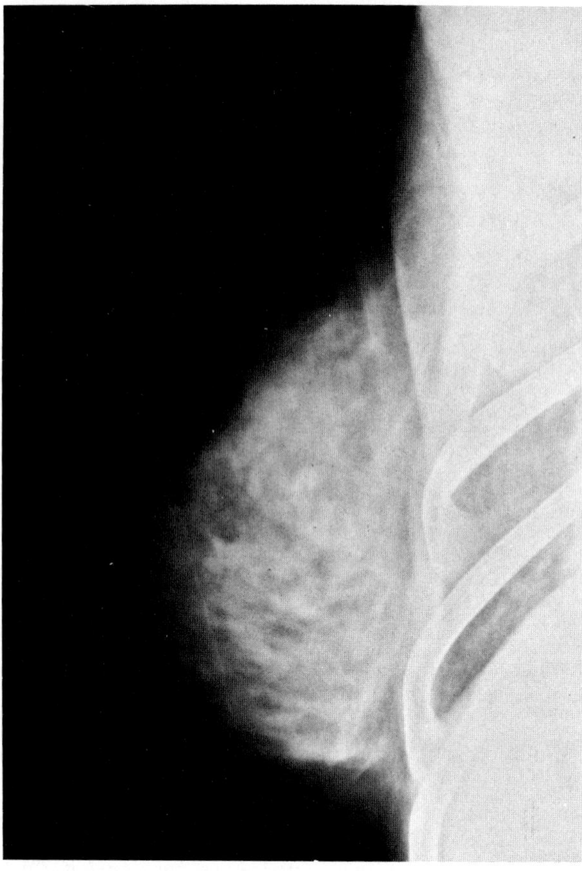

Figure 1-1. Mediolateral film mammogram by Stafford Warren in 1939. Moving grid diminished scattered radiation. Technical factors included 60 kVp, 70 ma, and 25-inch target-film distance. Loss of image detail resulted from exposure time of 2.5 seconds, use of dual par-speed intensifying screens, and lack of compression. Courtesy of Stafford Warren, M.D.

mography. Thus, some radiologists, like their forebears a generation before, are evaluating images of suboptimal quality.

Screen-film mammography currently requires considerably less radiation than does xeromammography for the same two-view examination (an average glandular dosage of 0.1–0.2 rad for screen-film mammography, versus 0.5–0.8 rad for positive-mode xeromammography, and 0.3–0.5 rad for negative-mode xeromammography).[31]

Compared with their first generation counterparts, the new dedicated units for screen-film mammography have even smaller focal spots, a longer and fixed source-to-image distance to reduce geometric unsharpness, more effective compression devices to eliminate motion and to separate mammary structures, moving grids to reduce scattered radiation, automatic exposure control for more consistent quality, configurations that promote easy and rapid positioning by permitting a patient to stand during exposures, and an alternate smaller focal spot for the production of magnified images. Hooded anodes and electrostatic lenses are further advances. Used with the newest rare-earth screen-film combinations, these x-ray systems provide greater image contrast and detail, and require less dosage than ever before. For use with older dedicated systems without a built-in grid, an ultrahigh-strip-density, stationary focused grid that fits inside a standard mammographic cassette is available.[19] Although grids reduce scattered radiation and thereby improve image detail in dense breasts, they also require an increase in dosage. Therefore, grids are recommended only for breasts that contain more than 50 percent dense fibroglandular tissue, and not for predominantly fatty breasts whose images are usually excellent and tend not to be improved with the use of grids.[66]

X-ray tubes for mammography utilize cathodes that generally follow the traditional design of a helical coil filament. An exception is an experimental cathode containing a ribbon-shaped filament, whose flat surface causes the distribution of its emitted electron field striking the anode to be uniform or flat rather than twin-peaked like the field from a helical coil filament. The uniform focal spot yields an improved modulation transfer function.[47]

One commercially available microfocal spot unit utilizes a cup-shaped cathode containing molybdenum beads heated by a tungsten filament and emitting a Gaussian-shaped field of electrons. Compared with standard screen-film mammography performed with dedicated units and with xeromammography, direct radiographic magnification of the breast with this microfocal spot unit using xeroradiographic or screen-film recording systems produces images with superior resolution and reduced effective noise.[33,62] Because magnification mammography requires considerably more radiation, however, its major role is to supplement standard mammography when the latter produces equivocal findings.[61] In the future, faster screen-film combinations should permit a significant reduction in dosage, with the magnification causing a concomitant reduction of the increased noise inherent in the faster image receptor.[5,9]

Xerox has recently introduced a dedicated mammography x-ray unit suitable for xeromammography or screen-film mammography of a standing or recumbent patient. The x-ray tube has a tungsten target with 0.3-mm and 0.6-mm focal spots. Aluminum filtration is used for xeromammography, paladium or molybdenum filtration and a stationary focused grid for screen-film mammography.

Although the competition between screen-film mammography and xeromammography to capture the market for mammographic equipment is intense, there is no significant difference in the ability of either one to detect cancer.[50] The efficacy of any mammographic technique is most dependent on the skill and experience of the technologist and the interpreter.

Risk Assessment

By a conservative risk analysis, an average dose of 1 rad to the breast would allow 13 annual mammographic examinations before the patient's risk is increased from the natural risk of 7 percent to 8 percent.[74] The midbreast dose for a typical mammogram in the National Cancer Institute/American Cancer Society-sponsored Breast Cancer Detection Demonstration Project (BCDDP) averaged 0.370 rad for Xerox units and 0.040 rad for screen-film units.[34] The average glandular dose, a more accurate standard, is approximately the same as the midbreast dose for the "hard" radiation of xeromammography performed with a tungsten target and twice the midbreast dose for the "soft" radiation of screen-film mammography performed with a molybdenum target. A complete two-view examination would therefore yield an average glandular dose of 0.740 rad for xeromammography and 0.160 rad for screen-film mammography. Under these conditions, an average glandular dose of 0.160 rad would result in one excess breast cancer per million women at risk per year. Put into everyday terms, and assuming the worst—that the one excess cancer is fatal—the risk (1 death/million persons/year) of a two-view mammographic study is about equivalent to the risk of traveling 400 miles by air, traveling 60 miles by automobile, smoking three-quarters of a cigarette, or being a 60-year-old woman for 20 minutes.

In fact, none of the risks identified in previous studies that found increased cancers due to radiation (atomic bomb exposure, therapeutic irradiation, or chest fluoroscopies) can be reasonably applied to current mammographic technology. However small the risk, technological advances in mammography must nevertheless continue to be directed toward reducing radiation exposure while maintaining the high quality of the images. Mammographers should be aware of their dosage and should be able to communicate this information when requested.

Quality Assurance

A major concern of mammography is the need to control radiation standards in general mammography practice. In 1975, Bicehouse reported on the surface exposures delivered by mammography units in 70 medical facilities in eastern Pennsylvania.[11] In this study, the surface exposures ranged from 0.25 roentgen to 47 roentgens! Obviously, some centers were using doses too low to obtain diagnostic images, while others were delivering excessive radiation. In response, the Bureau of Radiologic Health of the Food and Drug Administration developed a voluntary mammography quality-assurance program to minimize patient exposure while optimizing image quality. This ongoing joint federal-state program, called BENT (Breast Exposure: Nationwide Trends), operates in most of the 50 states and the District of Columbia.[37] The BENT program functions in 4 phases: groundwork, evaluation, follow-up surveys, and re-evaluation. Regional centers for radiologic physics mail to participating radiologists a thermoluminescent dosimetry card for each of their mammographic units. After exposure, the cards are returned for analysis. The radiologists receive a report of the exposure levels of their units. In the event of unusually high or low exposures, state physics personnel visit the facility and provide expert advice on improving mammographic techniques. Finally, the effects of the program are reassessed by means of subsequent dosimetry cards mailed months later.

Most mammographic facilities monitor their doses with thermoluminescent dosimeters (TLD). These also can be used to check the exposure timer and to compare the doses of different machines, different screen-film combinations, or different configurations of equipment.[57] A comparison of TLD and corrected ionization chamber doses has shown that for molybdenum target dedicated units, the two methods differ by no more than 5 percent, while for tungsten target xerox systems, the TLD dose is 6 percent higher at depth than the corrected ion chamber values.[69]

Another aspect of quality assurance that cannot be overemphasized is the need to maintain the highest standards of image processing. The following are the most common pitfalls in film processing[70]: processing mammographic film in a processor that is also used for other kinds of film; underdevelopment due to a temperature that is too low, a developing time that is too short, or developing solutions that are too old; light leaks in the darkroom and improper red filters leading to fogging of film; and a dust- or cigarette-ash-laden darkroom environment leading to screen artifacts. Some helpful hints: Processors should be cleaned at regular intervals to avoid a build-up of crystallized processing solutions on the rollers, with subsequent pressure artifacts on the processed films. The processing instructions of the film manufacturer should be scrupulously followed. Intensifying screens should be cleaned at frequent intervals. And the radiologist should perform daily quality control. A checklist of common processing problems is presented in Fig. 1-2.

Expected Future Trends

Because a further breakthrough in rare-earth screen technology is unlikely, film manufacturers probably will continue to direct their research efforts toward increasing the sensitivity of film emulsions in order to further decrease dose without diminishing diagnostic information (e.g., slicing silver halide grains into even finer "T-grains").

Xerox has recently introduced a black liquid toner development process that should provide improved image resolution and broad area contrast and significant exposure reduction through enhanced photoreceptor sensitivity. The new system combines conditioning and processing in a single unit. The black liquid toner has an average particle size less than half that of the conven-

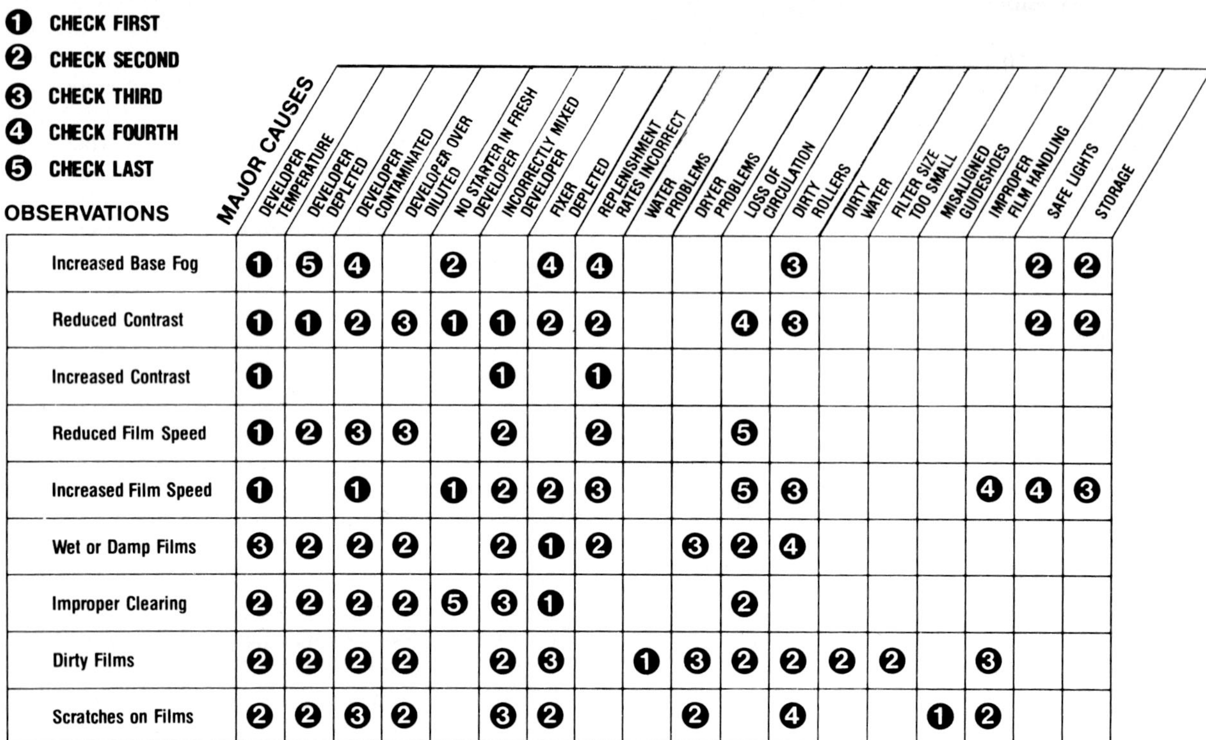

A GUIDE TO COMMON PROCESSING PROBLEMS

1 CHECK FIRST
2 CHECK SECOND
3 CHECK THIRD
4 CHECK FOURTH
5 CHECK LAST

OBSERVATIONS / MAJOR CAUSES	Developer Temperature	Developer Depleted	Developer Contaminated	Developer Over Diluted	No Starter in Fresh Developer	Incorrectly Mixed Developer	Fixer Depleted	Replenishment Rates Incorrect	Water Problems	Dryer Problems	Loss of Circulation	Dirty Rollers	Dirty Water	Filter Size Too Small	Misaligned Guideshoes	Improper Film Handling	Safe Lights	Storage
Increased Base Fog	1	5	4		2		4	4				3					2	2
Reduced Contrast	1	1	2	3	1	1	2	2			4	3					2	2
Increased Contrast	1					1		1										
Reduced Film Speed	1	2	3	3		2		2			5							
Increased Film Speed	1		1		1	2	2	3			5	3				4	4	3
Wet or Damp Films	3	2	2	2		2	1	2		3	2	4						
Improper Clearing	2	2	2	2	5	3	1				2							
Dirty Films	2	2	2	2		2	3		1	3	2	2	2	2		3		
Scratches on Films	2	2	3	2		3	2			2		4			1	2		

Figure 1-2. A guide to common processing problems. Courtesy of the DuPont Company.

tional blue powdered toner. The new development process is coupled with a new xeroradiography plate that features a more sensitive selenium alloy twice the thickness of the selenium layer on the older plate, and results in a 50 percent reduction in dose. Xerox predicts that the new system will require less preventive maintenance and fewer service calls than the previous system.

One potentially fruitful area for research is digital mammography.[28] Coupled with an intensifying screen below the breast, a detector array can transmit the signals emanating directly from the x-ray tube to a high-resolution, high-contrast television monitor, where contrast may be adjusted by digital manipulation. Alternatively, digital imaging can be coupled with a reusable selenium plate receptor, where the pattern of charges on the plate may be converted into digital form from which the image may be enhanced and stored in a computer. Digital imaging can also be coupled with a phosphor-coated plate. After x-ray exposure of the breast with dedicated mammography equipment, a scanning laser can ''read out'' the information on the plate and convert it to a digital format suitable for image enhancement. Due to its ability to window gray levels (as in computed tomography), laser digitization of films may permit the imaging of microcalcifications if the pixel size can be reduced to 50 square microns (10 line pairs/mm). Even if the definition of the microcalcifications were to be obscured because of a volume effect, the density of the digitized pixel might still be sufficient to become detectable when contrast was increased on the display monitor.[68] Since higher resolution systems are becoming available, digital mammography should soon attain clinical utility.

The addition of microfocal spot magnification to grids or to scanning double slits to reduce scattered radiation could also lead to future digital mammography systems that are both practical and effective. The image enhancement capabilities of digital systems combined with their lower dose requirements make them attractive for future research in breast imaging.

X-Ray Mammography for Cancer Screening

The first randomized control study to assess mammography in the periodic screening of asymptomatic women was that of the Health Insurance Plan of Greater New York (HIP). Beginning in 1963, enrolled women were offered annual screening by physical examination and mammography for 4 successive years. Evaluation after 7 years showed a 30 percent reduction in breast cancer mortality in the group offered screening compared with the control group. Fourteen years after the

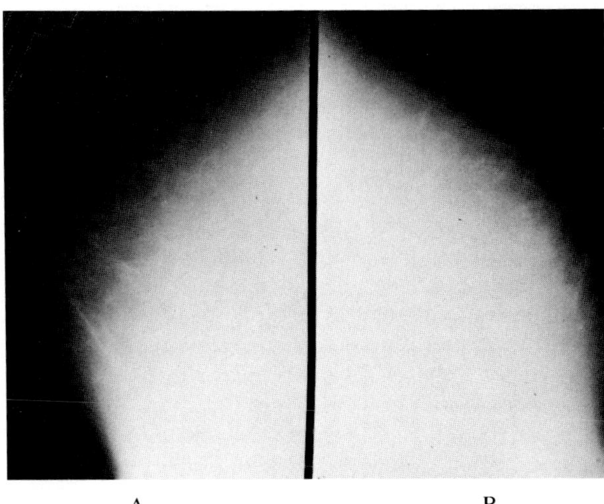

Figure 1-3. HIP right (A) and left (B) mediolateral film mammograms, *circa* 1963. Examination was performed with industrial film, no screens, 6-second exposure, and no compression. Although typical of state of the art in the early 1960s, detail is poor compared to that obtainable with current techniques and equipment. Patient had fatty breasts and was, therefore, excellent candidate for mammography. Nevertheless, carcinoma could be detected only by palpation. Courtesy of Philip Strax, M.D.

completion of screening, mortality was still reduced by 24 percent.[58] Survival was best for women whose cancers had been detected by mammography alone. However, largely because of the primitive state of mammography at the time, mortality was not reduced among the women under the age of 50 (Fig. 1-3).

In 1973, after the publication of the seven-year HIP results, the American Cancer Society and National Cancer Institute jointly initiated the Breast Cancer Detection Demonstration Project. Five consecutive annual screening examinations were undertaken using physical examination and mammography. Thermography was also used for the first two or three annual screenings, but was abandoned when shown to be ineffective. Although the BCDDP was not a controlled study and the population was self-selected, the accumulated data showed that mammography had undergone a striking technological advance since the HIP study and was far superior to physical examination in detecting cancer, especially early cancer. Mammography detected 91 percent of all cancers. The proportion of cancers detected by mammography alone was 42 percent (compared with 33 percent in the HIP study), while the proportion detected by physical examination alone was only 9 percent (compared with 44 percent in the HIP study). One-third of all detected cancers were noninfiltrating, or infiltrating but less than 1 cm in size; the majority of these cancers were detected by mammography alone. Only 20 percent of all detected cancers were associated with positive axillary lymph nodes, less than half the figure reported for all other newly diagnosed breast cancer cases in the United States during the same time period.[6,10]

Three recent reports of mammography screening confirm its effectiveness in reducing mortality from breast cancer. In one Dutch study, all female residents age 35 and over in the city of Nijmegen were invited to participate in single-view mammography screening every other year starting in 1975. All deaths from breast cancer that occurred in the invited group between 1975 and 1982 were ascertained and a case-control study was conducted. The 48 percent relative risk of dying from breast cancer among the women who had been screened compared with those not screened implied a reduction in breast cancer mortality of 52 percent in the screened population.[75]

A second Dutch study was conducted in the city of Utrecht, where all women age 50–64 were invited to be screened by mammography and physical examination. Screening was repeated at 12-, 18-, and 24-month intervals. A case-control evaluation carried out in the same manner as in the Nijmegen project revealed a reduction in breast cancer mortality of 70 percent among women who were screened.[16]

A Swedish screening study initiated in 1977 was designed as a randomized control prospective investigation. Of the enrolled women age 40 and over, one-half were offered screening at 24- to 33-month intervals by single oblique-view mammography, while the other half served as controls. After 7 years, a reduction in breast cancer mortality of 31 percent occured among the screened group compared with the control group. Although women under the age of 50 showed no mortality reduction, the number of deaths in that group was too small to give statistically significant results. The study showed that the rate of stage II and more advanced cancers was 25 percent lower among women who were screened than in the control group, while the rate of in situ and stage I cancers was much higher. Thus, the effectiveness of mammography in detecting cancer at an early stage was confirmed.[71]

Indications for X-Ray Mammography

The American Cancer Society and American College of Radiology have provided guidelines for mammography of asymptomatic women based on the present state of our knowledge of its benefits and hypothetical risks[1,3,4]:

1. A single baseline mammogram should be performed between ages 35 and 40. A small number of early cancers will be detected; more importantly, a single study will provide the essential baseline for assessing subtle changes in subsequent mammograms that may indicate cancer.
2. For women age 40–49, mammography with low-dose radiation factors should be performed every 1–2 years. The periodicity should be linked to an individual analysis of relative risk factors.

3. Women 50 years of age and older should have a mammogram every year.
4. Women with personal or strong family histories of breast cancer should consult their physicans about the need to begin mammography before age 40.

Mammography should be performed at any age when clinical findings indicate a suspicion of cancer. As useful as it is for examining a palpable breast lesion prior to its evaluation by the pathologist, mammography is even more valuable for evaluating both breasts preoperatively for mammographic signs of clinically occult cancer. Should ominous findings be detected in an area other than the area to be biopsied, a biopsy specimen of the mammographically suspicious area also should be obtained. Just as mammography should not be expected to replace a physical examination, physical examination of the breasts cannot replace mammography. A negative mammogram or a negative physical examination should never deter the biopsy of a suspicious lesion that has been detected by either method.

BREAST ULTRASONOGRAPHY

Historical Perspectives

The breast was one of the first organs evaluated by ultrasound when, over 30 years ago, Wild and Reid[79] and Howry et al.[35] examined palpable masses by A-mode technique and demonstrated the potential for differentiating cystic from solid lesions. Thereafter, contact scanning with conventional B-mode equipment was found useful by Kratchowil and Kaiser[45] in the evaluation of palpable masses. With the subsequent development of dedicated automated water path scanners by Deland,[18] and Jellins et al.,[38] Kobayashi,[40] and Kelly-Fry,[39] rapid systematic examination of the entire breast became possible.

State of the Art

Hand-held real-time ultrasound

The primary clinical indication for breast sonography currently rests with evaluation of the symptomatic patient. The most important clinical role for breast sonography is the differentiation of cysts from solid masses. In this endeavor, accuracy rates of 96–100 percent have been reported for sonography and far exceeded those of mammography and physical examination.[24,53,63] For palpable masses, any hand-held real-time unit having a transducer frequency no lower than 5 MHz is adequate to identify simple cysts and thereby avert unnecessary biopsies. The alternative of needle aspiration is, however, both diagnostic and therapeutic for masses that are cysts. The greatest usefulness of sonography is when cyst-solid differentiation is needed for a mammographically detected, nonpalpable, noncalcified mass of indeterminate origin for which aspiration is impractical. Sonography is useful in imaging palpable masses not detected by mammography, but needle aspiration often proves sufficient in this clinical setting. The exception is in the case of a breast containing cysts in such large numbers that needle aspiration is impractical.

The sensitivity and specificity of breast sonography for cancer detection are far lower than for cyst diagnosis. Sonographic differentiation of benign from malignant solid masses is not sufficiently reliable to direct clinical decisions.[36] All sonographically imaged solid masses must therefore be considered potentially malignant. Sonography is relatively ineffective in detecting carcinomas less than 1 cm in size. The vast majority of cancers detected mammographically solely by virtue of clustered calcifications are not imaged by ultrasound. Cancers are also difficult to detect sonographically in fatty breasts because the hypoechoic pattern of most malignancies is similar to that of normal fat. Because of these limitations, sonography functions most successfully as an adjunct to mammography and physical examination. Indeed, the combined use of x-ray and ultrasound mammography has been shown to improve the detection rate for breast cancer.[73]

Hand-held real-time breast sonography may be a useful adjunct to the x-ray mammogram in 3 groups of patients: those with palpable masses considered indeterminate on mammograms; those with dense breasts, localized signs, and inconclusive findings on mammograms; and those with nonpalpable indeterminate masses.[55]

Hand-held real-time units usually rely on multiformat camera images for permanent records. The radiologist, or a specially trained technologist, performs the examination. During scanning, the breast structures are depicted three-dimensionally. Phased array transducers currently are being used as an alternative to mechanical sectoring transducers. Limitations of phased array transducers result from three factors:

1. To form a focused beam, delays in firing elements of the array are computed from the known velocity of sound in tissue. An average velocity of 1540 m/sec is assumed. In the breast, however, velocities can vary from 1460 m/sec in fat, to 1580 m/sec in fibroglandular tissue,[44] producing a potential 8 percent focusing miscalculation that may cause blurring of the image. Refraction effects, due to these velocity changes, further defocus the beam.
2. While the lateral direction of the beam is focused electronically, array elements (except for annular arrays) are individually focused with an external lens in the slice thickness (or elevation) direction. A general-purpose ultrasound unit will probably focus its 5 MHz array at 4 cm in the slice thickness direction. Thus, even if the array is dynamically focused at 2 cm, the slice will be much thicker there than the 2 mm achieved by lateral-direction focusing. This may account for localization failure when

a dynamically focused phased array is used to evaluate small masses in the breast.[77]

3. If the array is poorly designed or has been damaged, grating lobes can cause artifactual echoes in anechoic lesions, causing them to simulate solid masses. Grating lobes can be diagnosed by imaging a fabric test object on edge when it is submerged in a water tank. Lobes are most likely to occur in high frequency arrays since they result from array elements being separated by more than half a wavelength from their neighboring elements.[26] For 5-MHz arrays, this requirement causes each element to be less than 0.4 mm in width.

Hand-held ultrasound-guided aspiration biopsy of nonpalpable lesions is gaining in popularity.[42] Because no harmful effects of breast sonography have been demonstrated, it may be used often and at closely spaced intervals to evaluate the response of multiple cysts to medical therapy.[65]

Advantages of hand-held real-time ultrasound units over automated units include improved resolution due to higher frequency whole-breast transducers and absence of compounding, ability to vary the amount of compression to assess tissue compliance and fixation, and usefulness in guiding needle aspiration biopsies. The disadvantage of decreased resolution in the near field can be overcome by attaching a water-path stepoff device to the transducer. Thus, the hand-held sonographic technique is useful when attention can be directed to a specific area of the breast. Although sonographic information may lead to fewer equivocal interpretations of x-ray mammograms, ultrasonography should not be used as a substitute for x-ray mammography.

Automated whole-breast ultrasound

Automated water-path instruments designed specifically for whole-breast examination make it possible to systematically examine the breast in its entirety, an essential feature when breast ultrasound is used to search for nonpalpable lesions.[48] Contemporary units use single or multiple transducers with frequencies of 3–5 MHz and achieve resolution on the order of 2 mm. In order to identify small lesions, it is necessary to scan at closely spaced intervals, which results in multiple sequential images. It is also desirable to compare images of both breasts at identical planes. This is usually accomplished by dual-videotape or videodisc playback of the examination.

The potential usefulness of automated breast sonography as a screening device has been suggested by reports of cancer detection rates approaching those of x-ray mammography.[13,20,41,51] X-ray mammography was, however, used in some of these series of cases only in the event of a palpable or sonographic abnormality, while in other series correlative clinical data were available for sonographic but not for x-ray mammographic interpretation. In still other series, the ability of sonography to differentiate solid from cystic masses was compared with the ability of x-ray mammography to specifically indicate malignancy. The accuracy of automated whole breast ultrasound relative to that of x-ray mammography has thus tended to be overestimated. Later reports have revealed a significant number of nonpalpable cancers detected by x-ray mammography and missed by sonography.[43,55,64] Persistent imaging problems have included unreliable imaging of fatty breasts, inability to depict microcalcifications (often the earliest x-ray sign of breast cancer) inconsistent detection of solid lesions less than 1 cm, inadequate differentiation between benign and malignant solid lesions, and excessive scan time, physician review time, and equipment cost.

Automated whole breast ultrasonography is least accurate in fatty breasts, the type in which x-ray mammography is most accurate in cancer detection. Ultrasound, however, is most accurate in breasts that are dense in x-ray mammograms. Ultrasound is thus helpful in the evaluation of uniformly dense breasts in which noncalcified cancers may go undetected by x-ray mammography. One area for which automated breast ultrasound has been proposed as the initial imaging procedure is the evaluation of asymptomatic women under the age of 35 in whom the breasts tend to be dense and the false-negative rate for mammography correspondingly high.[32] Another proposed application is the evaluation of tissue surrounding augmentation prostheses, where the effectiveness of x-ray mammography and physical examination is limited.[14]

Does automated whole breast sonography have a role to play in breast cancer screening? The primary purpose of x-ray mammography in breast cancer screening is the detection of clinically occult lesions. Breast sonography is currently limited in this regard by its inability to detect most malignancies presenting mammographically as clustered calcifications and by its poor reliability in detecting cancers smaller than 1 cm. Because of these deficiencies, automated breast sonography cannot yet be considered adequate for cancer screening. It should be considered an adjunct to x-ray mammography and physical examination rather than a substitute for them.[28]

Expected Future Trends

Application of automated breast sonography to the clinical setting is currently being evaluated by many individual researchers working independently. This has led to considerable variability in protocols, equipment, images, and diagnostic accuracy. Most subjects have been symptomatic. Data for an entirely asymptomatic population have yet to be acquired, primarily because sonography has failed to identify many of the nonpalpable cancers routinely detected by mammography. A multi-institutional study of image interpretation with properly controlled technical and biostatistical procedures would be highly desirable.

Ultrasonic computerized axial tomography (UCAT) is now under development in an attempt to provide quantitative data relative to the production of ultrasound images of the breast.[12,29] Related techniques such as backscatter and transmission computerized sonography, which combine data regarding the velocity and relative attenuation of sound through the breast, have also been attempted. Although UCAT appears promising, especially in fatty breasts, problems include image distortion produced by nonuniform refractive indices and the influence of surrounding tissues upon sound velocity through lesions, and diminished effectiveness of cancer detection in the dense breast.

Doppler systems are being used on an experimental basis to study the vascular physiology of the breast and breast tumors. The Doppler signal represents the velocity of the blood circulating within tissue. Preliminary work has shown that Doppler signals from carcinoma differ from those obtained from normal breast tissue.[7]

Basic investigations of the interactions of sonic waves with breast tissue of differing types and combinations must be continued. The effect of collagen, mucin, mucopolysaccharides, and other biologic substances on image formation and, specifically, on the sonographic appearance of cancer must be further defined.[15] The breast architecture adjacent to and remote from cancer must be analyzed. This will require correlation with x-ray mammography, specimen radiography, and pathology.[72]

Efforts must continue toward improving the resolution of existing dedicated breast ultrasound scanners. Pulse-echo scanners would benefit from high frequency transducers, provided they could maintain penetration sufficient to image the entire breast. UCAT resolution could be improved by reducing the distortion produced by the curved sonic beam within the breast. To test and calibrate ultrasonic imaging machines and to train ultrasonographers, an ultrasound anthropomorphic breast phantom is a necessity. Such a phantom, mimicking the various types of parenchyma, malignant tumors, cysts, benign masses, and calcifications, would require production in large quantities under conditions of careful quality control, and should be reasonably priced.

Economic Considerations

Hand-held real-time ultrasonography frequently results in a more timely or deferred biopsy, in comparison to an equivocal physical and/or mammographic examination without ultrasound clarification, and is therefore considered to be cost-effective. Because of the current high cost of automated ultrasonographic equipment and the long duration of each examination, the cost per examination may equal or exceed that of x-ray mammography. Although automated breast sonography sometimes provides clinically relevant information when used as an adjunct to physical examination and mammography and occasionally is the only method to detect a carcinoma, especially in a dense breast, the cost of the examination may preclude its routine use. Specific clinical situations for which the addition of an automated whole-breast sonographic examination may be cost-effective are still largely undefined. The most promising of such applications appears to be the evaluation of multiple palpable masses in radiographically dense breasts in which mammography has shown no abnormality. Automated whole-breast sonography may also be useful when the x-ray mammograms are significantly compromised by dense parenchymal tissue. Until technological improvements permit a substantial increase in the accurate detection of nonpalpable cancer, however, the role of sonography will be limited primarily to making cyst-solid differentiations. This can be performed most rapidly and least expensively with a hand-held real-time unit.

MAGNETIC RESONANCE IMAGING

Breast cancer can be imaged by magnetic resonance imaging (MRI), and image detail is improved with the use of surface coils. Although there is considerable overlap in T1 and T2 values between cancer and benign breast lesions,[54] the shape of the lesion and the change in its signal intensity with different radiofrequency pulse sequences may aid in differentiation.[23] Microcalcifications associated with carcinoma cannot be delineated on MRI.[17] Experimental intravenous paramagnetic agents such as gadolinium-DPTA, which highlight differences in signal intensity between regions of differing tissue perfusion, have been considered as potential adjuvants to extend the usefulness of MRI for breast cancer detection.[52,56] Intravenous injection and possible toxicity would, however, prevent the application of paramagnetic agents to widespread screening. Before a clinical role for MRI in breast cancer detection can be established, the question of cost effectiveness of expensive MRI technology will have to be confronted.

TRANSILLUMINATION LIGHT-SCANNING

Recent advances in this technique are based on the concept that breast cancer, because of its increased blood supply, absorbs more near-infrared and red electromagnetic radiation than does benign tissue. As a consequence, emphasis has shifted away from real-time viewing by the human eye, which is totally insensitive to near-infrared rays, and toward a hard copy made from infrared-sensitive photographic film.[49] Alternatively, a television camera that is sensitive to near-infrared radiation can display the image on a television monitor. Electronic contrast enhancement of the video image increases the likelihood of visualizing subtle lesions. Rapid, noninvasive, risk-free, and relatively inexpensive, transillumination of the breast has elicited increasing interest. In addition, transillumination has met with a high degree of patient acceptance. Several prospective controlled feasibility studies have, however, shown transillumination to be considerably less sensitive than x-ray mammography in the detection of nonpalpable cancer.[8,21,27,59]

THERMOGRAPHY

Thermography is ineffective in detecting clinically occult cancer, either as an independent examination or as a prescreener to determine which patients need mammography. Thermography cannot reliably differentiate benign from malignant breast disease.[28] In the Breast Cancer Detection Demonstration Project, the cancer detection rate of thermography was only 42 percent, a clinically unacceptable level, especially when compared with rates of 57 percent for physical examination and 91 percent for mammography.[6,10] Furthermore, thermography gave an unacceptably high number of false-positive examinations.

CONCLUSION

The underlying goal of all breast imaging procedures is to detect cancer. X-ray mammography places greatest emphasis on the disclosure of early, nonpalpable, curable cancer. Diagnostic ultrasonography stresses the differentiation of benign cysts from diagnostically indeterminate solid masses that require biopsy. Evolving experimental procedures such as transillumination light-scanning and magnetic resonance imaging are currently undergoing preliminary evaluation. Thermography is an older procedure that seems to operate at a high level of effectiveness only for advanced cancer. Since x-ray mammography is the technique that has proven most successful in detecting early breast cancer, it is the standard to which all imaging alternatives must be compared.

REFERENCES

1. ACS Report on the Cancer Related Health Checkup: Cancer of the breast: CA 30:224–229, 1980
2. American Cancer Society: 1986 Cancer Facts and Figures. New York: American Cancer Society, 1986, p10
3. American Cancer Society: Mammography guidelines 1983: Background statement and update of cancer-related checkup guidelines for breast cancer detection in asymptomatic women age 40 to 49. CA 33:25, 1983
4. American College of Radiology: Guidelines for mammography. ACR Bulletin 38:6–7, 1982
5. Arnold BA, Eisenberg H, Bjarngard B: Low-dose magnification mammography. Radiology 131:743–749, 1979
6. Baker LH. Breast Cancer Detection Demonstration Project: Five-year summary report. CA 32:196–225, 1982
7. Bamber JC, Sambrook M, Minasian H, et al: Doppler study of blood flow in breast cancer. In Jellins J, Kobayashi T (eds): Ultrasonic Examination of the Breast. Chichester, John Wiley and Sons, 1983, pp 371–378
8. Bartrum RJ Jr, Crow HC: Transillumination lightscanning to diagnose breast cancer: A feasibility study. AJR 142:409–414, 1984
9. Bassett LW, Arnold BA, Borger D, et al: Reduced dose magnification mammography. Radiology 141:665–670, 1981
10. Beahrs OH, Shapiro S, Smart C, et al: Report of the Working Group to Review the National Cancer Institute-American Cancer Society Breast Cancer Detection Demonstration Projects. J Natl Cancer Inst 62:639–698, 1979
11. Bicehouse HJ: Survey of mammographic exposure levels and technique used in Eastern Pennsylvania. Seventh Annual National Conference on Radiation Control, Hyannis, Massachusetts, April 27-May 2, 1975. DHEW Publication 76-8026
12. Carson PL, Meyer CR, Scherzinger AL, et al: Breast imaging in coronal planes with simultaneous pulse echo and transmission ultrasound. Science 213:1141–1143, 1981
13. Cole-Beuglet C, Goldberg BB, Kurtz, AB, et al: Ultrasound mammography. Radiology 139:693–698, 1981
14. Cole-Beuglet C, Schwartz G, Kurtz, AB, et al: Ultrasound mammography for the augmented breast. Radiology 146:737–742, 1983
15. Cole-Beuglet C, Soriano RZ, Kurtz, AB, et al: Ultrasound analysis of 104 primary breast carcinomas classified according to histopathologic type. Radiology 147:191–196, 1983
16. Collette HJA, Rombach JJ, Dey NE, et al: Evaluation of screening for breast cancer in a non-randomized study (the DOM Project) by means of a case-controlled study. Lancet 1:1224–1226, 1984
17. Dash N, Lupetin AR, Daffner RH: Magnetic resonance imaging in the diagnosis of breast disease. AJR 146:119–125, 1986
18. Deland FH: A modified technique of ultrasonography for the detection and differential diagnosis of breast lesions. AJR 105:446–452, 1969
19. Dershaw DD, Masterson ME, Malik S, et al: Mammography using an ultrahigh-strip-density, stationary, focused grid. Radiology 156:541–544, 1985
20. Devere C: Current status of ultrasonic breast scanning. Appl Radiol 9:145–149, 1980
21. Drexler B, Davis JL, Schofield G: Diaphanography in the diagnosis of breast cancer. Radiology 157:41–44, 1985
22. Egan RL: Experience with mammography in a tumor institution. Evaluation of 1000 studies. Radiology 75:894–900, 1960
23. El Yousef SJ, O'Connell DM, Duchesneau RH, et al: Benign and malignant breast disease: Magnetic resonance and radiofrequency pulse sequences. AJR 145:1–8, 1985
24. Fleischner AC, Muhletaler CA, Reynolds VH, et al: Palpable breast masses: Evaluation by high frequency hand-held real-time sonography and xeromammography. Radiology 148:813–817, 1983
25. Frazier TG, Copeland EM, Gallager HS, et al: Prognosis

and treatment in minimal breast cancer. Am J Surg 133:697–701, 1977
26. Gatzke RD, Fearnside JT, Karp SM: Electronic scanner for a phased-array ultrasound transducer. Hewlett-Packard Journal 34:10–13, 1983
27. Geslien GE, Fisher JR, DeLaney C: Transillumination in breast cancer detection: Screening failures and potential. AJR 144:619–622, 1985
28. Gold RH, Bassett LW, Kimme-Smith C: Breast imaging: State of the art. Invest Radiol 21:298–304, 1986
29. Greenleaf JF, Bahn RC: Clinical imaging with transmissive ultrasonic computerized thermography. IEEE Transactions on Biomedical Engineering 28:177–185, 1981
30. Gros CM: Méthodologie. Symposium sur le sein. J Radiol Electr 48:638–655, 1967
31. Hammerstein GR, Miller DW, White DR, et al: Absorbed radiation dose in mammography. Radiology 130:485–491, 1979
32. Harper AP, Kelly-Fry E, Noe S: Ultrasound breast imaging—the method of choice for examining the young patient. Ultrasound Med Biol 7:231–237, 1981
33. Haus AG, Paulus DD, Dodd GD, et al: Magnification mammography: Evaluation of screen-film and xeromammographic techniques. Radiology 133:233–226, 1979
34. Hempelmann LH: Mammography. NCRP Report no. 66. National Council on Radiation Protection and Measurements, 1980
35. Howry DM, Stott DA, Bliss WR: The ultrasonic visualization of carcinoma of the breast and other soft tissue structures. Cancer 7:354–358, 1954
36. Jackson VP, Rothschild PA, Kreipke DL, et al: The spectrum of sonographic findings of fibroadenoma of the breast. Invest Radiol 21:34–40, 1986
37. Jans RG, Butler PF, McCrohan JL Jr, et al: Status of film/screen mammography: Results of the BENT study. Radiology 132:197–200, 1979
38. Jellins J, Kossoff G, Buddee FW, et al: Ultrasonic visualization of the breast. Med J Aust 1:305–307, 1971
39. Kelly-Fry E: Breast Imaging. In Saggagha RE (ed): Ultrasound Applied to Obstetrics and Gynecology. New York, Harper & Row, 1980, pp 327–350
40. Kobayashi T: Ultrasonic diagnosis of breast cancer. Ultrasound Med Biol 1:383–391, 1975
41. Kobayashi T, Takatani O, Hattori N, et al: Differential diagnosis of breast tumors: The sensitivity graded method of ultrasonography and clinical evaluation of its diagnostic accuracy. Cancer 33:940–951, 1974
42. Kopans DB, Meyer JE, Lindfors KK: Breast sonography to guide cyst aspiration and wire localization of occult solid lesions. AJR 143:489–492, 1984
43. Kopans DB, Meyer JE, Lindfors KK: Whole-breast US imaging: Four-year follow-up. Radiology 157:505–507, 1985
44. Kossoff G, Jellins J: The physics of breast echography. Semin Ultrasound 3:5–12, 1982
45. Kratchowil A, Kaiser P: Die Darstellung der Erkrankungen der weiblichen Brust im Ultraschallschnittbildverfahren. In Bock J, Ossoining K (eds): Ultrasono Graphica Medica, vol. III. Vienna, Verlag der Wiener Medizinischen Akademie, 1969, pp 119–128
46. Martin JE: Xeromammography—An improved diagnostic method: Review of 250 biopsied cases. AJR 117:90–96, 1973
47. Matsui H, Katsuhiro O: A uniform focal spot x-ray tube with improved MTF and KW rating. Radiology 156:227–230, 1985
48. McSweeney MB, Murphy CH: Whole-breast sonography. Radiol Clin North Am 23:157–167, 1985
49. Ohlsson B, Gundersen J, Nilsson DM: Diaphanography: A method for evaluation of the female breast. World J Surg 4:701–705, 1980
50. Pagani JJ, Bassett LW, Gold RH, et al: Efficacy of combined film-screen/xeromammography. Preliminary report. AJR 135:144–146, 1980
51. Pluygers E, Rombaut M: Ultrasonic diagnosis of breast diseases. Tumor Diagnostik 4:187–194, 1980
52. Revel D, Brasch RC, Paajanen H, et al: Gd-DTPA contrast enhancement and tissue differentiation in MR imaging of experimental breast carcinoma. Radiology 158:319–323, 1986
53. Rosner D, Weiss L, Norman M: Ultrasonography in the diagnosis of breast disease. J Surg Oncol 14:83–96, 1980
54. Ross RJ, Thompson JS, Kim K, et al: Nuclear magnetic resonance imaging and evaluation of human breast tissue: Preliminary clinical trials. Radiology 143:195–205, 1982
55. Rubin E, Miller VE, Berland LL, et al: Hand-held real-time breast sonography. AJR 144:623–627, 1985
56. Runge VM, Clanton JA, Lukehart CM, et al: Paramagnetic agents for contrast-enhanced NMR imaging: A review. AJR 141:1209–1215, 1983
57. Servomaa A, Taivonen M: Mailed TL dosimeters for monitoring the output from diagnostic x-ray equipment. Med Phys 11:75–77, 1984
58. Shapiro S, Venet W, Strax P, et al: Ten- to fourteen-year effect of screening on breast cancer mortality. J Natl Cancer Inst 69:349–355, 1982
59. Sickles EA: Breast cancer detection with transillumination and mammography. AJR 142:841-844, 1984
60. Sickles EA: Mammographic detectability of breast microcalcifications. AJR 139:913–918, 1982
61. Sickles EA: Microfocal spot magnification mammography using xeroradiographic and screen-film recording systems. Radiology 131:599–607, 1979
62. Sickles EA, Doi K, Genant HK: Magnification film mammography: Image quality and clinical studies. Radiology 125:69–76, 1977
63. Sickles, EA, Filly RA, Callen PW: Benign breast lesions: Ultrasound detection and diagnosis. Radiology 151: 467-470, 1984
64. Sickles EA, Filly FA, Callen PW: Breast cancer detection with ultrasonography and mammography: Comparison using state-of-the-art equipment. AJR 140:843–845, 1983
65. Sickles EA, Filly RA, Callen PW: Breast ultrasonography. In Feig S, McLelland R (ed): Breast Carcinoma. Current Diagnosis and Treatment. New York, Masson Publishing USA; Chicago, American College of Radiology, 1983, pp 191–205
66. Sickles EA, Weber WN: High-contrast mammography with a moving grid: Assessment of clinical utility. AJR 146:1137–1139, 1986
67. Snyder RE, Kirch RL: Comparison study of xeromammography and low-dose mammography. In Gallager HS (ed): Early Breast Cancer Detection and Treatment. New York, Wiley, 1975, pp 199–204
68. Sommer FG, Smathers RL, Wheat RL, et al: Digital processing of film radiographs. AJR 144:191–196, 1985

69. Stanton L, Day JL, Brattelli SD, et al: Comparison of ion changers and TLD dosimetry in mammography. Med Phys 8:792–798, 1981
70. Tabár L, Dean PB: Screen/film mammography: Quality control. In Feig S, McClelland R (eds): Breast Carcinoma. Current Diagnosis and Treatment. New York, Masson Publishing USA; Chicago, American College of Radiology, 1983, pp 164–165
71. Tabár L, Gad A, Holmberg LH, et al: Reduction in mortality from breast cancer after mass screening with mammography. Randomized trial from the Breast Cancer Screening Working Group of the Swedish National Board of Health and Welfare. Lancet 1:829–832, 1985
72. Teubner J, Muller A, van Kaick G: Echomorophologie der Brustdruse. Vergleichende sonographische, radiologische, anatomische und histologische. Untersuchungen von Mamapraparaten. Radiologe 23:97–107, 1983
73. Texidor HS, Kazam E: Combined mammographic-sonographic evaluation of breast masses. AJR 128:409–417, 1977
74. Upton AC, Beebe GW, Brown JM, et al: Report of NCI Ad Hoc Working Group on the Risks Associated with Mammography in Mass Screening for Detection of Breast Cancer. J Natl Cancer Inst 59:479–493, 1977
75. Verbeek ALM, Holland R, Sturmans F, et al: Reduction of breast cancer mortality through mass screening with modern mammography. First results of the Nijmegen project, 1975–1981. Lancet 1:1222–1224, 1984
76. Warren SL: Roentgenologic study of the breast. AJR 24:113–124, 1930
77. Weber WH, Sickles EA, Callen PW, et al: Nonpalpable breast lesion localization: Limited efficacy of sonography. Radiology 155:783–784, 1985
78. Weiss JP, Wayrynen RE: Imaging system for low-dose mammography. J Appl Photogr Engr 2:7–10, 1976
79. Wild JJ, Reid JM: Further pilot echographic studies on the histologic structure of the living intact human breast. Am J Pathol 28:839–854, 1952
80. Wolfe JN: Xerography of the breast. Radiology 91:231–240, 1968

Section 2
Diagnosis

Richard H. Gold, M.D.
Lawrence W. Bassett, M.D.
Walter F. Coulson, M.D.

1

Mammographic Features of Malignant and Benign Disease

THE MAMMOGRAPHIC EXAMINATION

The ideal mammographic examination consists of the following: (1) an interview of the patient, in which a detailed history relating to breast diseases is obtained; (2) a thorough physical examination of the breasts and axillae; and (3) mammography. It is convenient to use line drawings of the breasts to record scars, moles, and abnormal physical findings (Fig. 1-1A). The location of lesions seen in mammograms may be similarly depicted in line drawings as an aid to the referring physician (Fig. 1-1B). Correlative information is essential for optimal mammographic interpretation. Just as mammography should not be expected to replace a physical examination, the physical examination should not be expected to replace mammography. A negative mammogram or negative physical examination should never deter biopsy of a suspicious lesion that has been detected by either method. Most false-negative diagnoses of properly performed and optimally processed mammograms result from obscuration of pathology in dense parenchyma.[9,20,26] Mammography cannot be relied upon to invariably distinguish benign from malignant disease. Therefore, biopsy, ultrasonography, or cyst aspiration should be performed for almost all solitary masses regardless of their mammographic appearance, the exception being a smoothly outlined mass containing the typical coarse calcifications of a fibroadenoma. Surgical intervention is particularly important in women over age 60 because in that age group twice as many solitary breast lesions are malignant as are benign. Subtle and indirect signs of cancer are most readily recognizable when previous mammograms are used for comparison. Because such comparisons are essential, radiologists are encouraged to retain mammograms for the lifetime of the patients. Since some cancers grow exceedingly slowly, a comparison should be made not only with the preceding examination, but, whenever possible, with examinations of several years past.

The radiologic examination includes mediolateral and cephalocaudal views of both breasts. These views are made at right angles to each other, thus permitting the mammographer to make a three-dimensional assessment that allows suspicious lesions to be localized not only by breast quadrant, but also by clockface location and relative depth. The mediolateral view may include the axilla, but a special view of the axilla itself is not routinely obtained because it results in more radiation exposure than the other views and seldom provides information about the lymph nodes that is not readily obtainable through palpation. Lymph node metastases arising from mammary carcinoma rarely exhibit telltale radiographic evidence of calcifications. Moreover, the apparent size of lymph nodes displayed mammographi-

BREAST CANCER DETECTION
ISBN 0-8089-1842-7

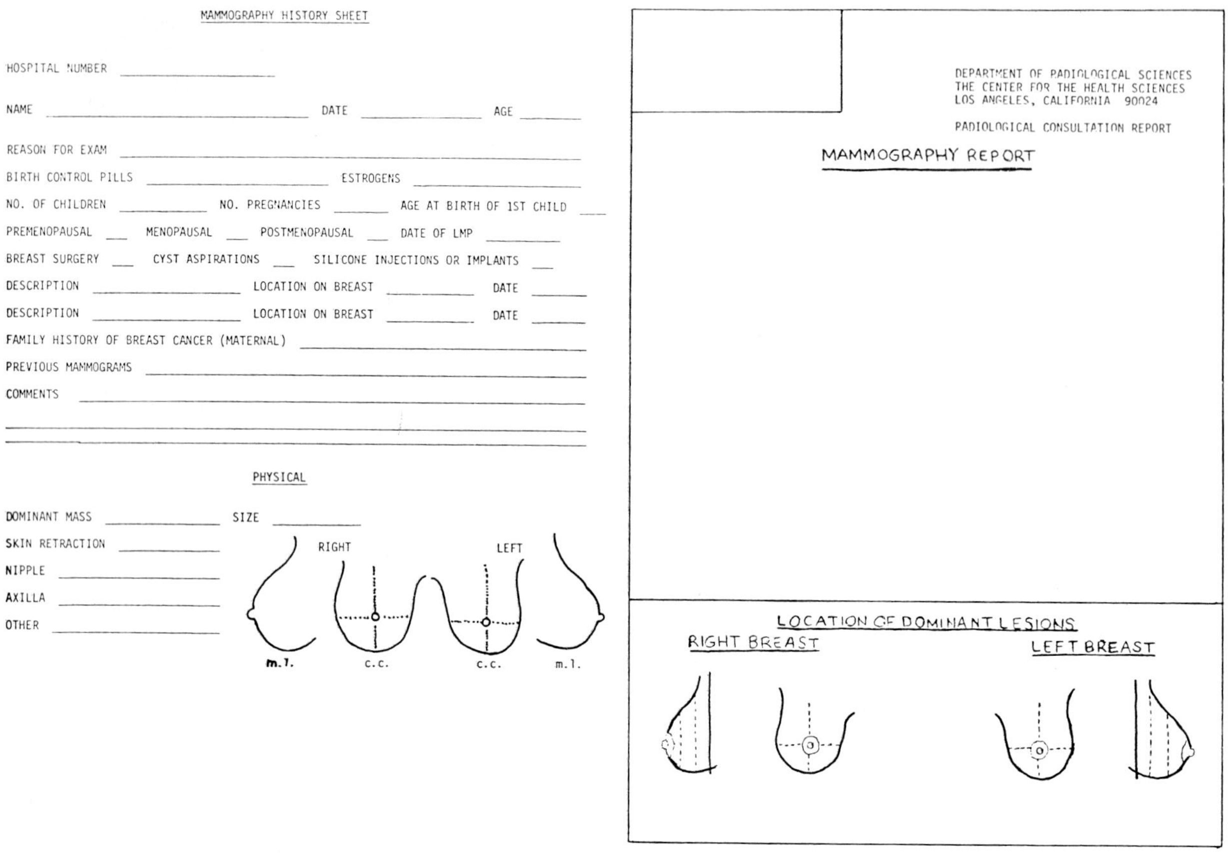

MAMMOGRAPHY HISTORY SHEET

HOSPITAL NUMBER ______

NAME ______ DATE ______ AGE ______

REASON FOR EXAM ______

BIRTH CONTROL PILLS ______ ESTROGENS ______

NO. OF CHILDREN ______ NO. PREGNANCIES ______ AGE AT BIRTH OF 1ST CHILD ______

PREMENOPAUSAL ___ MENOPAUSAL ___ POSTMENOPAUSAL ___ DATE OF LMP ______

BREAST SURGERY ___ CYST ASPIRATIONS ___ SILICONE INJECTIONS OR IMPLANTS ___

DESCRIPTION ______ LOCATION ON BREAST ______ DATE ______

DESCRIPTION ______ LOCATION ON BREAST ______ DATE ______

FAMILY HISTORY OF BREAST CANCER (MATERNAL) ______

PREVIOUS MAMMOGRAMS ______

COMMENTS ______

PHYSICAL

DOMINANT MASS ______ SIZE ______

SKIN RETRACTION ______

NIPPLE ______

AXILLA ______

OTHER ______

RIGHT LEFT

m.l. c.c. c.c. m.l.

A

DEPARTMENT OF RADIOLOGICAL SCIENCES
THE CENTER FOR THE HEALTH SCIENCES
LOS ANGELES, CALIFORNIA 90024

RADIOLOGICAL CONSULTATION REPORT

MAMMOGRAPHY REPORT

LOCATION OF DOMINANT LESIONS

RIGHT BREAST LEFT BREAST

B

Figure 1-1. Forms for history, physical examination, and mammography report. A. Form for breast history and physical examination contains line drawings of breasts to record scars, moles, and abnormal physical findings. B. Below space for mammography report are line drawings of the breasts that may be used to depict lesions seen in mammograms as aid to referring physician.

cally is a poor measure of metastatic involvement: small nodes may harbor metastases while large ones may be free of tumor. Indeed, Kalisher et al.[21] have determined that a lymph node, as recorded mammographically, must be more than 2.5 cm in its greatest diameter, and dense rather than fatty, before it can be considered suspicious of containing metastasis (Fig. 1-2). The presence of indurated or fixed axillary lymph nodes, as felt by the hand of the examining physician, is far more conclusive evidence of metastasis, albeit advanced, than the radiographic image of the nodes. Some screen-film mammographers add an oblique view, or substitute it for the mediolateral view, as the former shows the posterior portion of the breast and the base of the axillary tail to better advantage.[2] Logan has described the technique and positioning for the oblique view in her chapter on screen-film mammography.

ANATOMY OF THE BREAST

The breast, a modified sweat gland, contains from 12 to 24 lobes of glandular tissue radiating from the nipple and located between the superficial and deep layers of the superficial fascia. Each lobe drains through a separate lactiferous or secretory duct, and each duct has a separate orifice in the nipple. The lobes are separated from each other by sheaths of fibrous connective tissue. With advancing age or childbearing, the glandular tissue atrophies, undergoing transformation to fat; the connective tissue sheaths then become visible in mammograms (Fig. 1-3). The major ducts branch within the lobes to form smaller, intralobar ducts, which further branch and terminate in lobules. In contrast to the relatively radiolucent fatty breasts of older women, the breasts of adolescents have an almost homogeneous, exaggerated radiopacity because they contain only a small amount of fat in relation to the predominant fibroglandular tissue.

The suspensory ligaments of Cooper are toothlike projections of breast parenchyma covered by fibrous connective tissue that extend from the skin to the superficial layer of superficial fascia. Carcinoma may evoke fibrosis in the vicinity of the suspensory ligaments, causing them to shorten, a condition that is the basis for skin retraction associated with underlying carcinoma (Fig. 1-4). Similarly, this desmoplastic reaction in response to a carcinoma may thicken the walls of the nearby ducts, increasing their prominence in mam-

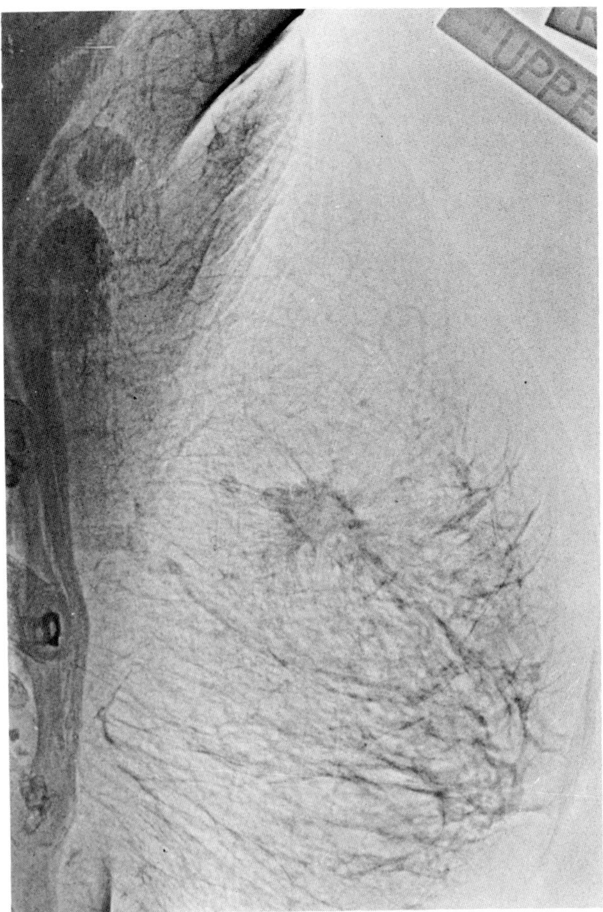

Figure 1-2. Mediolateral xeromammogram depicting spiculated carcinoma and axillary lymph node metastases. Lymph nodes are round rather than oval, greater than 2.5 cm in largest diameter, and dense rather than fatty—combination of features characteristic of metastasis. Presence of indurated or fixed axillary lymph nodes as felt by the hand of physician is nevertheless far more conclusive evidence of metastasis than radiographic image.

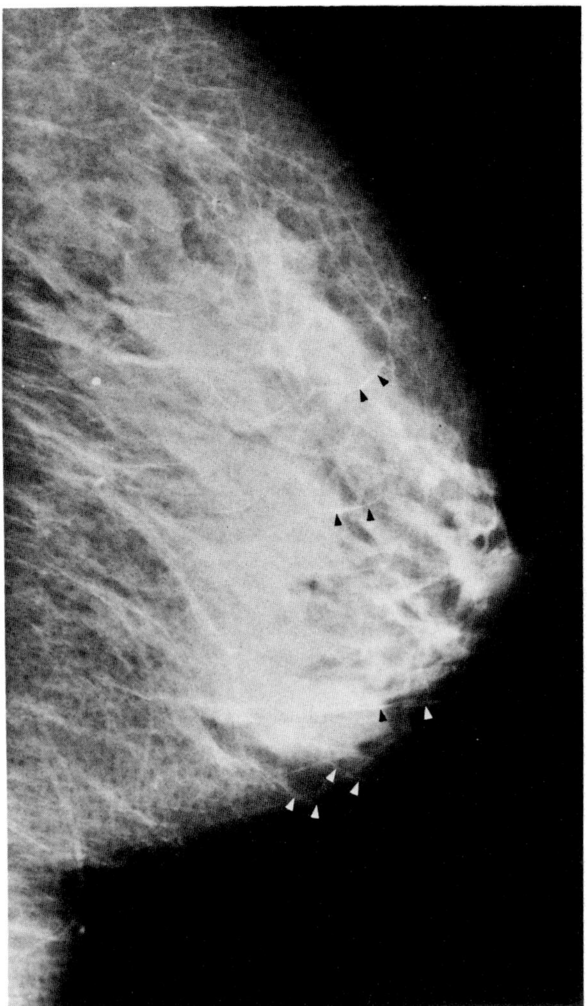

Figure 1-3. Mediolateral film mammogram illustrating normal breast of postmenopausal woman with two children. Ligaments of Cooper are outlined by arrowheads.

mograms, and eventually causing them to shorten, with subsequent nipple retraction (Fig. 1-5).

The breast tissue is normally distributed in a bilaterally symmetric pattern. Asymmetry may result from fibrocystic changes, prior surgical excision, or, most importantly, deposition of fibrous connective tissue in response to a carcinoma (Figs. 1-6 and 1-7). Such asymmetry is easiest to detect when the mammograms are so arranged for viewing that the right and left breasts appear to be mirror images of each other.

MAMMOGRAPHIC FEATURES OF CANCER

While the experienced physician can palpate a centrally located breast mass as small as 1 cm in diameter, mammography can disclose the presence of far smaller carcinomas. Surely, one of the most rewarding experiences in the professional life of a radiologist is the discovery through mammography of an early carcinoma—a lesion not yet symptomatic or palpable, still localized, and hence potentially curable. When mammography was in its infancy, mammographers took great pains to recognize certain "primary" and "secondary" signs of malignancy. The primary signs included a mass of relatively high density, with peripheral spiculations and numerous tiny calcifications, larger by palpation than by mammography. The secondary signs included skin thickening and/or retraction, nipple retraction, venous engorgement, fibrous tissue proliferation, and axillary node enlargement. All too often, however, these signs reflected cancer that was locally advanced. Today, mammographers place greater emphasis on less obvious signs that may signify early cancer.

If early cancer is defined as cancer that is asymp-

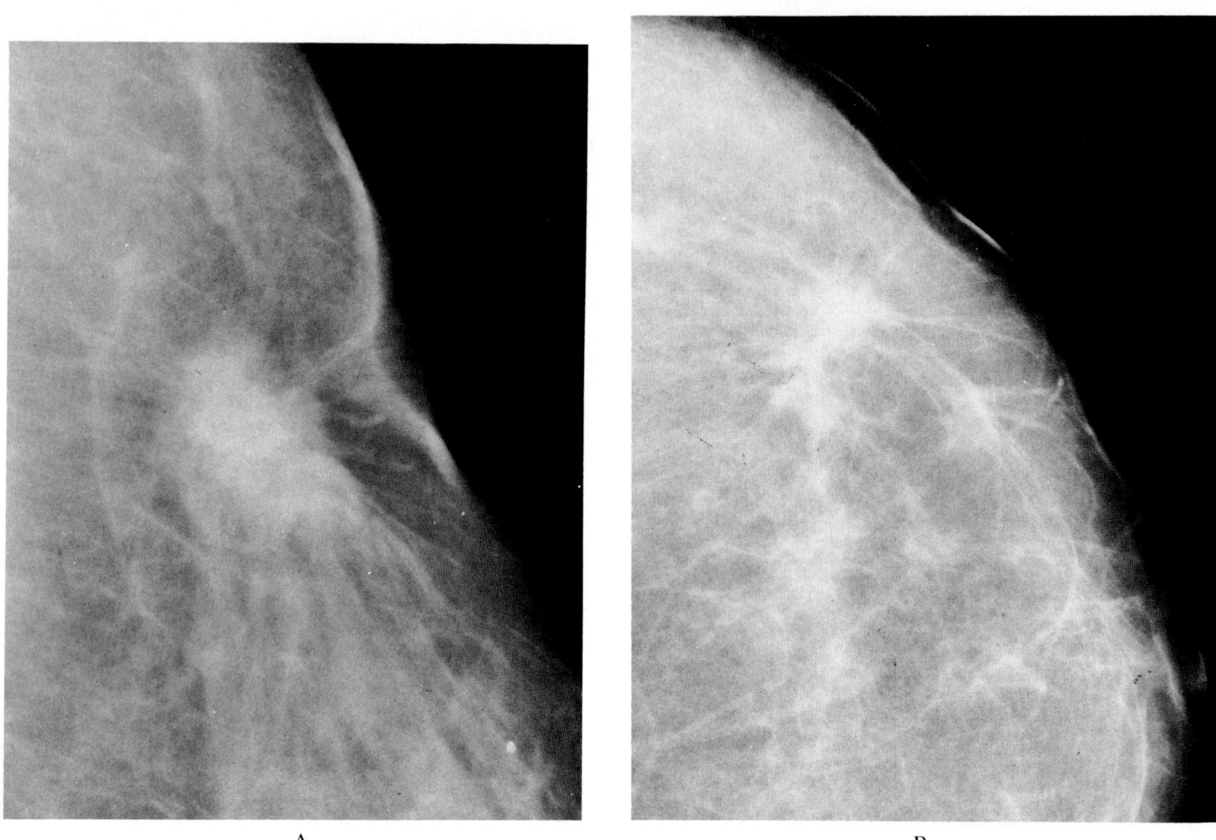

A B

Figure 1-4. Skin retraction associated with underlying carcinoma. A. Ligaments of Cooper are thickened and shortened because of elaboration of fibrous connective tissue in response to carcinoma. This desmoplastic process causes retraction of overlying skin. B. Two foci of skin retraction overlying multicentric carcinoma.

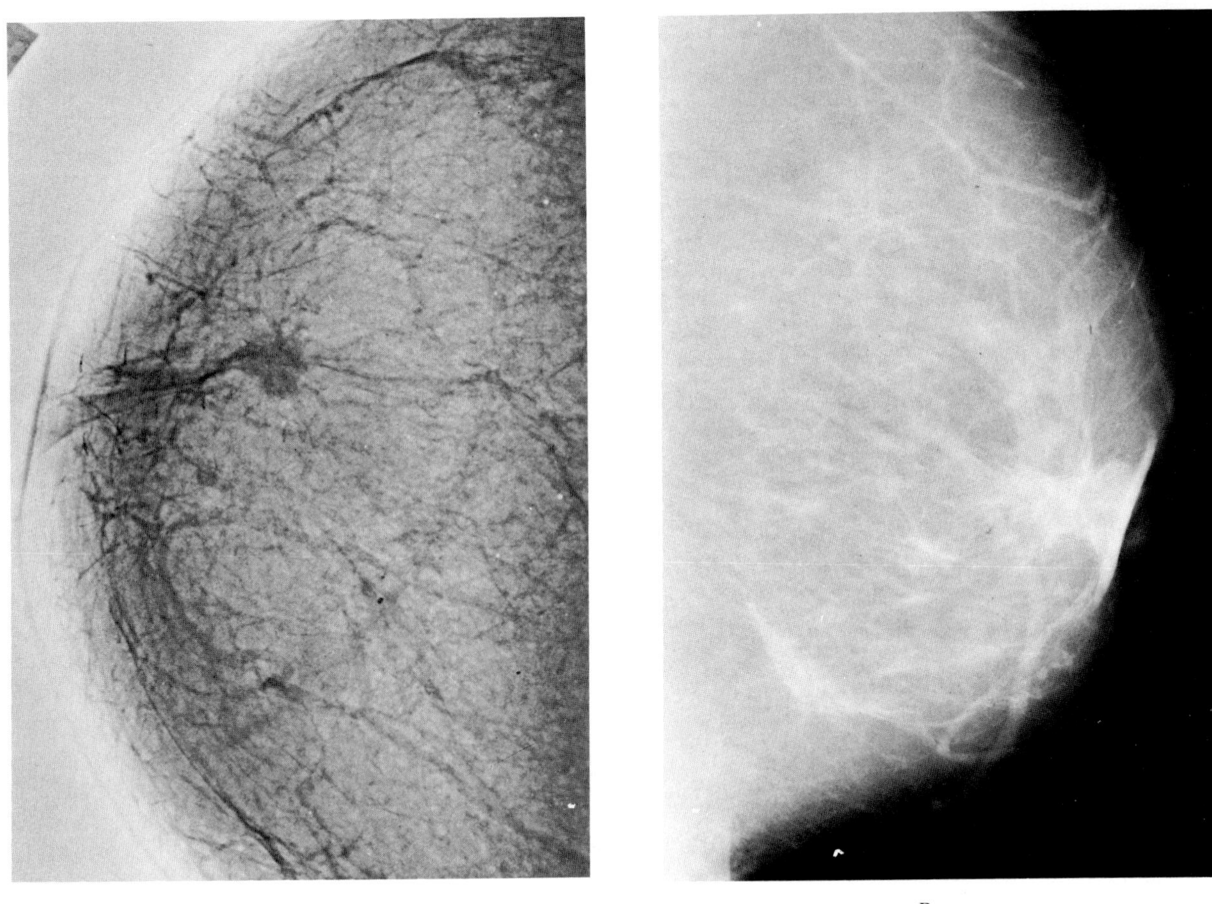

A B

Figure 1-5. Desmoplastic response to carcinoma with resultant thickening of duct walls and secondary retraction of nipple. A. Cephalocaudal view shows thickening of ducts between spiculated carcinoma and nipple. Localized focus of duct prominence such as this may sometimes be only sign of underlying carcinoma. B. Mediolateral view of more advanced lesion in another patient. Nipple has undergone extensive retraction into spiculated tumor.

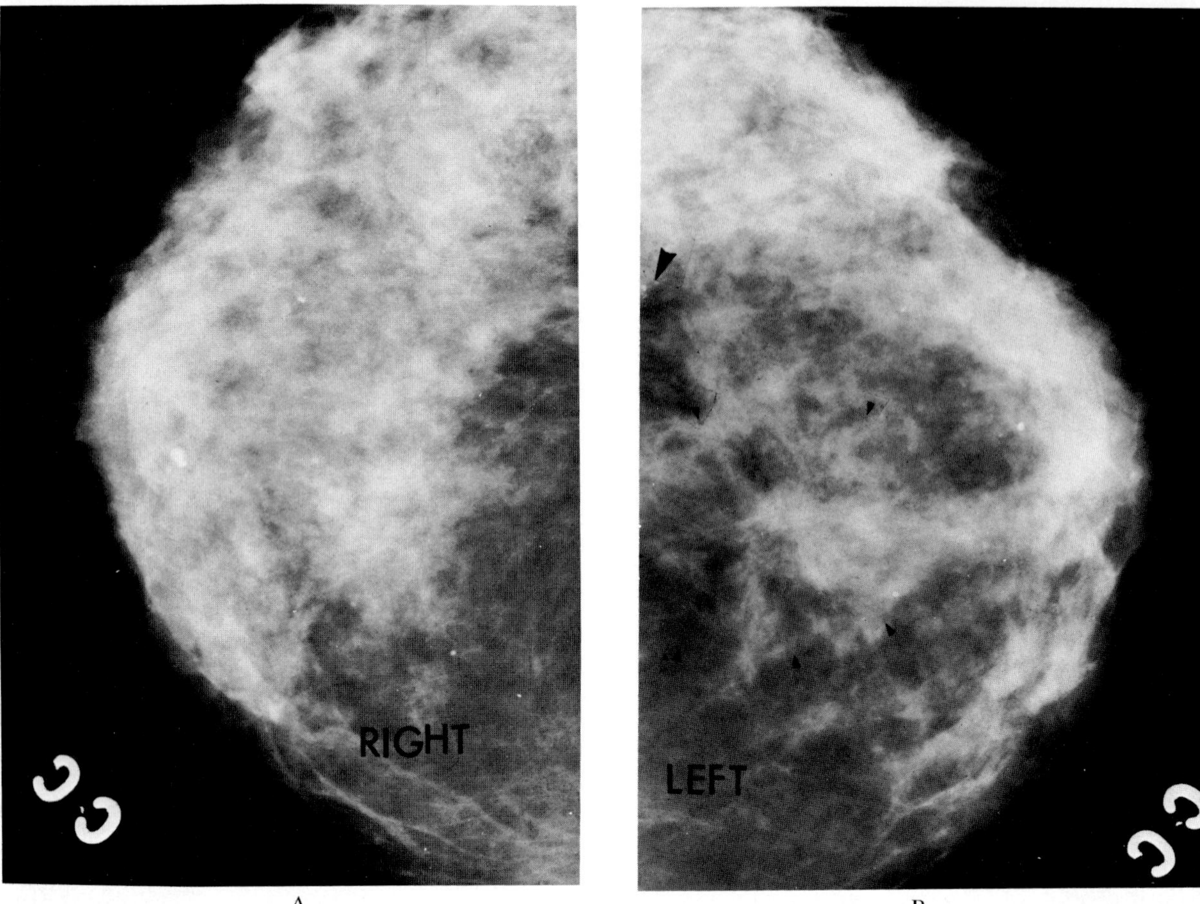

A B

Figure 1-6. Bilateral asymmetry as clue to presence of underlying malignancy. A. Right breast. Diffuse nodularity, scattered calcifications, and occasional cysts represent features of fibrocystic changes with sclerosing adenosis. B. Left breast. Area of duct prominence and fibrillary fibrous connective tissue proliferation (encircled by small arrowheads) signifies carcinoma that was nonpalpable. Cluster of tiny calcifications (large arrowhead), although suspicious for carcinoma, was actually within focus of benign sclerosing adenosis. Obvious asymmetry is more easily detectable when cephalocaudal and mediolateral views are arranged for viewing in such a way that they appear to be mirror images of each other.

tomatic, too small to be palpable, without metastases, and without clinical signs, the mammographic signs associated with such lesions include the following: (1) a circumscribed cluster of microcalcifications (Fig. 1-9); (2) a segmental prominence of one or more ducts (Figs. 1-5A and 1-9); and (3) a localized distortion of breast architecture (Figs. 1-6B and 1-8)—the latter two features reflecting a desmoplastic reaction. Indeed, if the cancer is less than 1 cm in greatest diameter as measured pathologically, any or all of these signs may be manifest in the absence of mammographic evidence of a mass. Moskowitz has described certain indirect radiological signs that may imply the presence of early breast cancer and has expressed his confidence in their individual worth and importance for patient management (Table 1-1).[33] These criteria, some of which are extremely subtle, may not assure the diagnosis, but their use will substantially increase the number of early cancers detected.

An analysis by Sickles of the mammographic presentation of 300 nonpalpable breast cancers disclosed that clustered calcifications were the primary mammographic abnormality in 42 percent of cases, but only 23 percent of the 300 cases exhibited the rod, curvilinear, and branching shapes that are characteristic of malignancy. Thirty-nine percent of the cancers presented mammographically as dominant masses, but only 16 percent manifested spiculated or knobby margins typical of carcinoma. Almost 20 percent of the cancers were detected primarily by indirect mammographic signs of malignancy (Table 1-1). Sickles reminds us that in order to take full advantage of the capabilities of mammography, we radiologists must search diligently not only for the classic mammographic features of

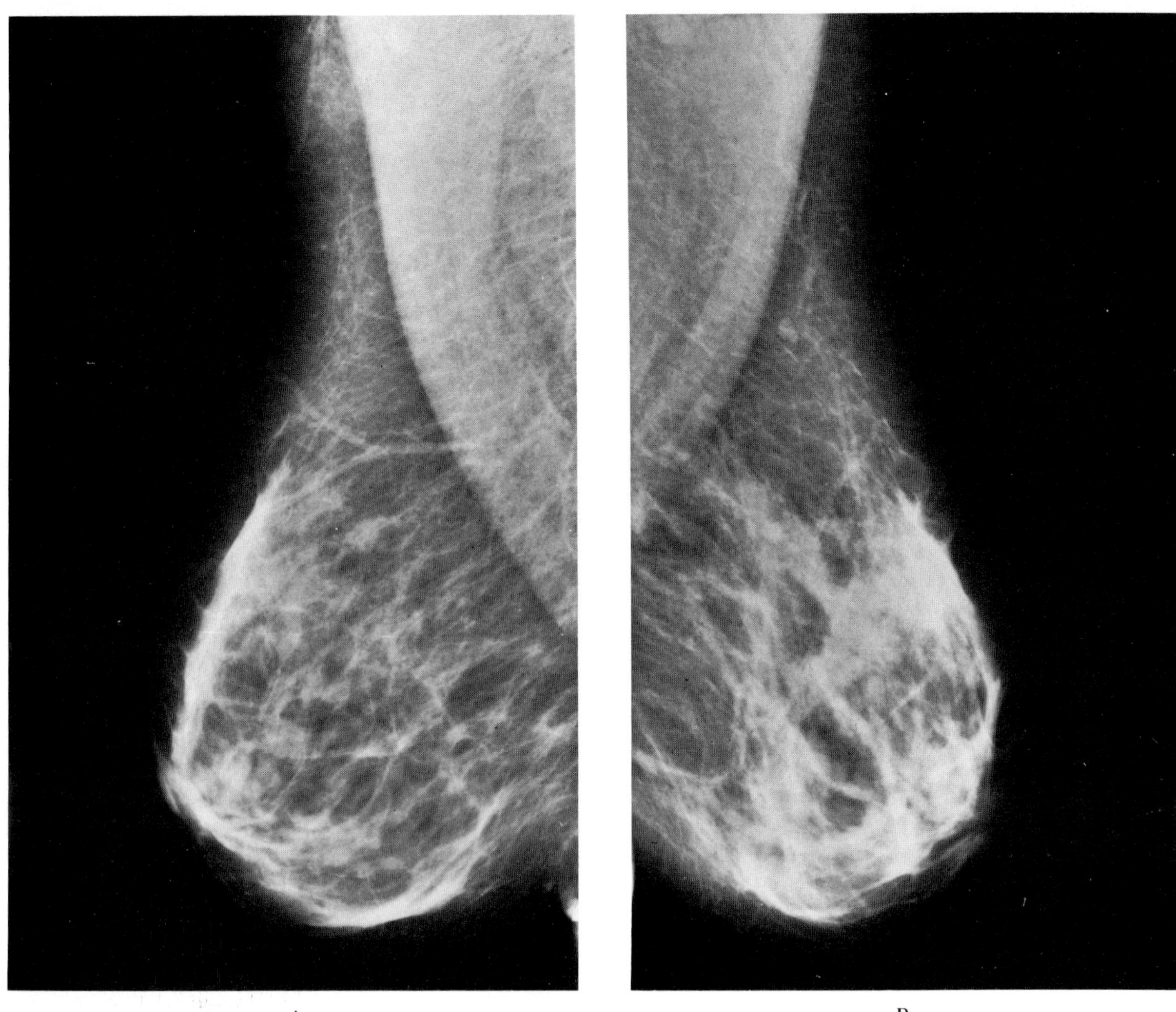

Figure 1-7. Mammograms of woman, age 34. Mediolateral oblique projections of right (A) and left (B) breasts and cephalocaudal projections (C and D) reveal asymmetrical increase in density in upper hemisphere of left breast which led to biopsy. E. Histologic section reveals intraductal (in situ) carcinoma characterized by proliferating ductal epithelial tumor cells encroaching upon and partially obliterating duct lumens. Marked periductal fibrosis accounts for increased density seen on mammograms. Infiltrates of chronic inflammatory cells are present in surrounding stroma (hematoxylin and eosin strain, original ×160). F. Higher power view showing cellular atypia and foci of abnormal nuclei. Mitotic figures are numerous. Proliferating neoplastic cells have hyperchromatic nuclei and abundant cytoplasm. Ductal basement membranes as well as myoepithelial cell layers are intact, indicating that cancer was intraductal and noninvasive.

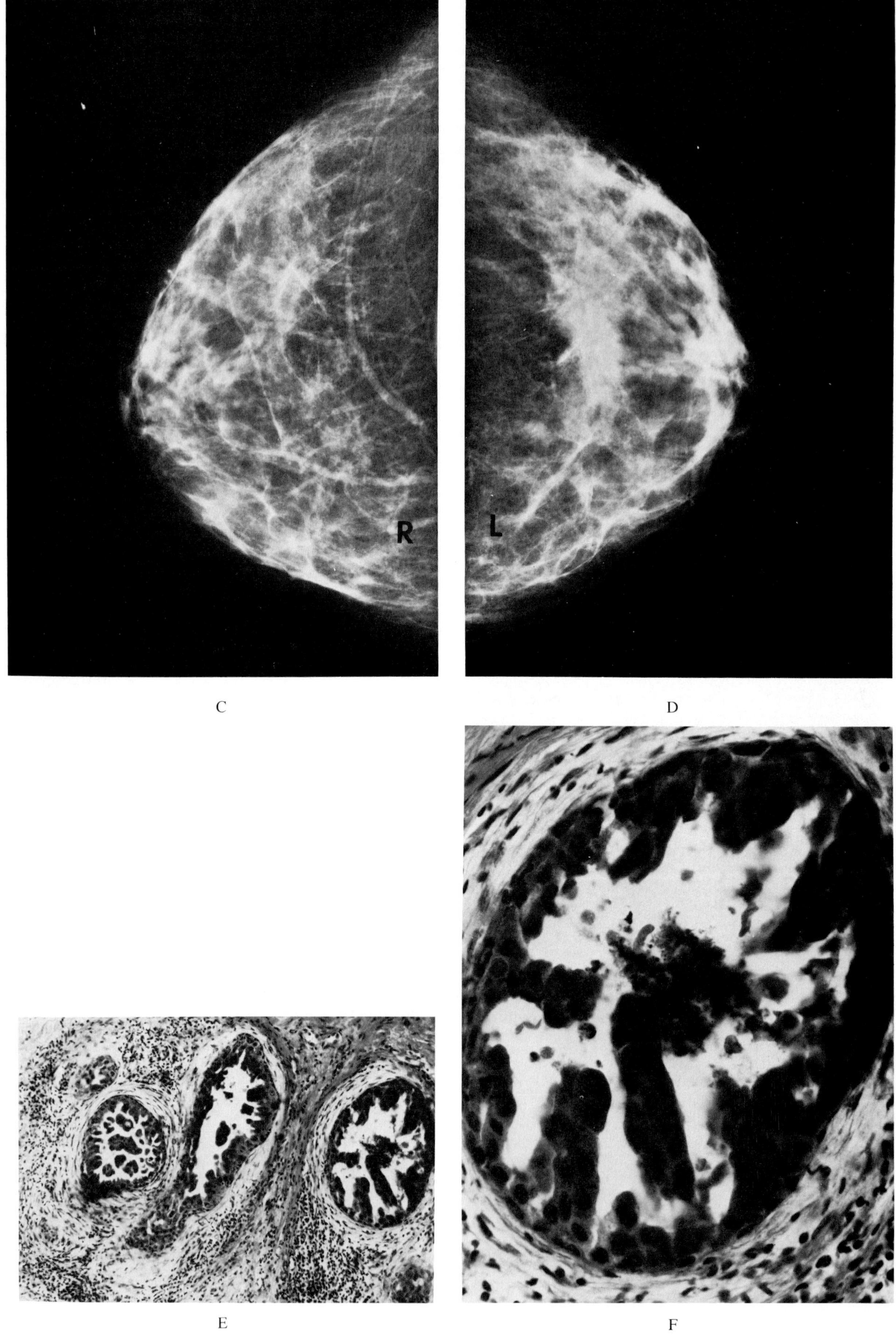

C D
E F

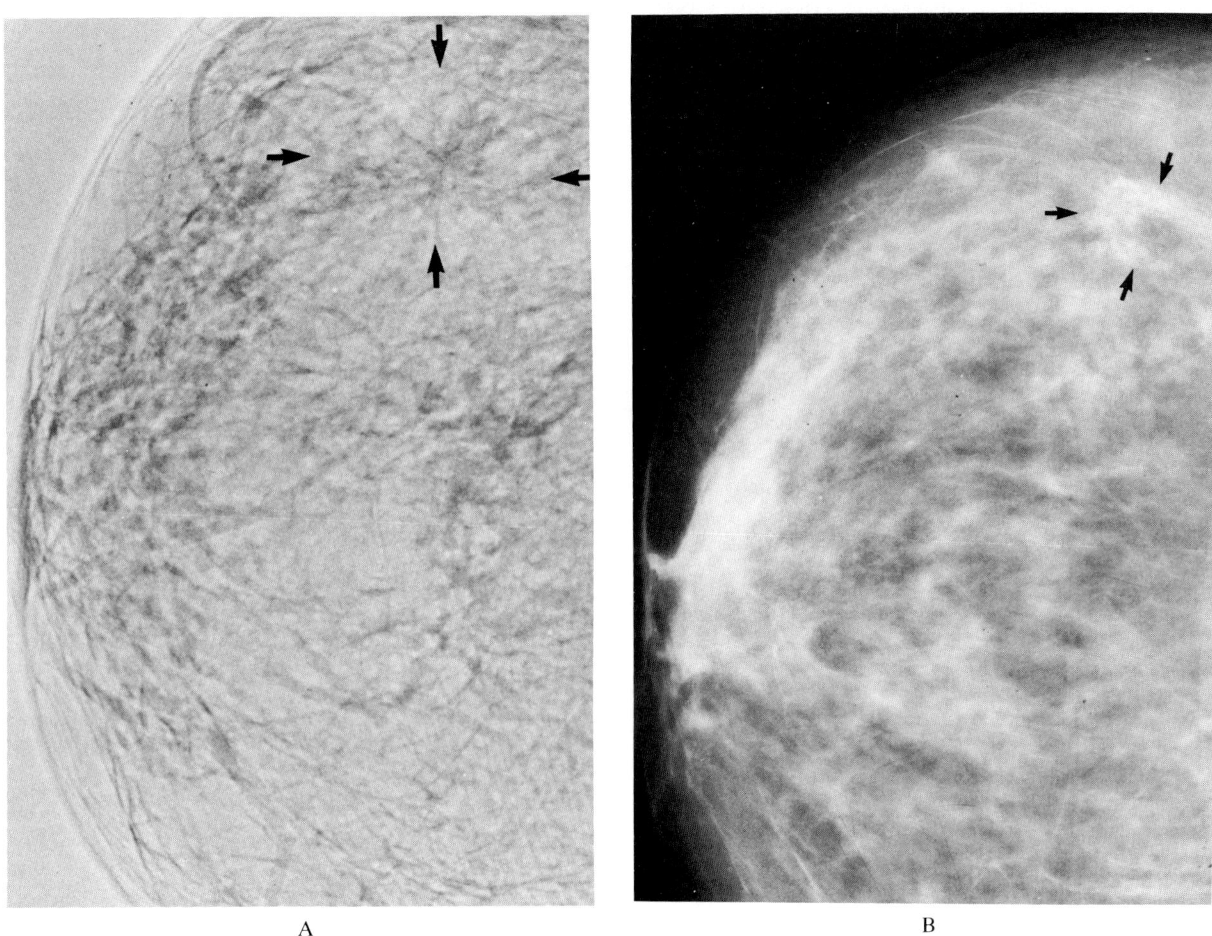

Figure 1-8. Subtle localized distortion of breast architecture as only sign of carcinoma. A. Localized distortion in form of subtle spicules (arrows) representing desmoplastic response to nonpalpable carcinoma. B. Boomerang-shaped focus of nonpalpable desmoplastic reaction (arrows) secondary to early carcinoma.

Table 1-1
Indirect Radiological Signs of Breast Cancer

Signs	Degree of Confidence in Diagnosis of Cancer*	Preferred Management
1. Calcifications		
a) Linear, semitranslucent, sharply marginated, arranged in a linear or branching array	8–10	Biopsy
b) Small, punctate, angular, interspersed among larger irregular calcifications, localized in one or more clusters	7–9	Biopsy
c) Innumerable small, irregular calcifications clustered in an area less than 1 cm	6–8	Biopsy
d) Isolated cluster(s) of small calcifications, irregular or smooth, solid or hollow, 150–200 μ, 5 or more per cluster per cm diameter circle	1–3	Localize and describe for M.D. to include degree of confidence in a diagnosis and consider for biopsy; if biopsy is not performed, reexamination 6 mo. later may be appropriate; if there is no change, yearly examinations can be done
2. Asymmetry: a density within the breast that does not have a counterpart on the opposite side and can be localized three-dimensionally		
a) Palpable abnormality of any kind, described by clinician	7–9	Biopsy
b) No palpable abnormality	1–2	Check again 30–60 days later at a different point in the patient's menstrual cycle. If the abnormality persists, offer biopsy; if biopsy is not done, patient should be rechecked clinically at monthly intervals and have another mammogram in 6 mo. to see if there is any progression
3. Neo-density: this represents any newly developing, not previously demonstrable density		
a) Classical sign of carcinoma	9–10	Biopsy
b) Classically benign findings	1–2	Either check again at a different point in the menstrual cycle within 6 wk. or consider immediate aspiration or biopsy or ultrasound to establish the cystic or solid nature of the lesion; if solid, excisional biopsy is necessary
c) Nonspecific neo-density	1-2	If physical examination is negative, check again in 3–6 wk.; if it persists, the patient should be offered biopsy
4. Benign-appearing dominant mass of over 1 cm	1–2	If palpable and solid, if should be biopsied; if palpable and cystic, or not palpable, it should be rechecked in 6 weeks. If it is not changed, its cystic or solid character should be established by ultrasound or aspiration and/or biopsy

5. Unilateral duct dilatation	<1	If there is no discharge, check again 1 year later with appropriate breast self-examination. If there is a discharging duct, it should be considered for injection and/or biopsy
6. Localized architectural distortion	2–6 (depending upon the type of distortion)	Offer biopsy
7. Central nipple ulceration	1	Call to the attention of the patient's physician, who may have overlooked a saucerized area of Paget disease which is filled in with debris. Biopsy is recommended

* Degree of clinical confidence = scale of 1–10, with 10 the most confident.
From Moskowitz M: Screening is not diagnosis. Radiology 133:267, 1979. With permission.

malignancy, but especially for the more subtle and indirect signs that are less specific in predicting the presence of cancer.[35]

Carcinoma may remain intraductal (in situ) for years (Figs. 1-7 and 1-9) before penetrating the basement membrane and becoming infiltrative. Most carcinomas are classified as the infiltrating ductal type. Most of these are further subdesignated *scirrhous carcinoma* because of the prominent desmoplastic reaction they incite, resulting in a characteristic rock-hard induration. The key mammographic feature distinguishing infiltrating carcinoma from most benign breast masses is the irregular margin of the former (Figs. 1-9 through 1-11). This irregularity reflects spicules of fibrous connective tissue and cords of tumor cells aggressively infiltrating the surrounding tissue. Carcinomas that infiltrate less aggressively appear more circumscribed, but still demonstrate knobby, irregular, or indistinct margins (Fig. 1-12).[14] On palpation, highly infiltrative carcinomas feel two or three times larger than their mammographic dimensions. The less-infiltrating carcinomas with minimal desmoplastic reaction exhibit the same dimensions on palpation as appreciated in mammograms—an identical characteristic of benign masses.

Lobular carcinoma, a less common variety, is difficult to detect mammographically because it is found most often in fibrocystic breasts and tends not to form a distinct mass. Moreover, the calcifications associated with lobular carcinoma tend to occur in smaller numbers and are more scattered in distribution than the calcifications of scirrhous carcinoma.

Comedocarcinoma, also uncommon, frequently results in a characteristic branching pattern of calcifications (Fig. 1-13). The tumor forms exuberant plugs of cells within the ducts. The debris of the necrotic centermost cells may calcify, accounting for the branching pattern of calcifications following the ramifications

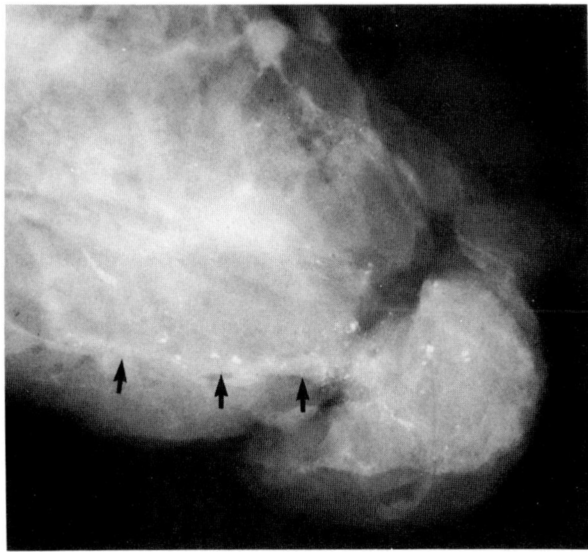

Figure 1-9. Biopsy specimen radiograph of intraductal carcinoma revealing branching calcifications that are punctate, linear, and irregular in shape. Prominent duct (arrows) has resulted from increased fibrous connective tissue in duct wall, along which calcifications have spread.

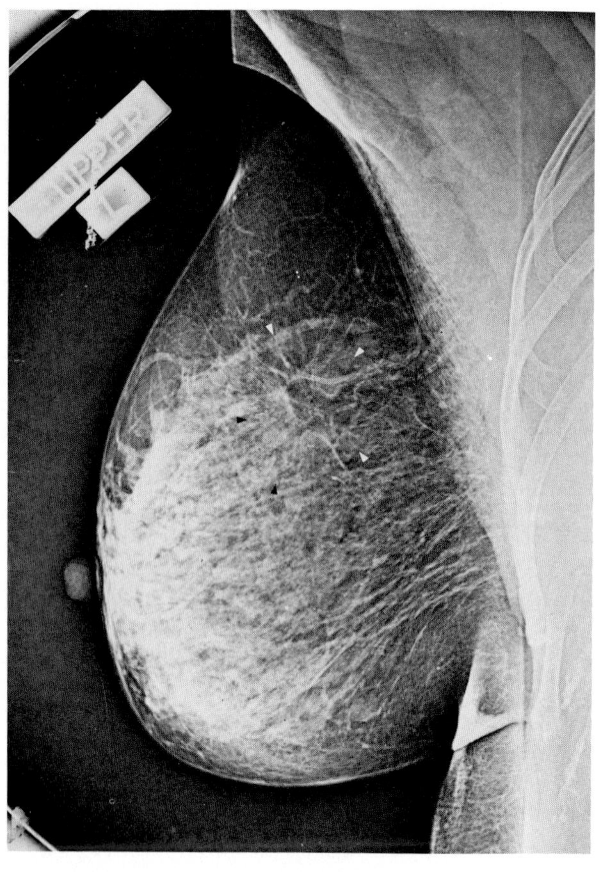

A

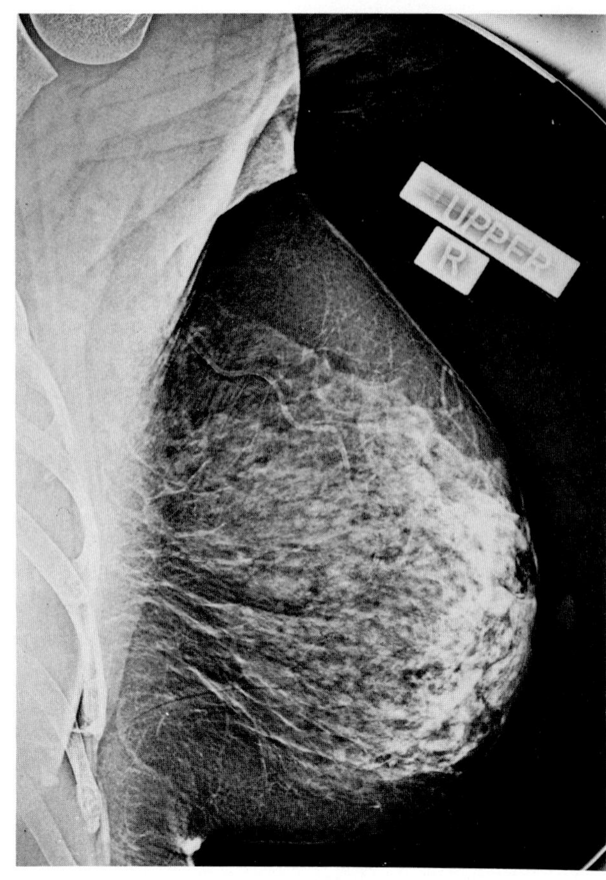

B

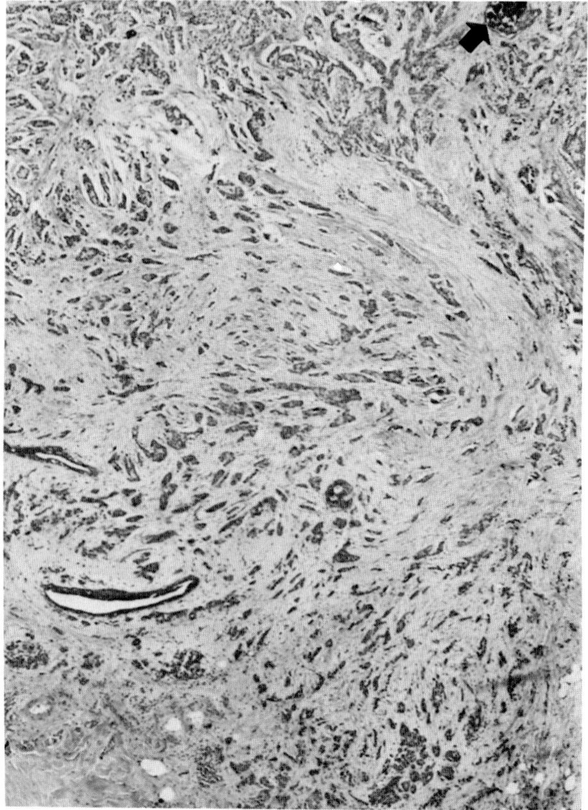

C

Figure 1-10. A. Carcinoma of left breast characterized by architectural distortion in forms of radiating spicules (arrowheads). B. Comparison view of right breast enhances detection of abnormality. C. Histologic section. Infiltrating duct carcinoma with radiating pattern of productive fibrosis, leading to designation of scirrhous or stellate carcinoma. Focal calcification is present (arrow) (hematoxylin and eosin stain, original ×55).

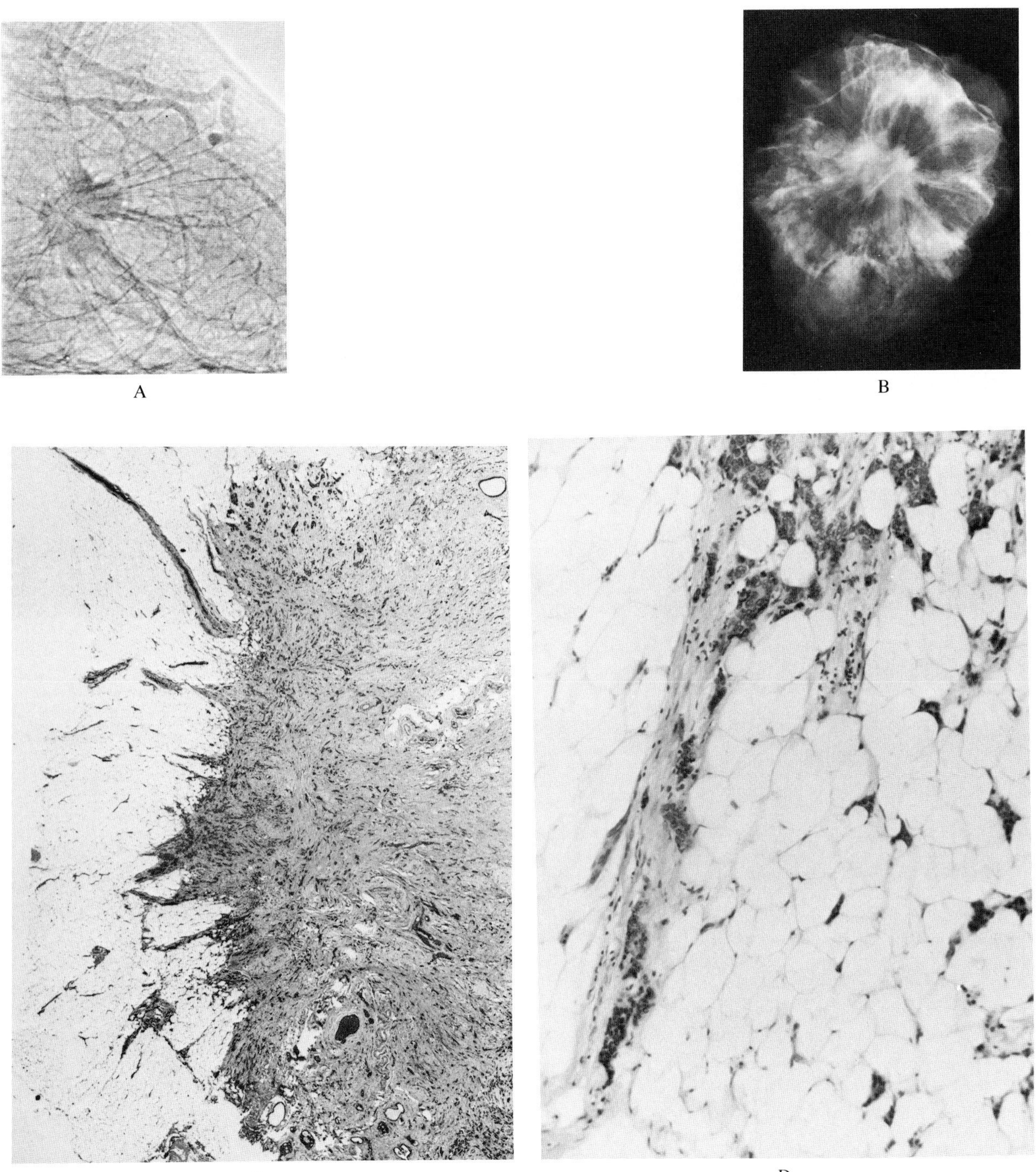

Figure 1-11. Examples of scirrhous carcinoma. A. Highly infiltrative carcinoma characterized by extensive spiculation along periphery. Central core or nucleus of lesion (not including spicules) measured 3 cm in greatest diameter. B. Specimen radiograph of 1-cm highly infiltrative scirrhous carcinoma surrounded by cysts and foci of fibrocystic changes. Scirrhous carcinomas typically have irregular margins and peripheral tendrils radiating into surrounding fat. C. Histologic section shows a strikingly irregular boundary between carcinoma on right and mammary fat on left (hematoxylin and eosin stain, ×10). D. Higher magnification reveals infiltration of mammary fat by small nests of tumor cells accompanying fibrous tendrils (hematoxylin and eosin stain, original ×100).

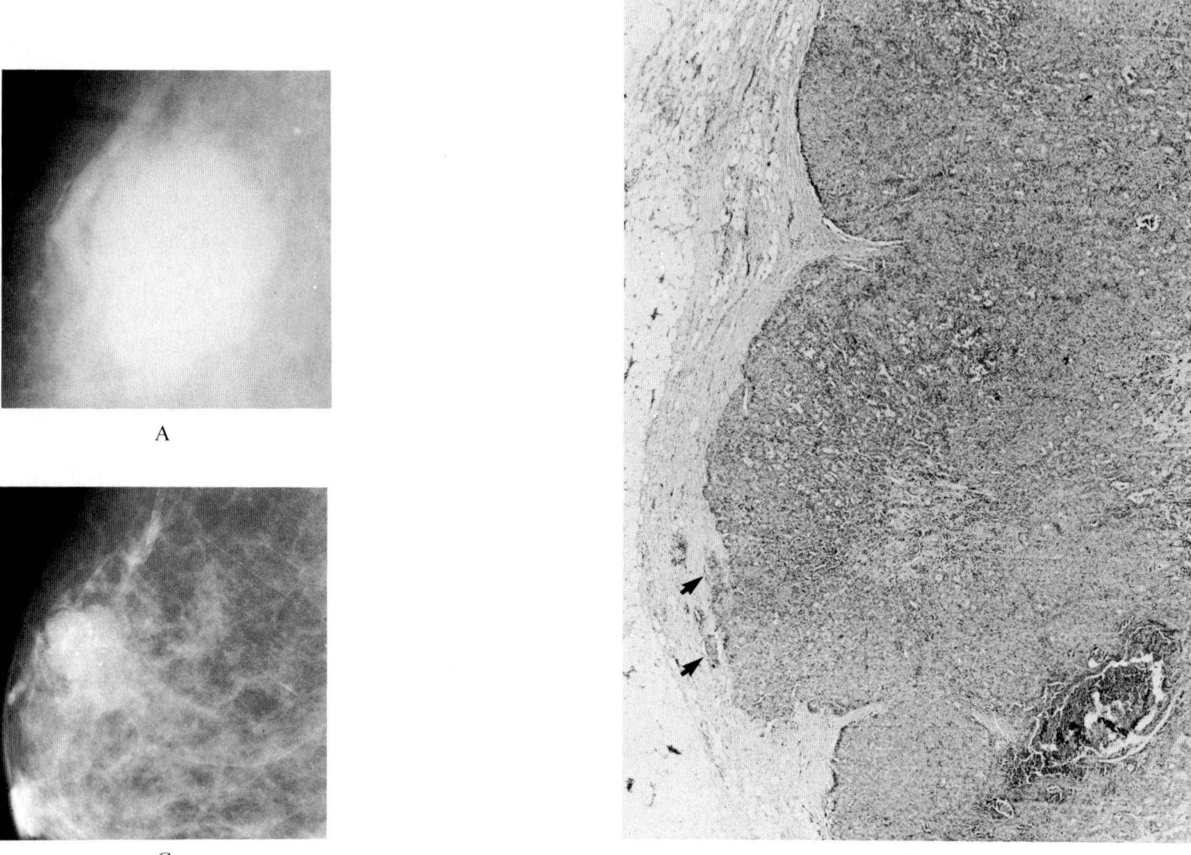

A

C

B

Figure 1-12. Slightly infiltrative carcinoma characterized by irregular margin without spiculation. A. Mammographic image of lesion 3 cm in greatest diameter. Absence of perfectly smooth margin in presence of sufficient fat to delineate border implies that lesion may be malignant. B. Histologic section reveals that tumor, along much of its margin, is sharply demarcated from thin layer of collagen that surrounds it. Small fingerlike extensions of tumor nevertheless extend into surrounding fibrous tissue (arrows) (hematoxylin and eosin stain, original ×20). C. Infiltrating duct carcinoma combining characteristics of highly infiltrative and mildly infiltrative lesions. Anterior surface of lesion is smooth and lobulated, while posterior surface appears indistinct and highly infiltrative. Lesion contains less than 10 flecks of rather coarse but irregularly shaped calcification. Relative paucity in number of calcifications should not be significant factor against diagnosis of malignancy. Calcifications are recognizable mammographically in no more than one half of all breast carcinomas and although characteristically very numerous, they may be few. Irregularity of shape of calcifications is a far more significant point in favor of their malignant origin.

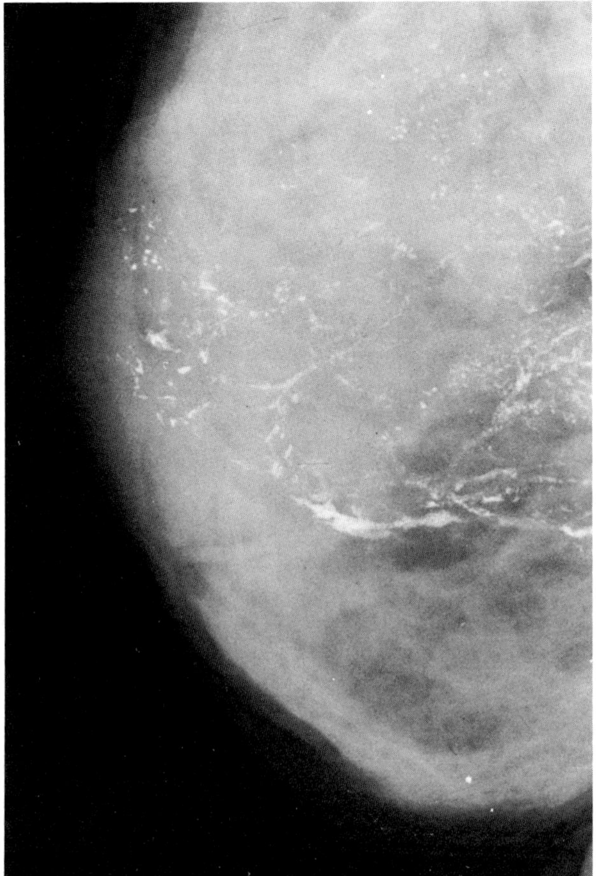

Figure 1-13. Characteristic branching pattern of calcifications of comedocarcinoma. Lesion, although extensive, was not palpable and was completely intraductal.

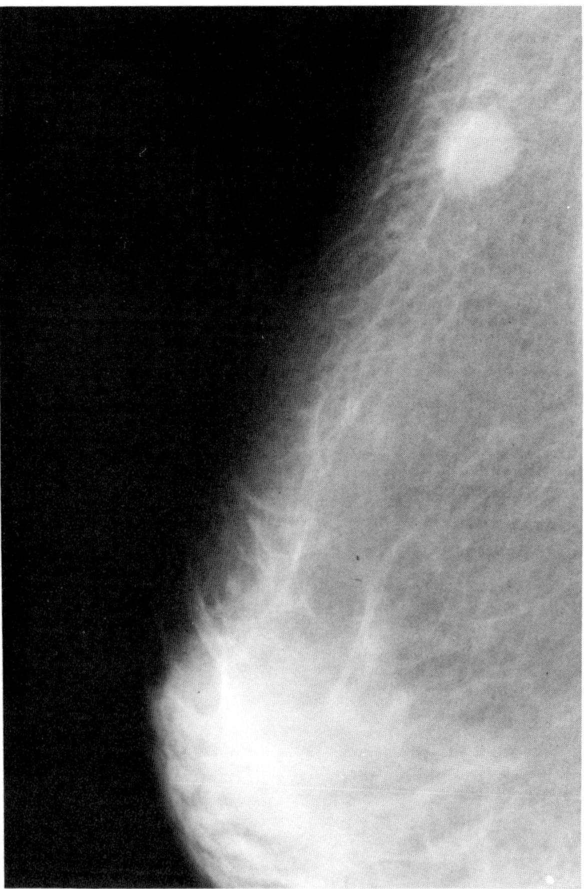

Figure 1-14. Metastasis to breast from squamous cell carcinoma of lung. Metastases from extramammary malignancies are characteristically round and well circumscribed and may mimic benign lesions.

of the ducts. Since comedocarcinomas frequently extend throughout much of the duct system and may remain entirely intraductal (noninvasive) and nonpalpable, mammography may be the only method for detection.

Tubular carcinoma, a rare, unusually well-differentiated type, is associated with a low incidence of metastasis. Well-formed but haphazardly arranged carcinomatous tubules within a fibrous stroma are characteristic pathologic features.[7] Mammographically, the lesion often presents as a small (average diameter 1 cm) stellate mass that may contain microcalcifications, an appearance identical to that of scirrhous carcinoma.[10]

In contrast to the infiltrative character of most carcinomas, the majority of benign masses—cysts and fibroadenomas—appear sharply circumscribed. Occasionally, however, a carcinoma is so well circumscribed as to resemble a benign lesion, both clinically and mammographically. Metastases to the breast from extramammary malignancies are also characteristically well circumscribed and may mimic benign lesions (Fig. 1-14).[5] It is therefore prudent to perform needle aspiration, excision biopsy, or ultrasonography of all solitary breast masses in women who are at risk for cancer, regardless of mammographic features (except in cases of the typical calcifying fibroadenoma).

Examples of well-circumscribed carcinomas include *papillary carcinoma* (Fig. 1-15), *medullary carcinoma* (Fig. 1-16), and *colloid (mucinous) carcinoma* (Fig. 1-17).[28]* Careful inspection of technically optimal mammograms usually reveals that the margins of these well-circumscribed carcinomas are not smooth throughout but rather are partially irregular or indistinct. Because they incite little desmoplastic reaction, these carcinomas, like most benign breast masses, tend to feel the same size to palpation as they appear in mammograms. Fortunately, these cancers are less aggressive, grow more slowly, metastasize later, and thus have a more favorable prognosis than scirrhous or infiltrative lobular carcinomas.

* pp 55–57

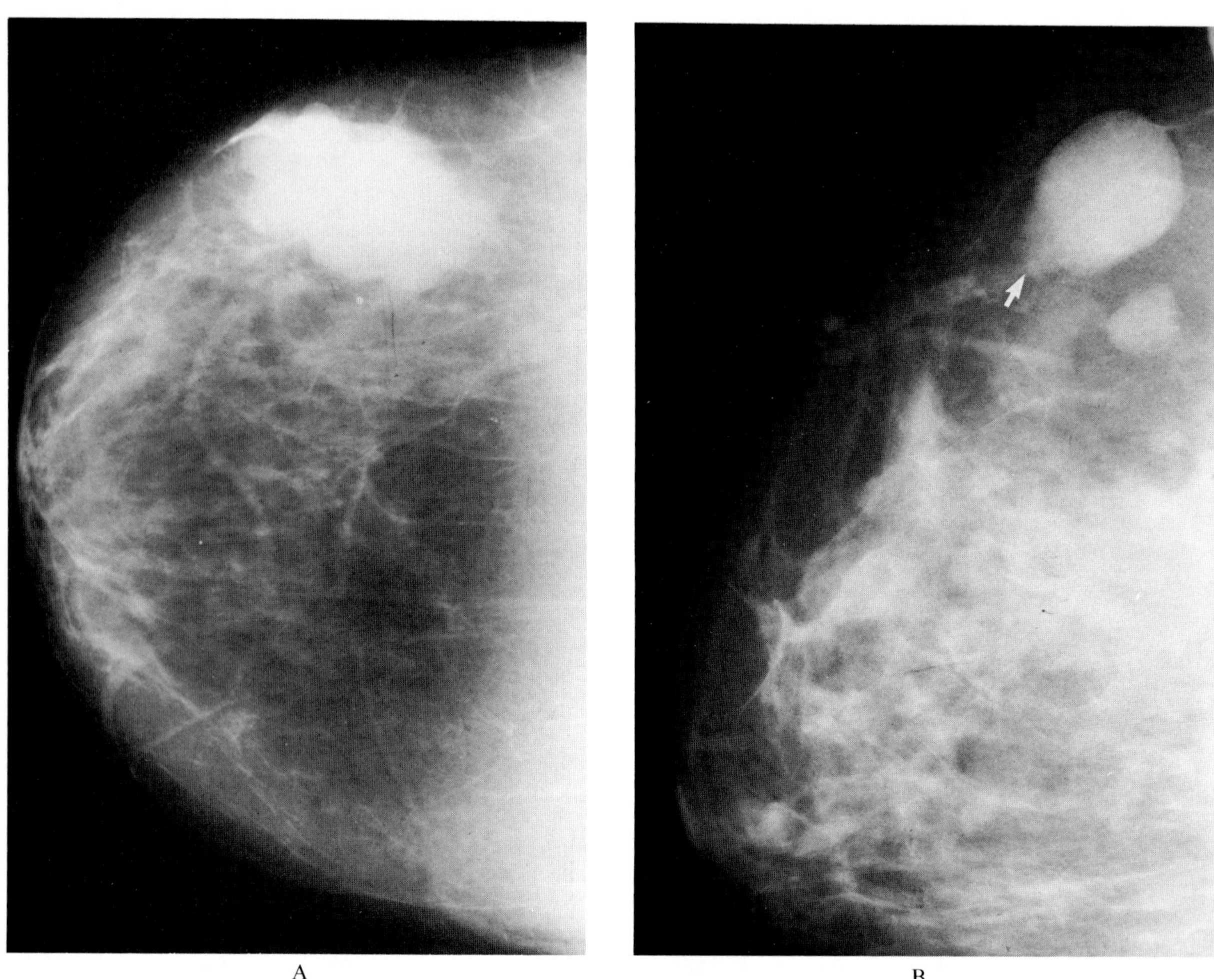

Figure 1-15. Papillary carcinomas. A. Papillary carcinoma characterized by irregular, indistinct margin but without spiculation, an example of less aggressive, well-circumscribed carcinoma with more favorable prognosis than scirrhous carcinoma. B. Another papillary carcinoma, smoothly delimited except anteriorly, where its margin has indistinct, infiltrative appearance (arrow). Smaller nodules nearby represent benign intraductal papillomas.

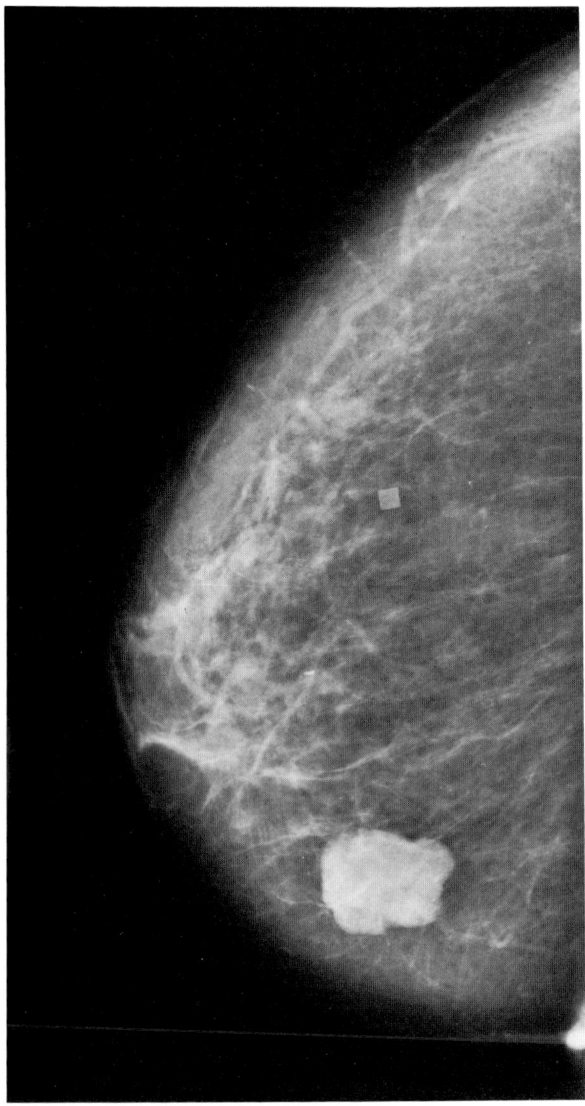

Figure 1-16. Medullary carcinoma. Lesion has lobulated, well-circumscribed appearance, without peripheral spiculations of highly infiltrative scirrhous carcinoma. A thermoluminescent dosimetry chip is present on skin of upper hemisphere.

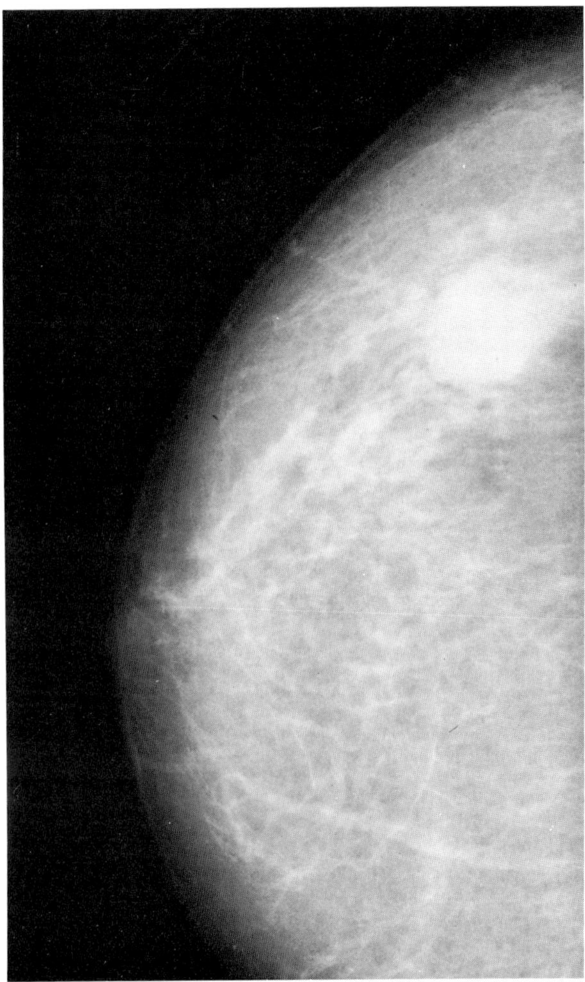

Figure 1-17. Colloid (mucinous) carcinoma, another example of well-circumscribed carcinoma. This lesion has indistinct anterior, superior, and posterior margins, but not characteristic spiculation of scirrhous carcinoma. Well-circumscribed carcinomas, such as colloid, papillary, and medullary carcinomas, tend to grow more slowly, metastasize later, and thus have more favorable prognosis than scirrhous or infiltrative lobular carcinomas.

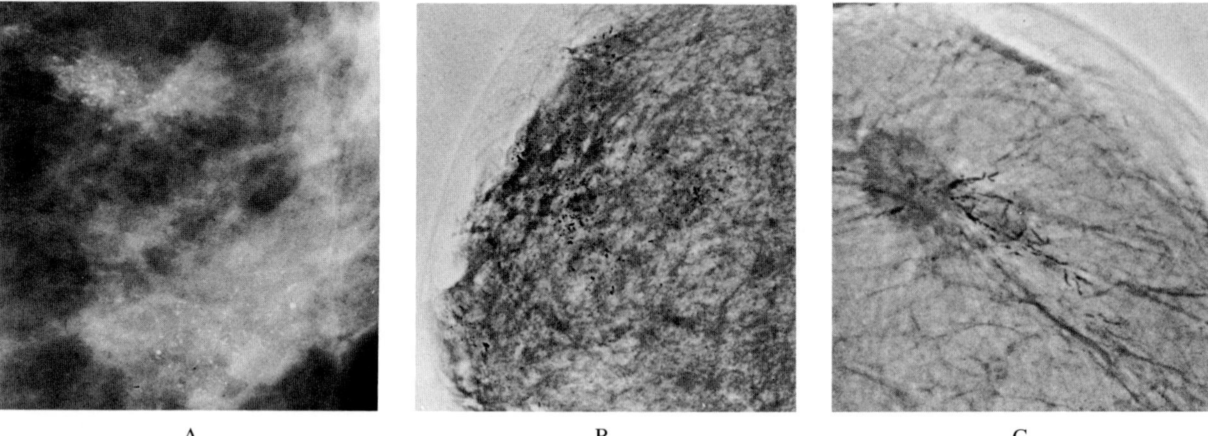

Figure 1-18. Features of malignant calcifications. A. Multicentric carcinoma characterized by separate foci of numerous, polymorphic, finely stippled, lacy, branching, and bizarrely shaped calcifications of varying size. B. Extensive carcinomatous infiltration characterized by microcalcifications too numerous to count and variable in size and shape. C. Carcinoma calcifications featuring branching pattern.

CALCIFICATIONS

Calcifications characteristic of carcinoma tend to be numerous, tiny, clustered, polymorphic, finely stippled, angular, lacy, rod-like, curvilinear, irregularly shaped, bizarre, or branching, and of varying size (Figs. 1-18 and 1-19).[30,34] Calcifications in benign conditions tend to be larger, rounder, fewer in number, and less variable in size. Cancers exhibit mammographic evidence of calcification in approximately half of cases. Certain benign breast conditions—sclerosing adenosis (Figs. 1-20A through C), fat necrosis, and apocrine metaplasia (Fig. 1-20D)—may manifest microcalcifications similar to those seen in malignancy. In these benign disorders, however, the calcifications are usually rounder, fewer in number, and more scattered in distribution than the calcifications of carcinoma. Intraductal papillomas may contain a rosette pattern of several small calcifications that may resemble those of malignancy. Scattered, large ring-shaped, or coarse linear calcifications reflect calcified inspissated cellular and lipid debris of benign secretory disease (Figs. 1-20E and F).[12] Fibroadenoma, the most common solid benign tumor of the breast, may hyalinize and calcify with advancing maturity; these foci of calcifications tend to be large and amorphous (Fig. 1-20G). Calcified arteries appear as broken parallel lines of calcium (Fig. 1-20H). The skin may contain tiny round homogeneous or ring-shaped calcifications (Fig. 1-20I) similar to those of secretory disease. Dermal deposits of calcium may be confirmed through the use of a lead skin marker (Fig. 1-21). The marker, when placed directly over the calcifications on one mammographic projection, will closely overlie or be superimposed upon them in any other projection if they are in the skin.[22] The wall of a cyst may occasionally calcify in a typical curvilinear fashion (Fig. 1-20J). Milk of calcium within tiny benign cysts has been described.[36] Following primary radiotherapy for carcinoma, typical malignant calcifications may disappear (Fig. 1-22) and benign-appearing calcifications may appear (Fig. 1-23)[4,24] The skin may contain tiny, round, homogeneous or circular calcifications similar to those of secretory disease. Tattoo pigments (Fig. 1-24) and deodorant residues are often radiopaque and may simulate malignant calcifications. One or more benign calcifications of secretory disease may be drawn into a focus of carcinoma by its accompanying desmoplastic response (Fig. 1-25). In this situation, fat necrosis may be considered in the differential diagnosis, but carcinoma must be excluded by biopsy.

PREOPERATIVE NEEDLE LOCALIZATION AND SPECIMEN RADIOGRAPHY

All clusters of calcifications suspicious of malignancy should be biopsied, even though some will be found to result from benign disease—usually sclerosing adenosis. Similarly, any alteration of breast architecture that could signify a malignant desmoplastic reaction requires a biopsy, although benign disorders such as sclerosing adenosis and fat necrosis can manifest an identical fibrous connective tissue response. The indication and techniques relating to preoperative needle localization and specimen radiography are described in detail in the chapter by Kalisher and Hutter. For the detection, excision, and evaluation of possible early, nonpalpable cancer, the surgeon, mammographer, and pathologist must work together as a team. Preoperative needle localization of a nonpalpable lesion requires a specimen radiograph after the biopsy to confirm that the lesion has actually been excised and to localize the suspicious area in the biopsy specimen for the pathologist.

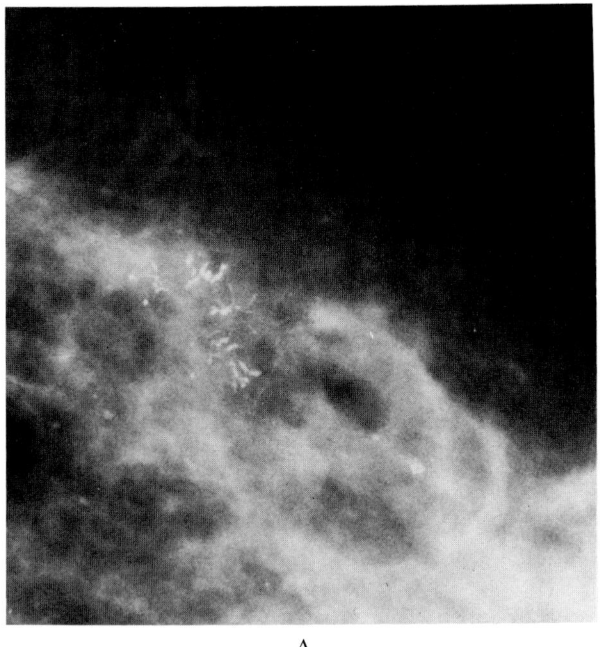

A

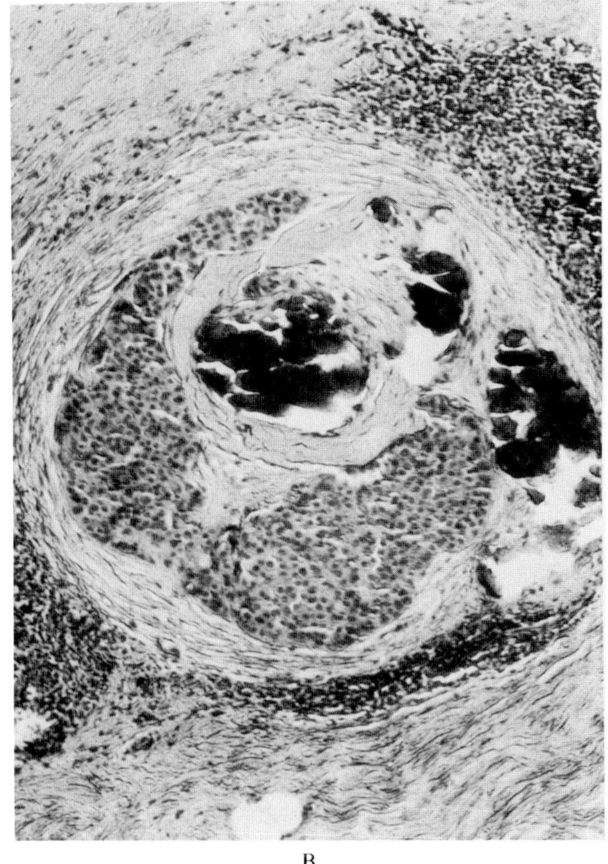

B

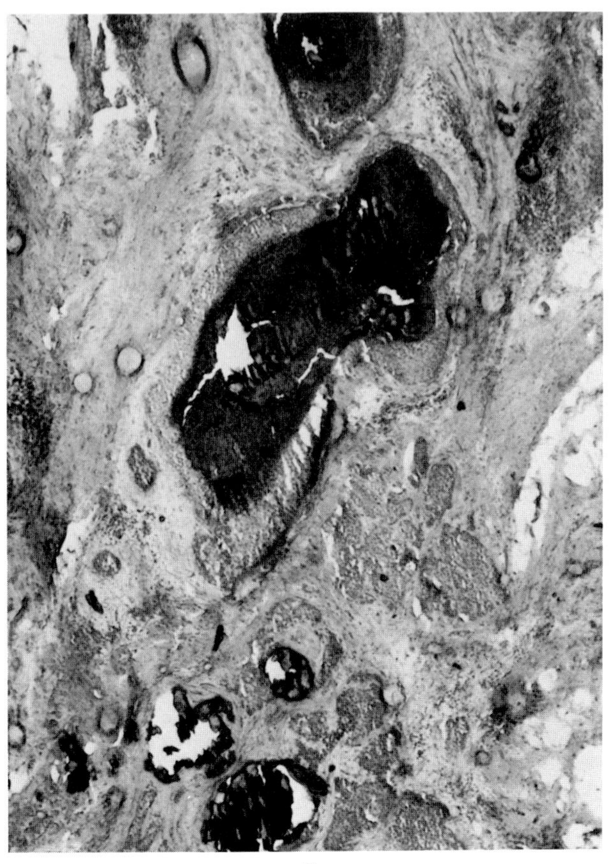

C

Figure 1-19. A. 2-cm cluster of irregularly shaped, linear and curvilinear calcifications in a branching array, characteristic of carcinoma. The patient was an asymptomatic woman, age 60, referred for screening mammography. B. Medium-power histologic section. Ductal carcinoma in situ, comedo pattern, in which central necrotic core of cells is extensively calcified (hematoxylin and eosin stain, original ×55). C. High-power histologic section. Metaplastic bone formation in center of field implies lesion has been present for many years (hematoxylin and eosin stain, original ×110.

Figure 1-20. Features of benign calcifications. A. Highly magnified calcifications in focus of sclerosing adenosis. Although shape of calcifications is rounder than that usually associated with malignancy, biopsy was necessary to exclude that possibility. B. Scattered microcalcifications of varying size and shape. Their great number and arrangement in clusters was suspicious for malignancy. C. Histologic section. A focus of calcifications was excised following needle localization. The tissue represents benign proliferative breast disease. A lobule exhibits microcystic blunt duct adenosis. The tubular profiles are lined by epithelium and myoepithelium and contain microcalcifications (arrows), (hematoxylin and eosin stain, original ×110). D. Highly magnified cluster of hundreds of punctate calcifications, many of which are round, implying benign disease. Others are irregular or bizarre in shape, suggesting malignancy. Biopsy revealed apocrine metaplasia, a benign condition. E. Scattered ring-shaped calcifications of secretory disease. F. Coarse, homogeneous rod-shaped calcifications of secretory disease. G. Large, amorphous calcification in hyalinized, completely calcified fibroadenoma. H. Broken parallel lines of calcium in wall of artery. I. Ring-shaped calcifications in skin, similar in appearance to those of secretory disease. J. Curvilinear calcification within wall of cyst.

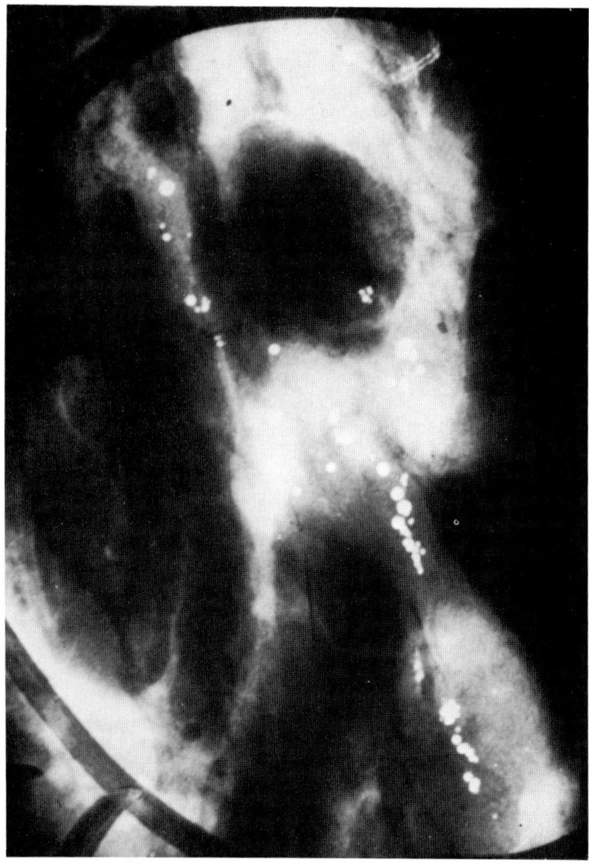

A

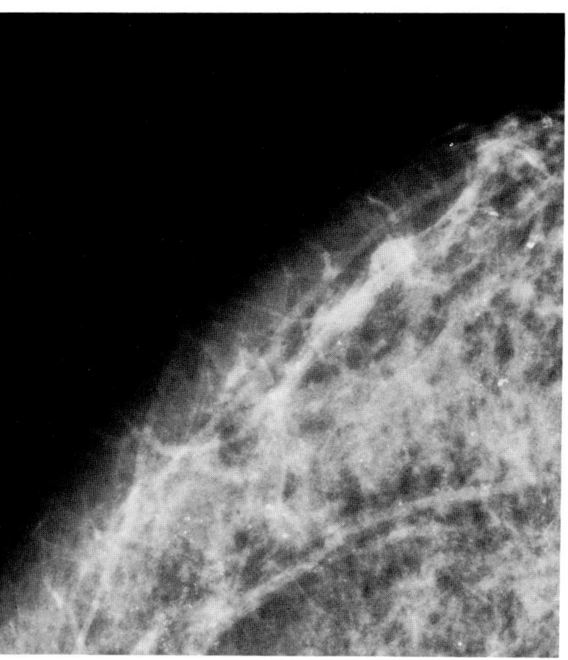

B

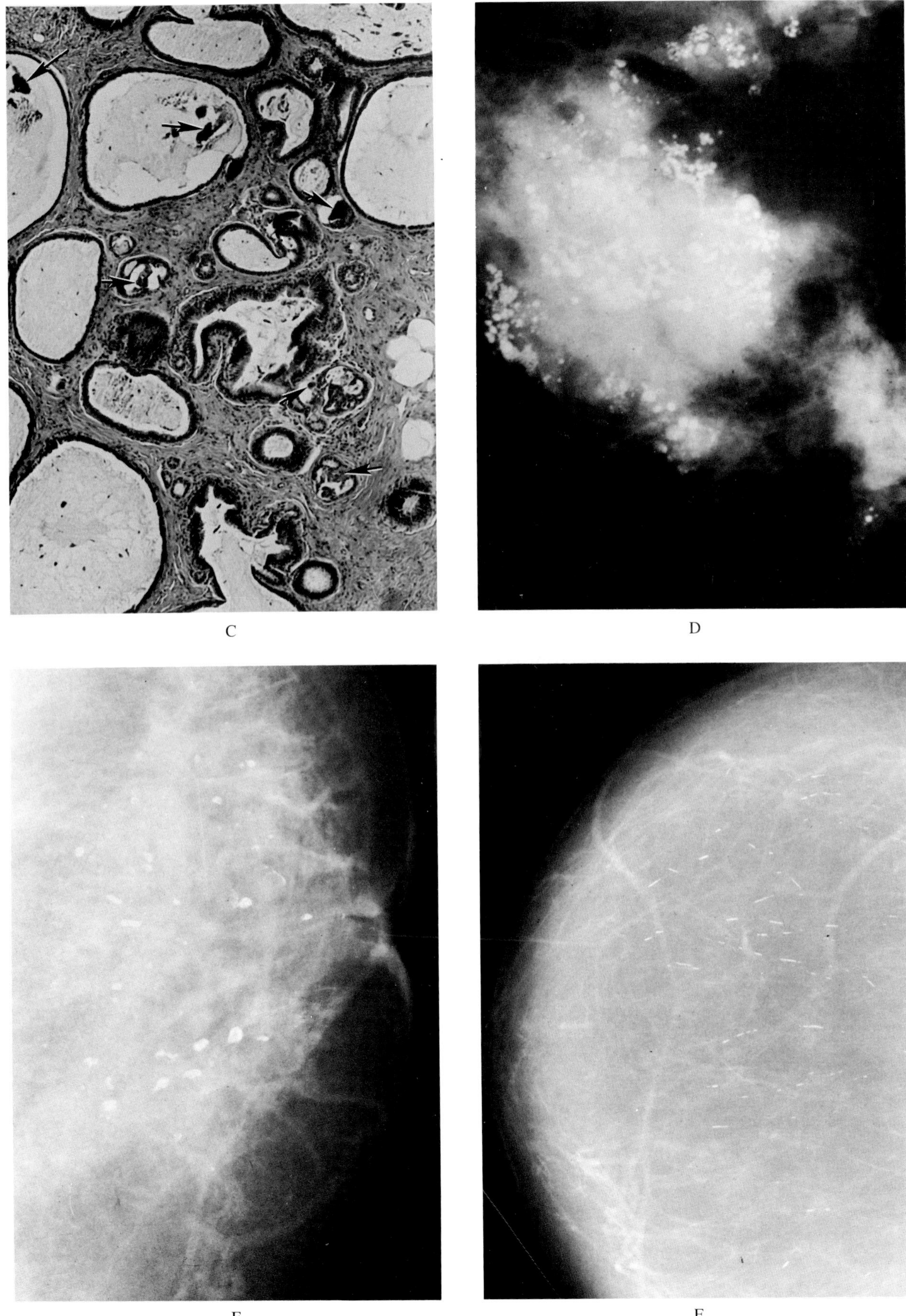

C

D

E

F

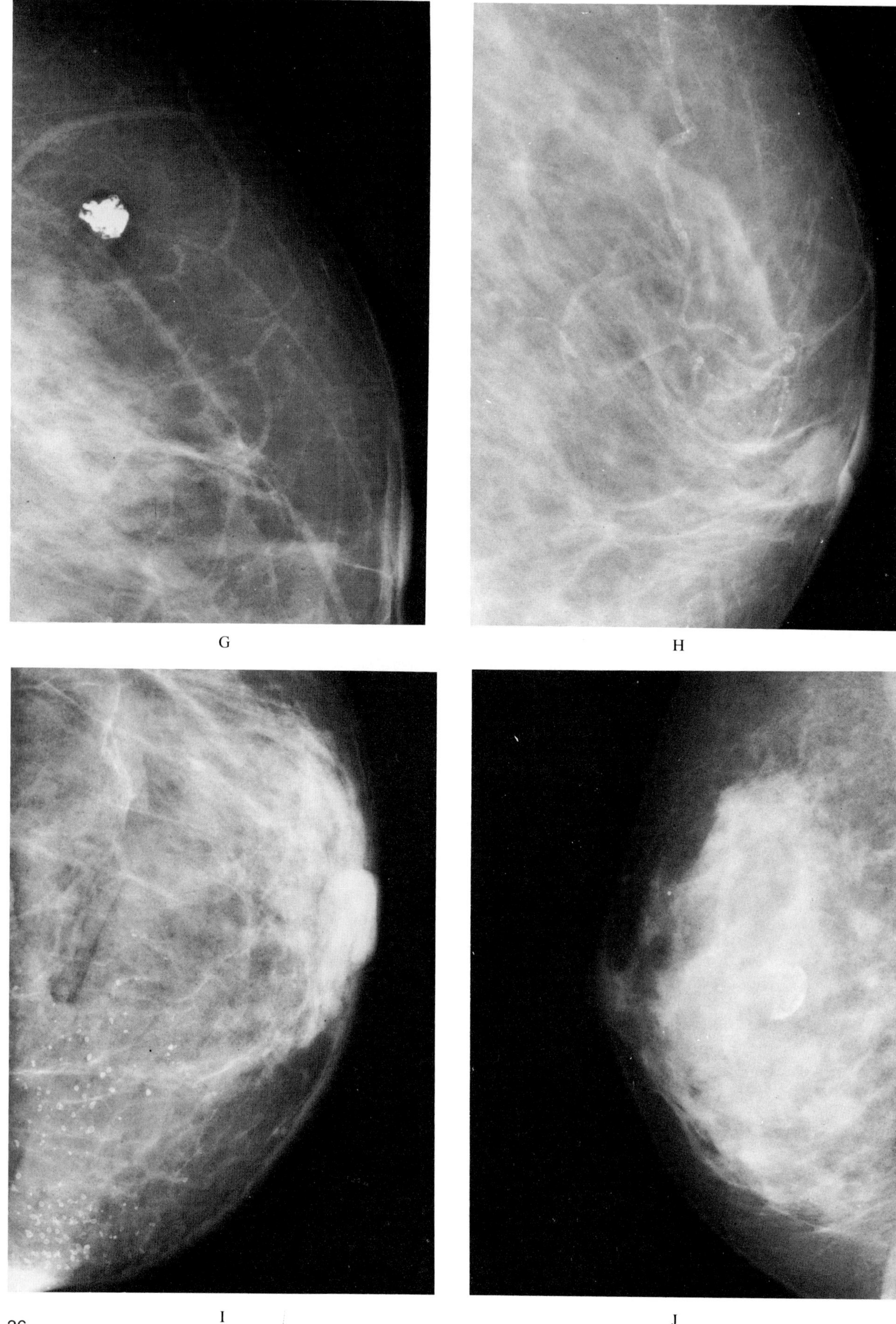

G H

I J

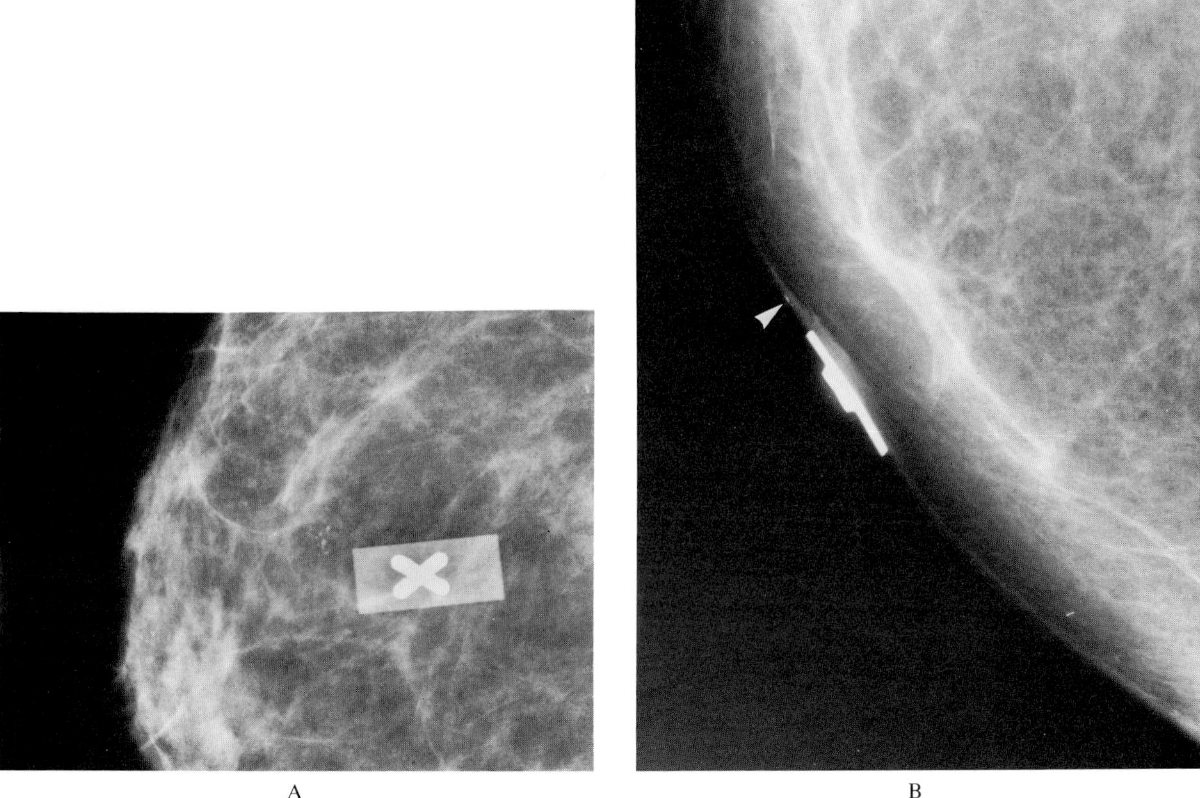

A B

Figure 1-21. Dermal calcifications proven by lead skin-marker technique. A. Mediolateral view. Marker placed on skin overlying cluster of calcifications seen on previous mammogram. B. Cephalocaudal view shows that marker remains in close proximity to calcifications, now depicted in skin.

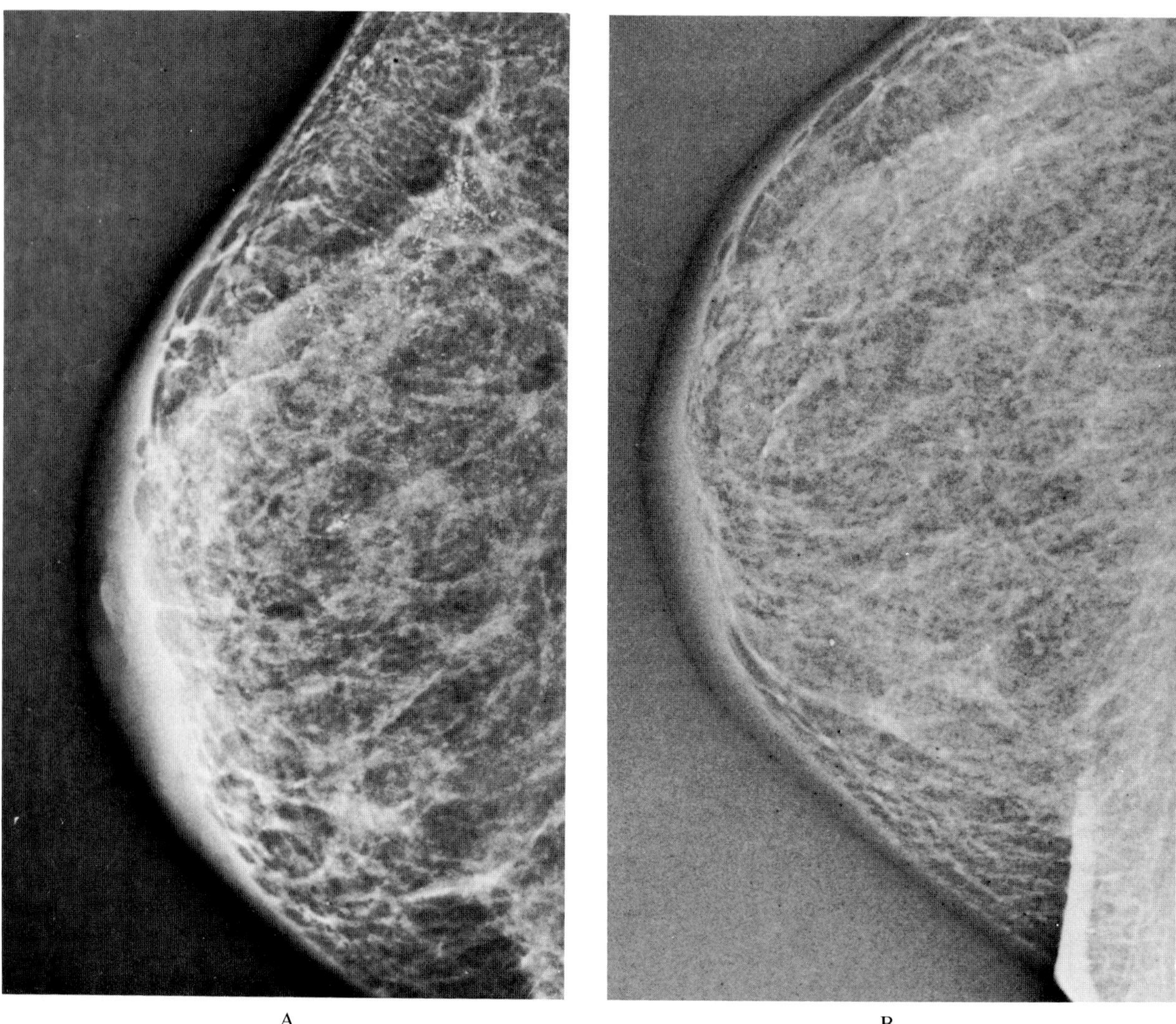

Figure 1-22. Disappearance of malignant calcifications following radiation therapy of inoperable inflammatory carcinoma. A. Characteristic cluster of calcifications in upper hemisphere signifies carcinoma. Patient had diffuse skin thickening and hot, red breast typifying inflammatory carcinoma. Biopsy of overlying skin and subcutaneous tissue revealed plugs of tumor cells in subdermal lymphatic channels. B. Six months following radiation therapy, calcifications have almost completely resolved.

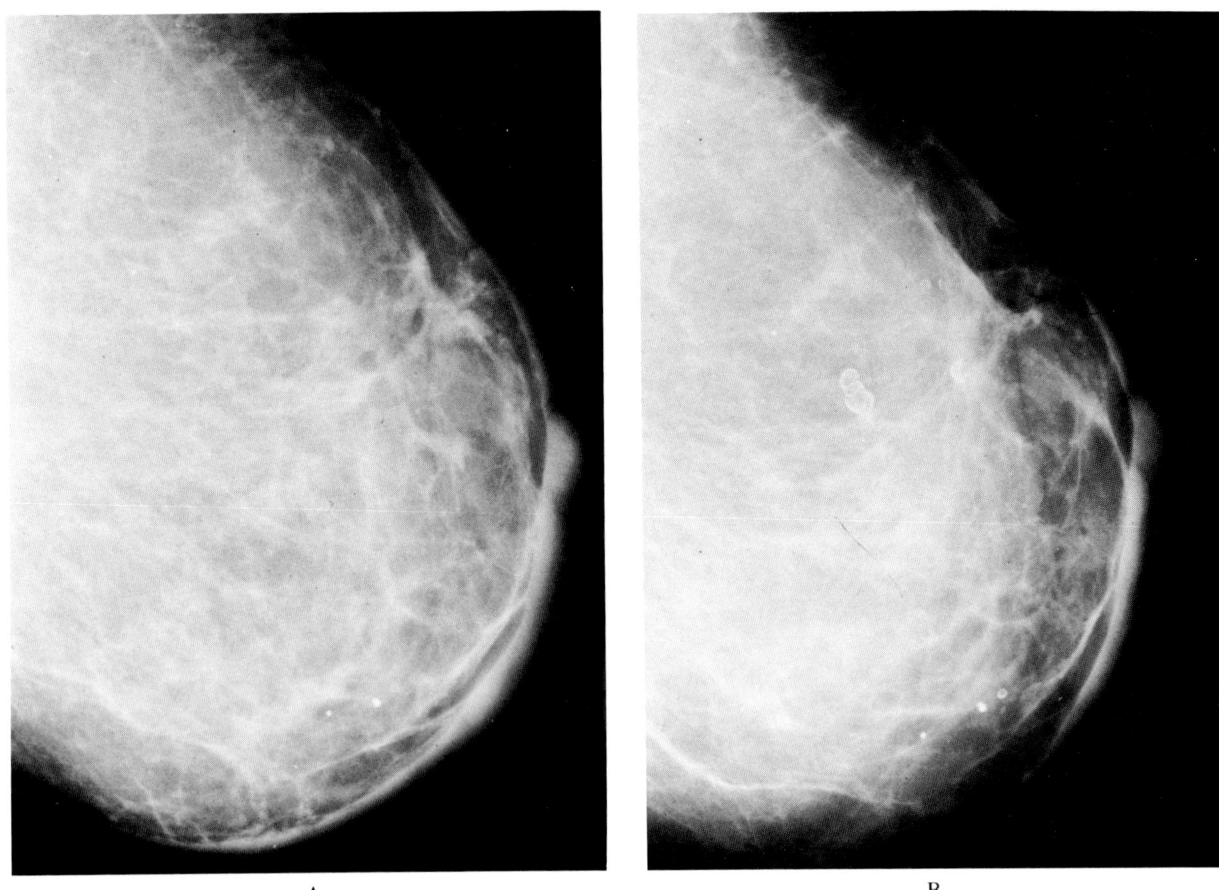

Figure 1-23. Benign calcifications appearing after excision biopsy and radiation therapy for carcinoma. A. Course of radiation therapy, just completed, has resulted in diffuse thickening of skin of breast. Two calcifications of secretory disease are present in lower hemisphere. B. One year following completion of radiation therapy. Several new ring-shaped calcifications are present centrally. Formation of such benign-appearing calcifications following radiation therapy and/or surgery is not unusual. Should calcifications be small, care must be taken not to ascribe them to recurrent tumor.

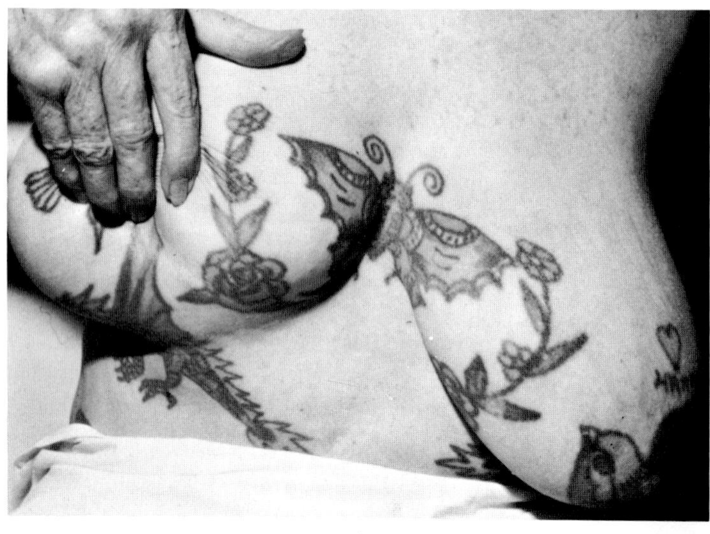

A

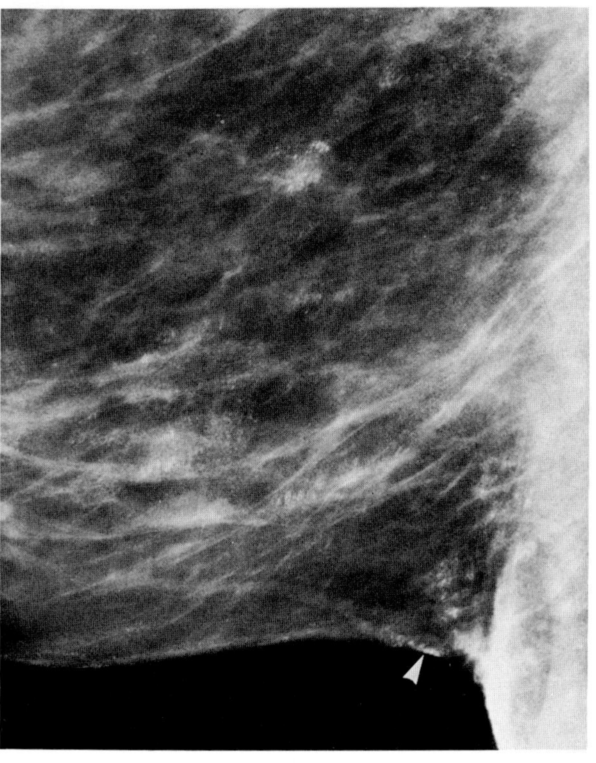

B

Figure 1-24. Tattoo pigment mimicking calcifications. A. Photograph of tattooed breasts. B. Radiopaque pigment has stippled appearance similar to microcalcifications but follows tattoo design. Note pigment in skin tangential to x-ray beam (arrowhead).

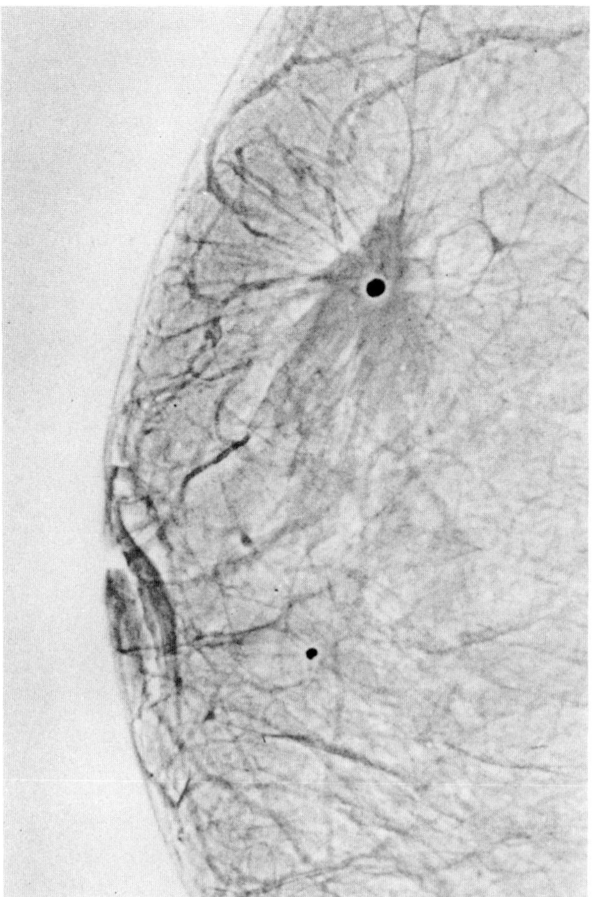

Figure 1-25. Cephalocaudal view disclosing single coarse, round calcification of benign secretory disease within center of carcinoma. Calcification was drawn into tumor by accompanying desmoplastic reaction and was shown to be in center of tumor on mediolateral view as well.

OBSTACLES TO THE MAMMOGRAPHIC DETECTION OF CANCER

The capability of mammography to reveal the shadow of a carcinoma, an alteration in architecture, or any lesion, benign or malignant, is largely dependent upon the presence of sufficient fat to serve as a contrasting radiolucent background.[9] Mammography may disclose an obvious carcinoma only a few millimeters in diameter in a breast in which fibroglandular tissue has been replaced by fat (Fig. 1-26). But in very dense breasts packed with radiopaque tissue, as in young nulliparous, pregnant, or lactating women, and in breasts manifesting severe fibrocystic changes, even a large carcinoma may be obscured by the dense surrounding tissues (Fig. 1-27).[14,20] Mammography thus should be considered of limited value in women with severe fibrocystic changes, or during pregnancy or lactation. Nevertheless, any rapidly enlarging mass during pregnancy is an indication for mammography. The low-energy mammography x-ray beam is primarily absorbed by the breast and underlying film holder and does not reach the abdomen or pelvis.

The radiographic density of injected silicone is even greater than that associated with fibrocystic changes, pregnancy, or lactation and may mask the presence of underlying calcifications that may be the sole clue to malignancy (Fig. 1-28).[32] Retromammary implants for the purpose of augmenting the size of the breasts prohibit optimal compression during the x-ray exposure, making visualization of the anteriorly displaced breast tissue less than ideal (Fig. 1-29). Retromammary saline implants (silastic-fabric sacs filled with saline) are less dense than silicone gel implants and tend to be more readily compressible, factors which result in improved visual detail.[19] Needless to say, when faced with increased density, the mammographer should alert the referring physician to the difficulty of detecting cancer in such breasts.

Normal intramammary lymph nodes are usually nonpalpable and are found in the upper-outer quadrant of the breast, near the chest wall. They tend to be less than 1 cm in diameter, often manifest a bean or kidney shape with a distinctive hilar notch, and are often partially replaced by fat. Should, however, an intramammary lymph node enlarge and its fat content be displaced or replaced by inflammatory or neoplastic change, the node may clinically and mammographically resemble a primary carcinoma.[23]

A mole on the skin of the breast may simulate an intramammary lesion in the mammogram (Fig. 1-30).

A surgical scar, particularly of recent origin, may resemble a desmoplastic reaction of carcinoma (Fig. 1-31).[37] Palpation is useful in excluding carcinoma in the region of a known scar. A scar is usually only palpable as a minimal, vague thickening, while most infiltrating carcinomas feel two or three times larger than their mammographic images and are usually rock hard. Moreover, follow-up mammograms will disclose a gradual decrease in the size and prominence of scar tissue.

CYSTS, FIBROADENOMAS, CYSTOSARCOMA, LIPOFIBROADENOMAS, LIPOMAS, SCLEROSING ADENOSIS, ABSCESS, FAT NECROSIS, AND PLASMA CELL MASTITIS

Cysts (Fig. 1-32) result from dilatation of terminal ducts. Because the fluid within a cyst is under tension, its wall tends to be displaced equally in all directions. A cyst, therefore, has a smooth, sharp border and, as shown by air insufflation, a thin wall with a smooth lining. Cyst fluid, once completely aspirated, rarely reaccumulates. If an attempt at aspiration fails, the possibility of a solid tumor must be considered, and the mass should then be

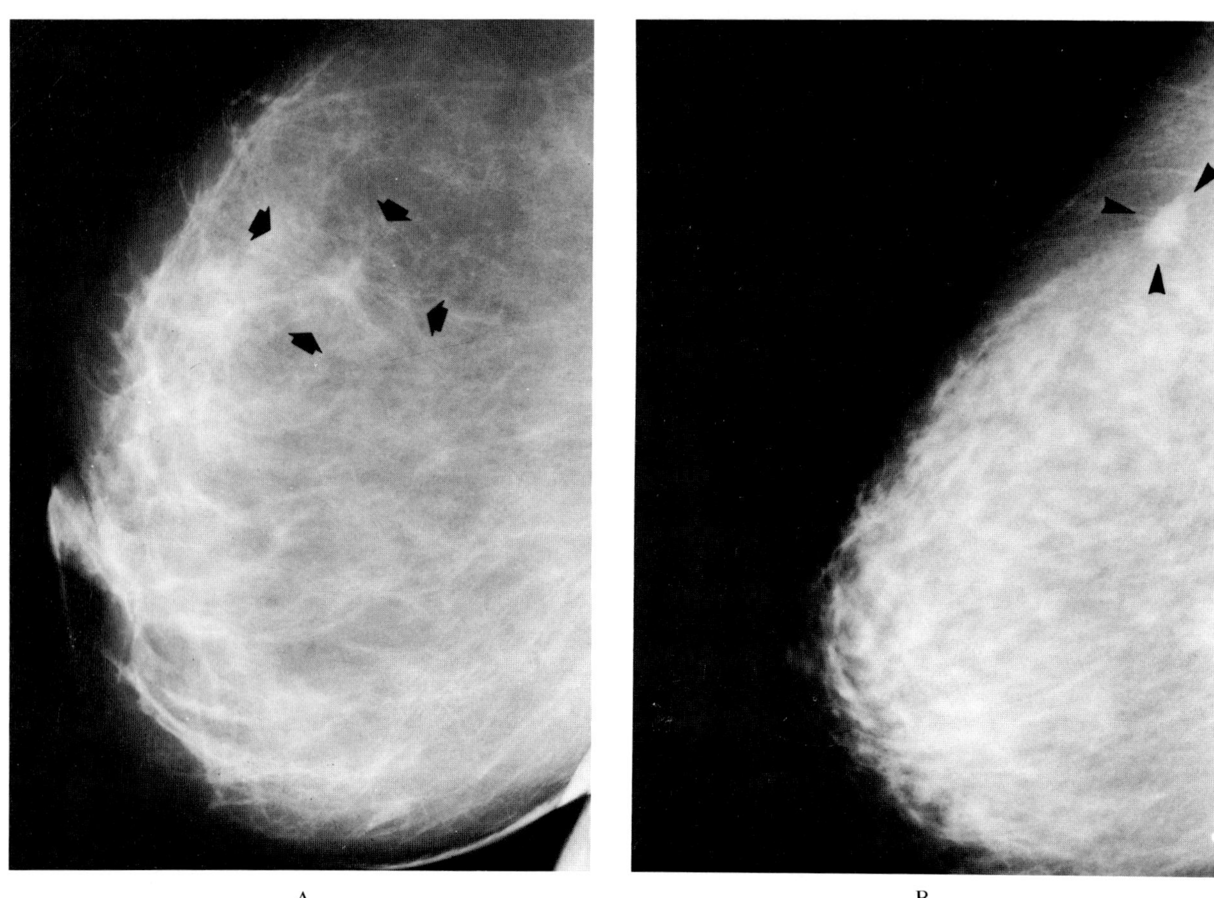

A B

Figure 1-26. Importance of radiolucent background of fat in detection of carcinoma. A. A 1-cm spiculated carcinoma (arrows), easily detected because it is surrounded by fat. B. 1-cm carcinoma (arrows) characterized by spiculated border. Lesion is located in relatively fatty part of breast. Were lesion more central in location, it might have been obscured by superimposed dense parenchyma.

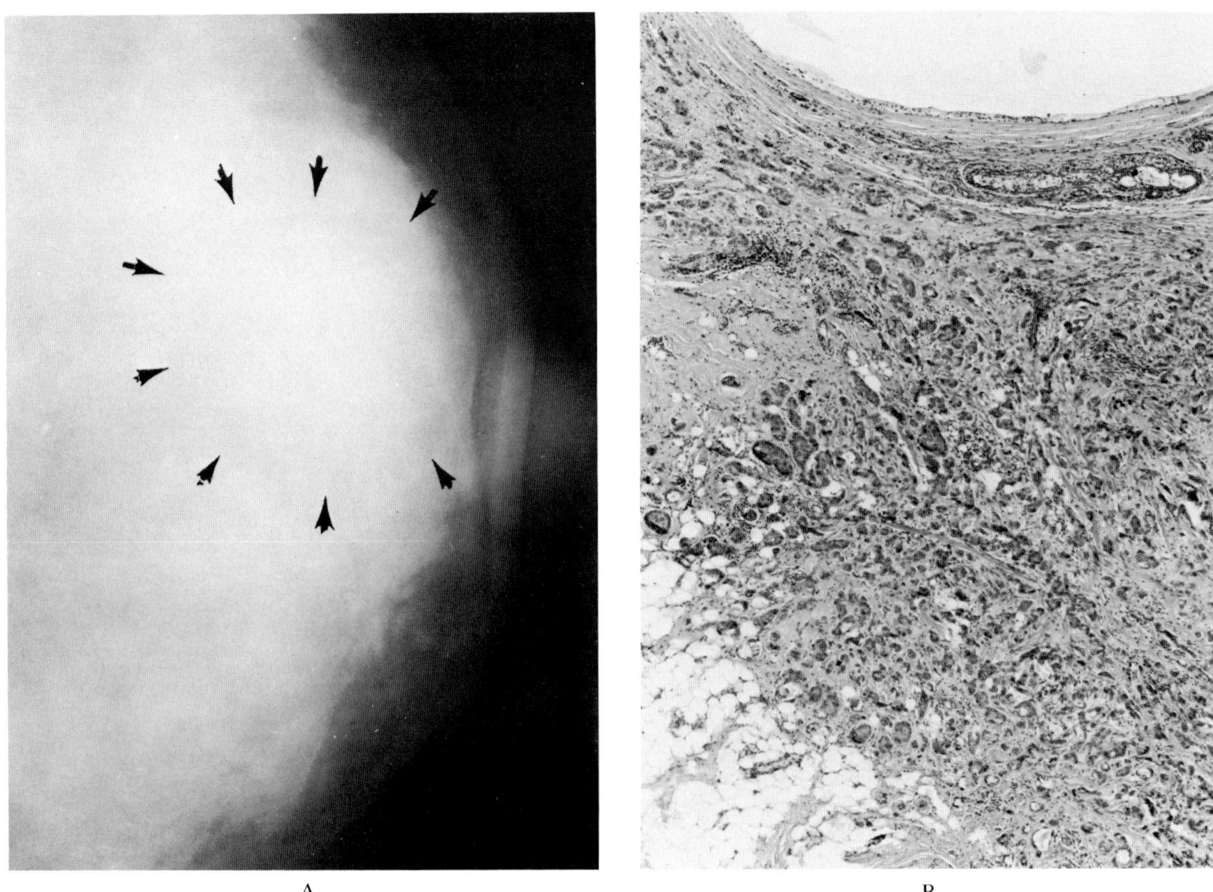

Figure 1-27. Example of difficulty in detecting carcinoma in breasts packed with radiopaque tissue in place of fat. A. Breast with dense parenchyma containing 2-cm benign cyst surrounded by radiolucent halo (arrows) and carcinoma that is completely obscured. Lack of fat in such breasts leads to extreme difficulty in detecting carcinoma. B. Histologic section. Macrocyst formation (upper part of field) and duct ectasia coexist with cords and nests of carcinoma cells (lower two-thirds of field) infiltrating mammary fat (lower left-hand corner) (hematoxylin and eosin stain, original ×40).

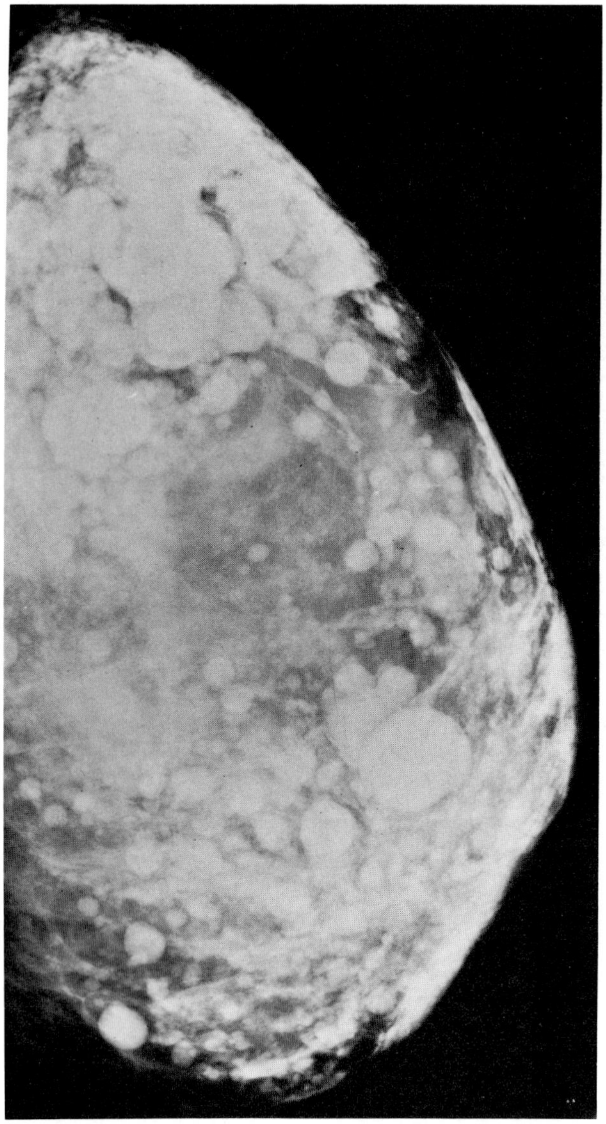

A

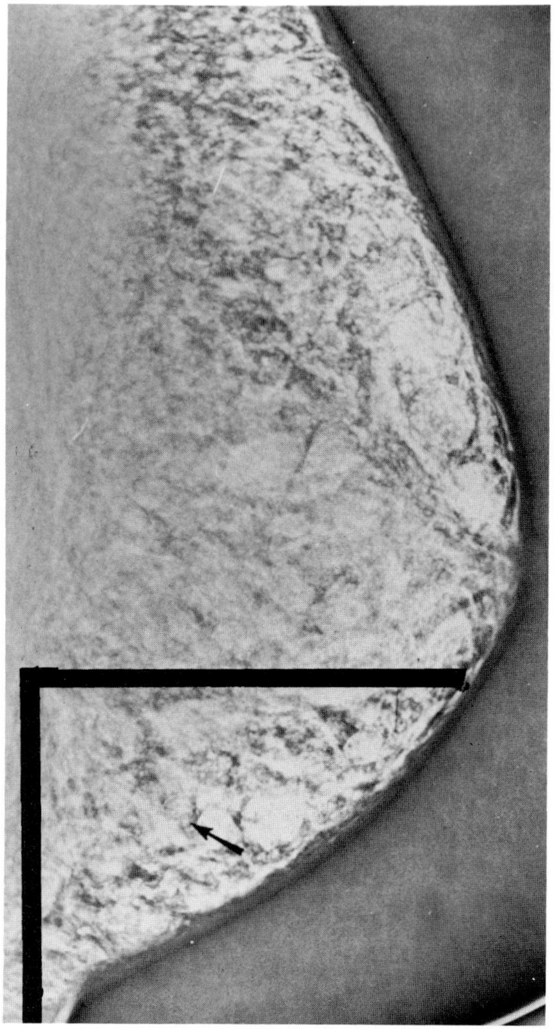

B

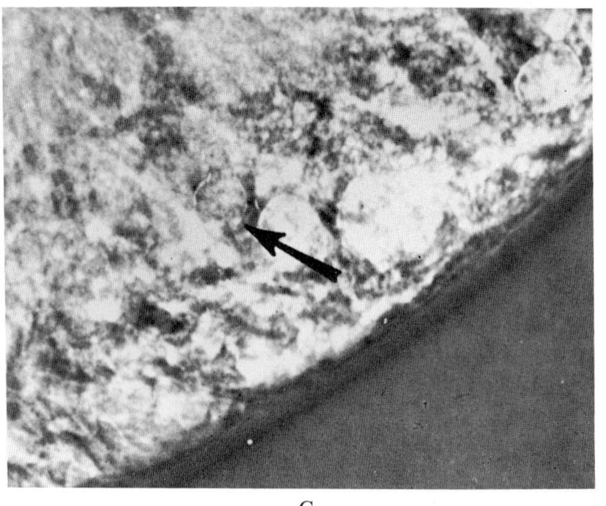

C

Figure 1-28. Injected silicone. A. Mediolateral screen-film mammogram. Density of injected silicone is even greater than that associated with fibrocystic changes, pregnancy, or lactation and may mask underlying malignant calcifications. B. Another breast containing injected silicone depicted by xeromammography in negative mode. Arrow points to small focus of fat necrosis represented by lipid-filled cyst with calcified wall. C. Close-up view of fat necrosis. Despite this astute observation, chance of detecting any pathology, let alone malignancy, in breast of this striking density is small.

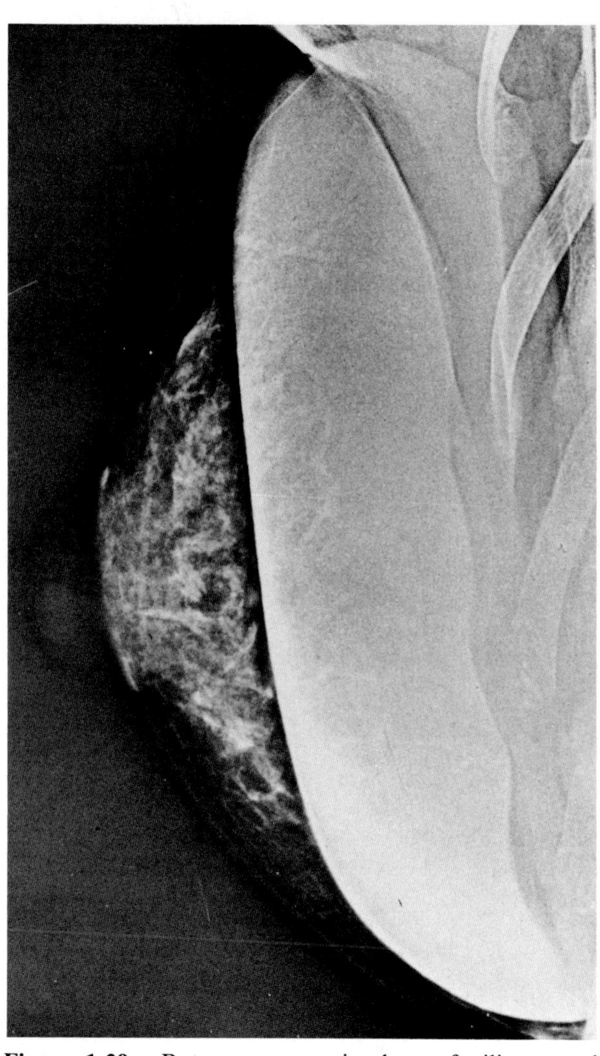

Figure 1-29. Retromammary implant of silicone gel depicted by negative-mode xeromammography.

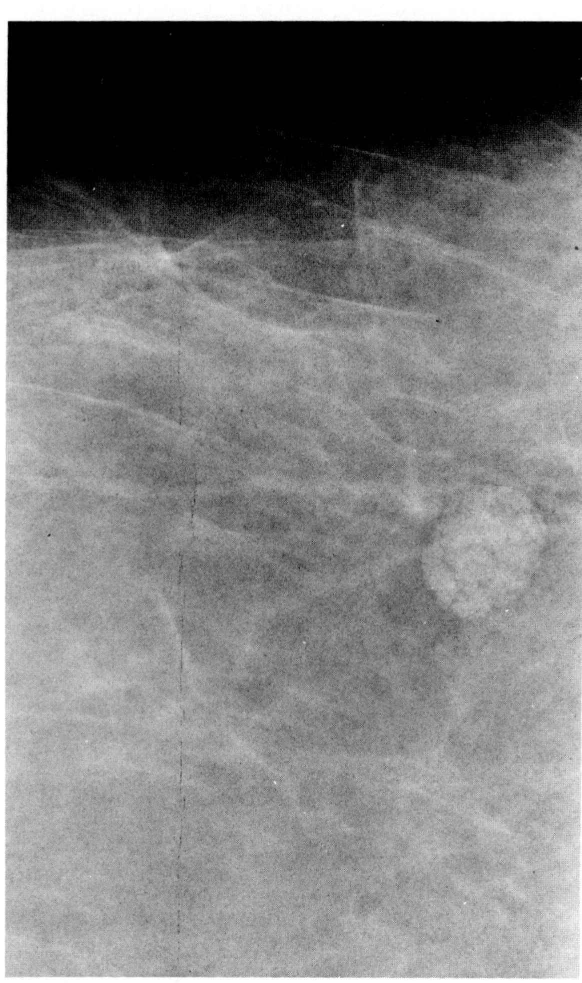

Figure 1-30. Skin mole masquerading as intramammary lesion. Verrucous surface and outer perimeter are outlined by air.

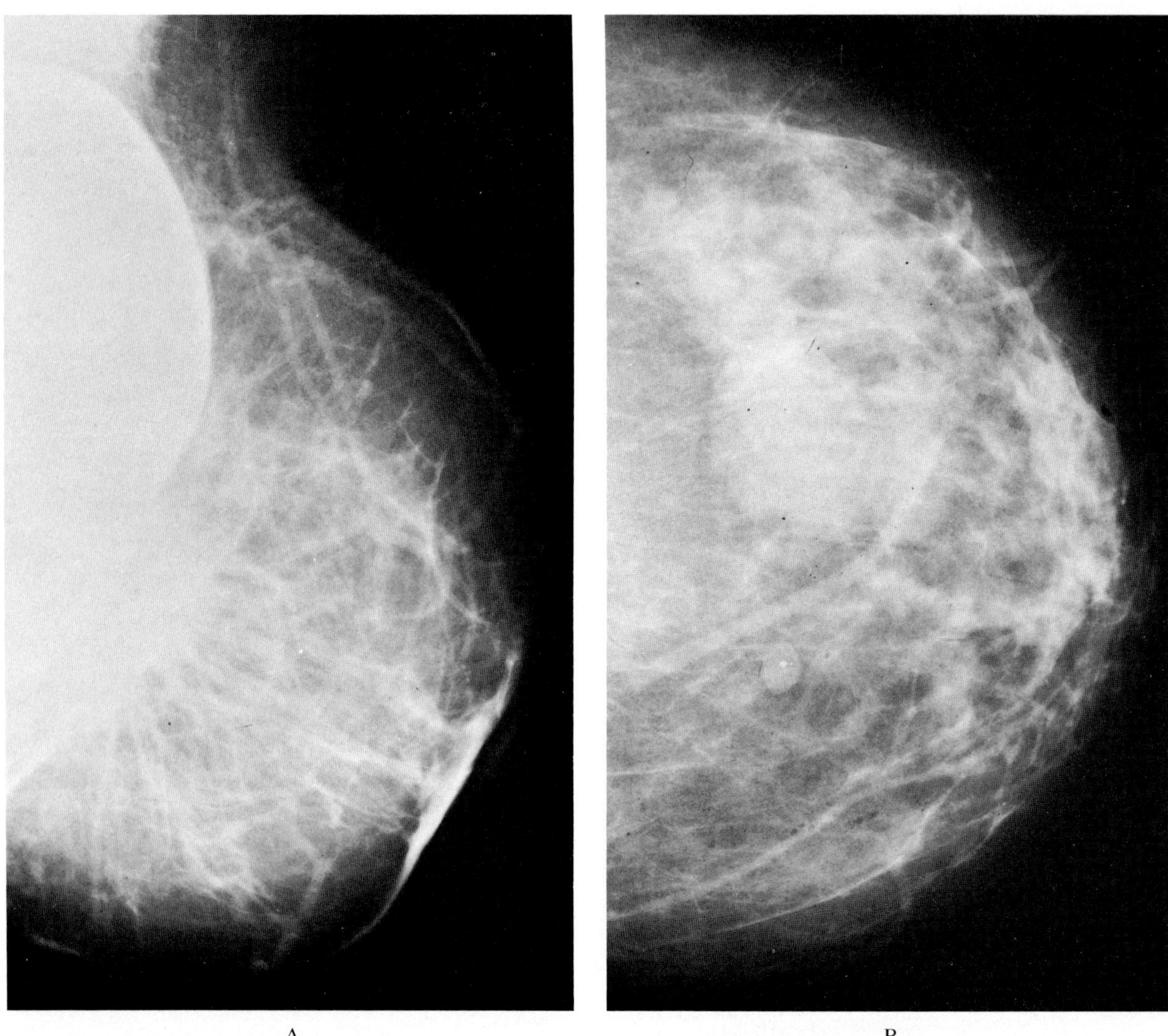

A B

Figure 1-31. Surgical scars resembling scirrhous carcinoma. A. Suspected infiltrating carcinoma with typical spiculations anterior to silicone-gel implant. Biopsy revealed only scar tissue. B. Large focus of nodularity that correlated with palpable mass. Pathologic diagnosis: fibrocystic changes. C. One year later, spiculated shadow has appeared. Palpation revealed only vague thickening rather than expected rock-hard mass characteristic of scirrhous carcinoma. On this basis, diagnosis of scar was made. D. One year later, scar had completely resolved without further surgical intervention.

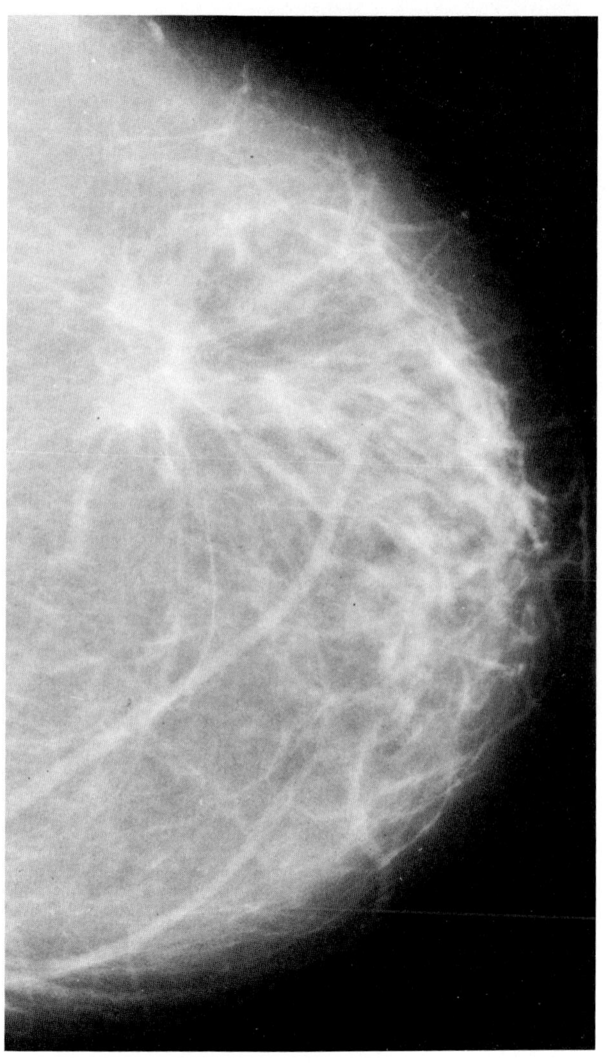
C

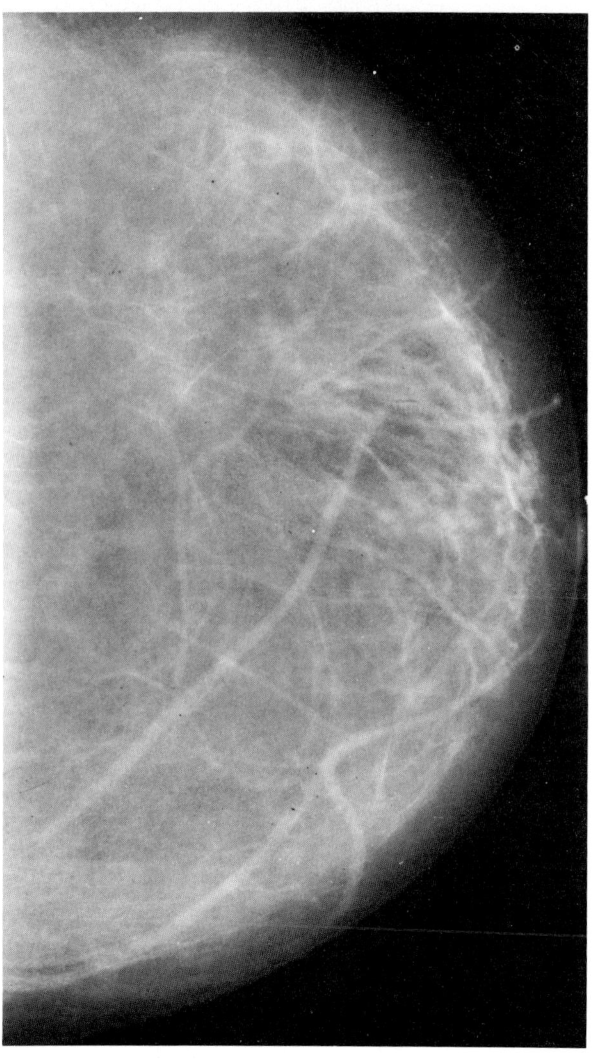
D

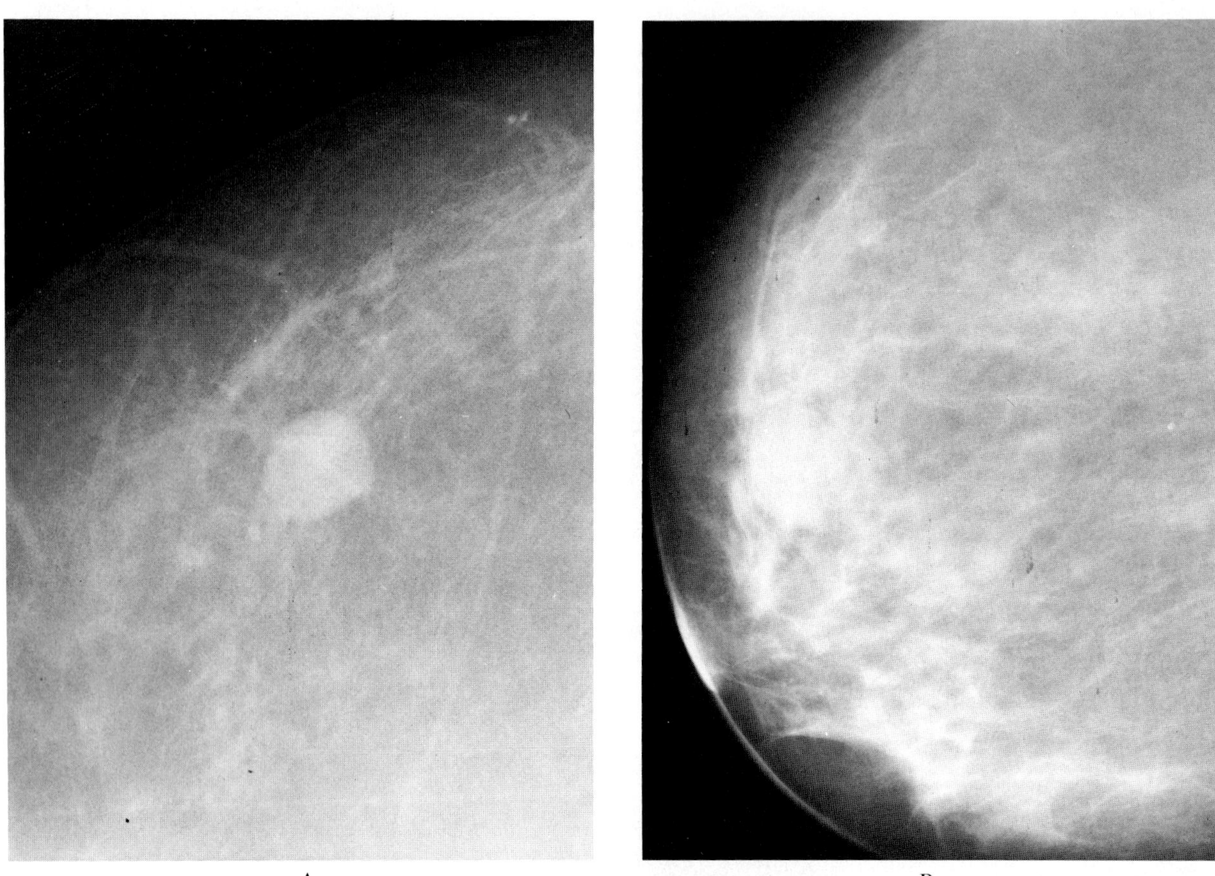

A B

Figure 1-32. Cysts. A. Cyst, 2 cm in greatest diameter. Because fluid within cyst is under tension, wall tends to be displaced equally in all directions, resulting in characteristic smooth, sharp border. B. Cyst surrounded by typical thin, radiolucent halo, an effect that may also be seen with fibroadenoma. C. Biopsy-specimen radiograph more clearly reveals smooth, sharp border and radiolucent halo seen in B. Absence of lobulations is more in keeping with cyst, whereas lobulated border is more characteristic of fibroadenoma. D. Multiple cysts. E. Aspiration of this cyst was inadvertently incomplete. Insufflation was then performed through same needle. As shown here, cyst characteristically has thin wall with smooth lining. Thickening of wall or nodularity of inner surface could represent intracystic papilloma or papillary carcinoma. One month later, cyst fluid had reaccumulated because of incomplete aspiration at initial attempt.

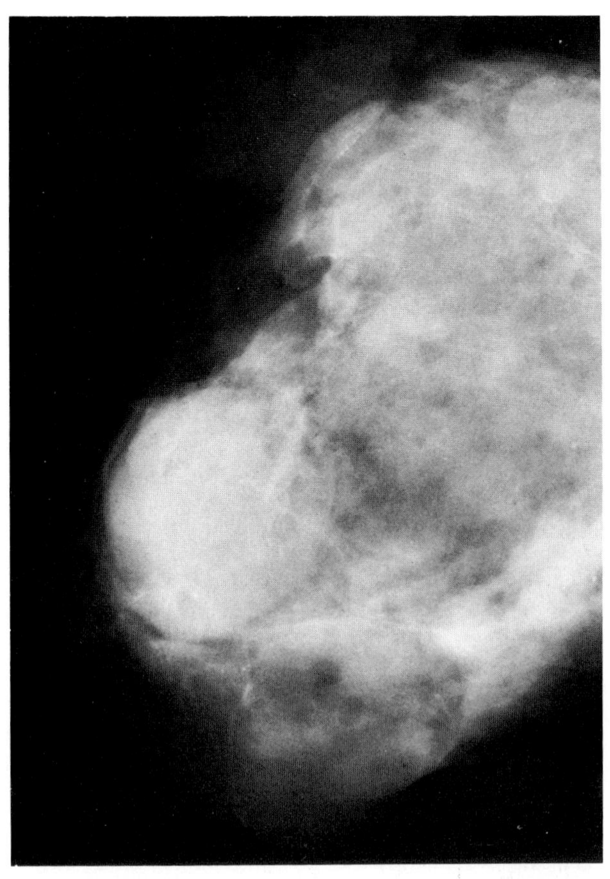

C

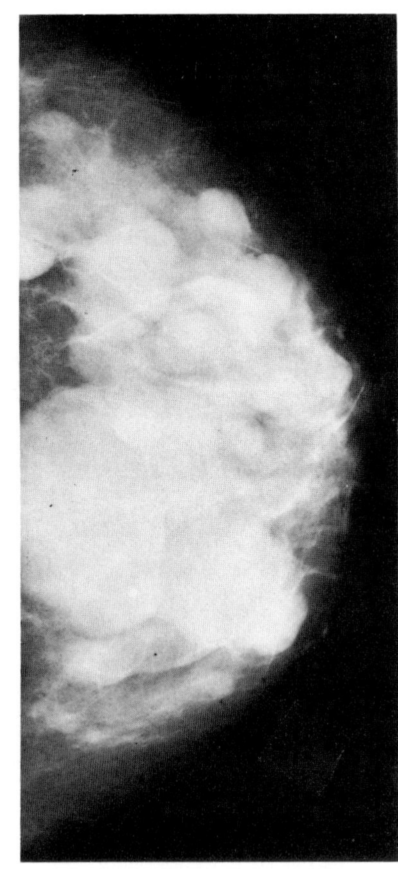

D

E

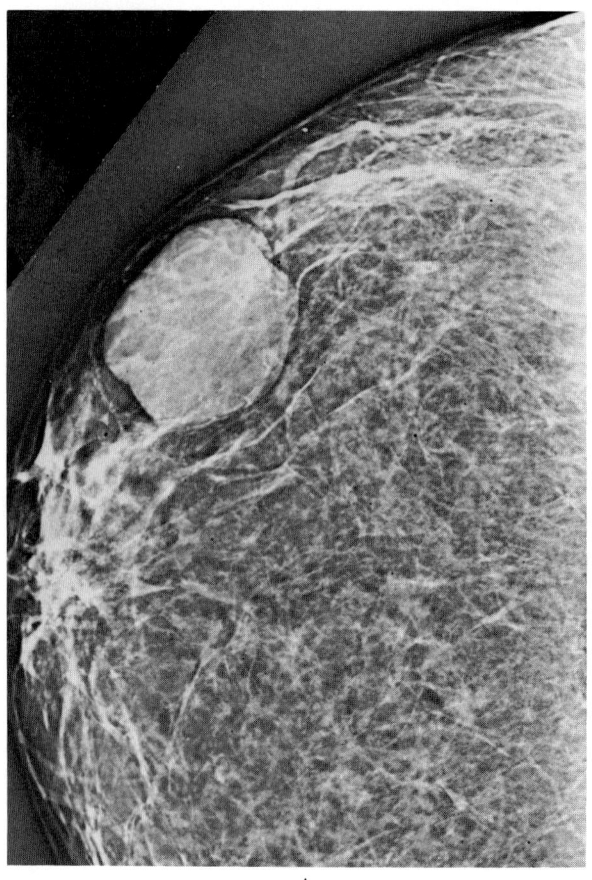

A

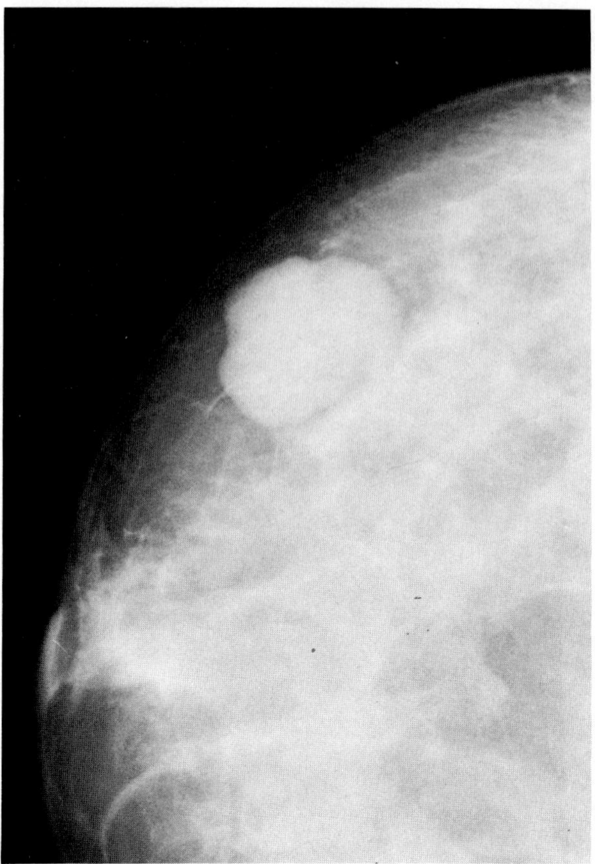

B

Figure 1-33. Fibroadenomas. A. Typical smooth, lobulated margin of fibroadenoma, most common solid benign tumor of breast. B. Another fibroadenoma characterized by lobulation. C. Fibroadenoma with smooth, nonlobulated border, mimicking cyst. D. Typical coarse calcification within hyalinizing fibroadenoma. E. Two fibroadenomas, upper one calcified and lower one not. Border of upper lesion is obscured by surrounding dense parenchyma. F. Fibroadenoma in pregnancy. Lesion was responsive to hormonal stimulation of pregnancy and grew at rapid rate during second and third trimesters. Surrounding radiolucent halo can also be seen with cysts. G. Low-power histologic appearance of typical fibroadenoma consisting of hypocellular fibrous connective tissue stroma that envelops ramifying tubules or clefts lined with epithelium.

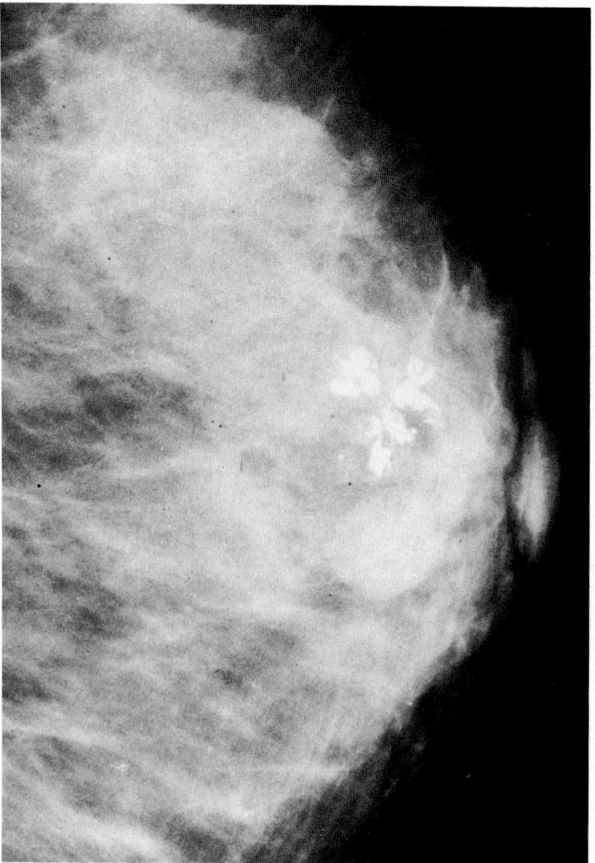

E

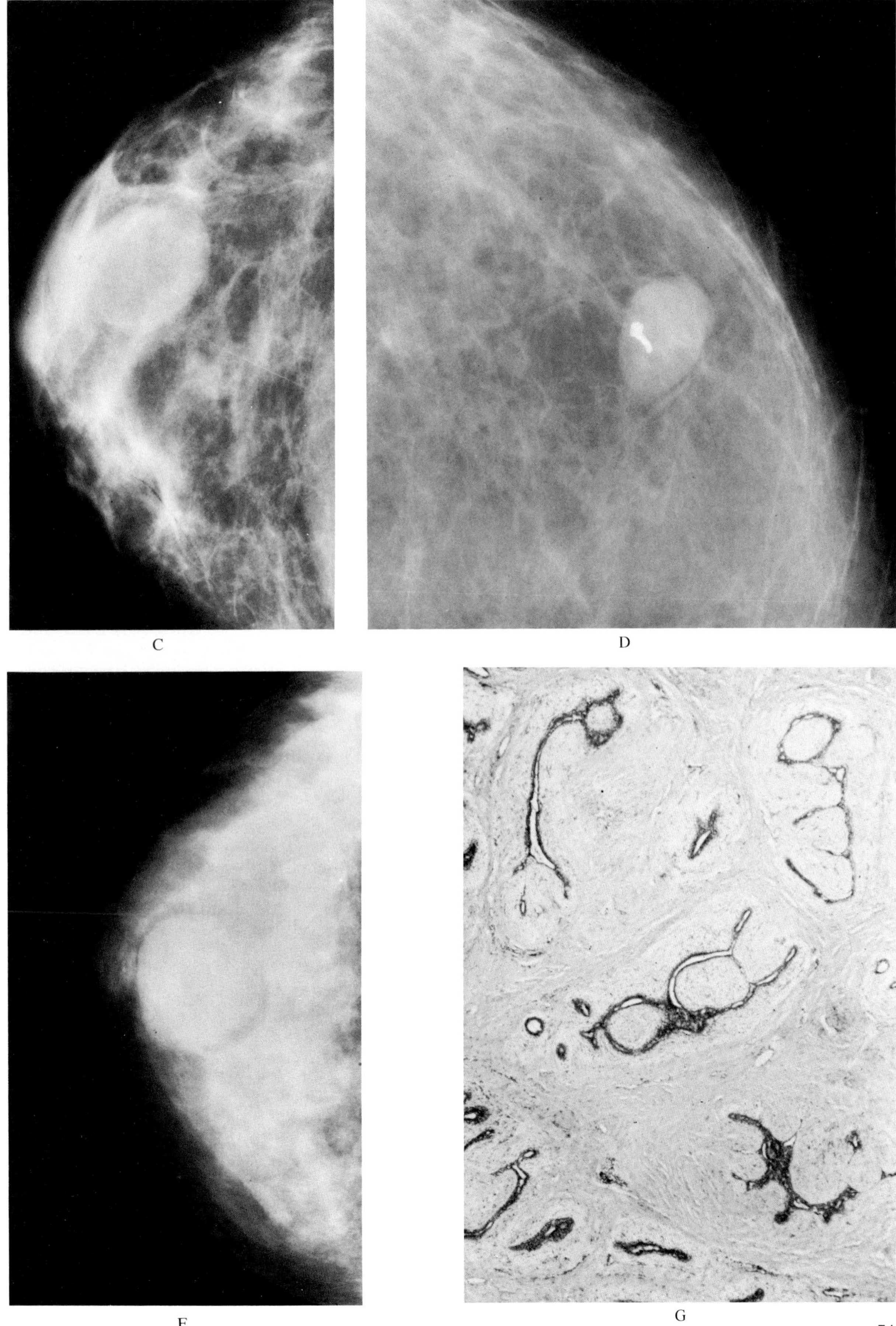
C
D
F
G

biopsied. Although intracystic papillomas and papillary carcinomas may result in a bloody aspirate, this is not invariably the case. Some mammographers prefer to insufflate the aspirated cyst with air to seek irregularities in the normally smooth inner contour of the cyst wall that imply an intracystic tumor.[38]

Fibroadenomas (Fig. 1-33) are the most common solid benign tumor of the breast. Fibroadenomas consist of an encapsulated fibrous connective tissue stroma that envelops ramifying canaliculi or tubules lined with epithelium.[28†] While cysts are usually round or oval, fibroadenomas are often lobulated while maintaining a smooth margin (Figs. 1-33A and B). With advancing age, a fibroadenoma may undergo hyalinization and develop characteristic coarse calcifications (Figs. 1-20G, 1-33D and E).

Both cysts and fibroadenomas may be surrounded by a thin radiolucent halo (Figs. 1-32C and 1-33F), which has been ascribed alternately to compressed fat or a Mach effect. On the other hand, a lack of surrounding fat caused by dense parenchymal tissue may obscure the margin of a cyst or fibroadenoma, leading to failure of visualization or, more importantly, to its being misdiagnosed as an infiltrating carcinoma. Although a fibroadenoma is usually innocuous, lobular carcinoma, usually in situ, may rarely arise within it.[27] Similarly, papillary carcinoma may occasionally arise in the wall of a cyst.

Cystosarcoma phylloides (Fig. 1-34) is a rare tumor that bears pathologic similarities to fibroadenoma, except for a more cellular, hyperplastic stroma. Mammographically it tends to be well-circumscribed but may invade adjacent normal tissue to a limited extent and may then undergo hematogenous metastasis.[27‡] A wide margin of surrounding normal breast tissue should therefore be excised with the cystosarcoma. The tumor may contain cystic cavities filled with clear or semisolid bloody fluid, and fatty elements as well. The histologic classification of a cystosarcoma as benign or malignant is based on the histology of the stromal portion of the tumor. Mammographically, it sometimes manifests coarse calcifications similar to those of fibroadenoma.

Lipofibroadenomas (adenolipomas, fibroadenolipomas, hamartomas) (Fig. 1-35) have pathognomonic mammographic features of a nonhomogeneous mass containing mottled densities corresponding to fat, epithelium, and connective tissue.[16] A rare lesion, its mammographic appearance has been alternately described as a slice of sausage or a cauliflower. As befits its benignity, the borders are sharply circumscribed. Because of the abundant fat content, even large lipofibroadenomas may be difficult to palpate.

Lipomas (Fig. 1-36) may be difficult to detect mammographically because they may be surrounded by fat of equivalent density. They usually are characterized by a discrete radiolucent mass with a thin wall of fibrous connective tissue.

Sclerosing adenosis (Fig. 1-37) is the most commonly occurring benign disorder that can mammographically mimic malignancy. This disorder is one of many conditions included in the spectrum of breast diseases known as fibrocystic changes. The latter probably result from an exaggeration and distortion of cyclic changes that normally occur during the menstrual cycle. In the fibrocystic breast, involution of these changes cannot keep pace with their proliferation. Fibrocystic changes are characterized by their pleomorphism; variable morphologic patterns occur not only in different regions of the same breast, but even in different areas of the same low-power microscopic field. At least four histologic patterns occur at differing rates and with so much overlap that it is usually impossible to detect one pattern in the absence of the others. The patterns are: (1) cysts, (2) stromal fibrosis, (3) proliferation of duct epithelium, and (4) adenosis or lobular hyperplasia. Fibrocystic changes occur clinically in 50–80 percent and histologically in 90 percent of women. Seventy percent of women with fibrocystic changes have nonproliferative lesions that are not potentially precancerous. The remaining 30 percent have proliferative changes that double their risk for breast cancer, as compared with the risk of other women in the general population. Women at highest risk for cancer are those with atypical ductal or lobular hyperplasia; their risk is up to 5 times that of women without such changes. Fortunately, only 4 percent of all women with histologic evidence of fibrocystic changes exhibit atypical hyperplasia.[18] According to the results of a 1985 consensus development meeting convened by the Cancer Committee of the College of American Pathologists, women with the following histologic lesions are *not* at increased risk for invasive carcinoma when compared to women who have not had a biopsy: sclerosing or florid adenosis, apocrine metaplasia, cysts, duct ectasia, fibroadenoma, fibrosis, mild hyperplasia (more than 2 but fewer than 4 epithelial cells in depth), mastitis, and squamous metaplasia. The following lesions imply slightly increased risk (1.5–2 times): hyperplasia, moderate or florid, solid or papillary; and papilloma with a fibrovascular core. The following implies a moderately increased risk (5 times): atypical ductal or lobular hyperplasia (borderline lesion).[17]

Sclerosing adenosis evolves in 2 stages within mammary lobules: an early stage of florid proliferation of epithelial cells and a late stage of stromal fibrosis with resultant loss of lobular boundaries. The proliferating cells may be compressed and distorted to such an extent that they appear to stream into and infiltrate the mammary stroma.[39] The disorder usually appears mammographically as an ill-defined, widespread, mottled, and nodular process, or, after coalescence of the nodules, as an extensive homogeneous soft-tissue density with indistinct margins.[14] Flecks of calcium, which tend to be fewer in number, rounder in shape, but similar in

† pp 45–46

‡ pp 117–123

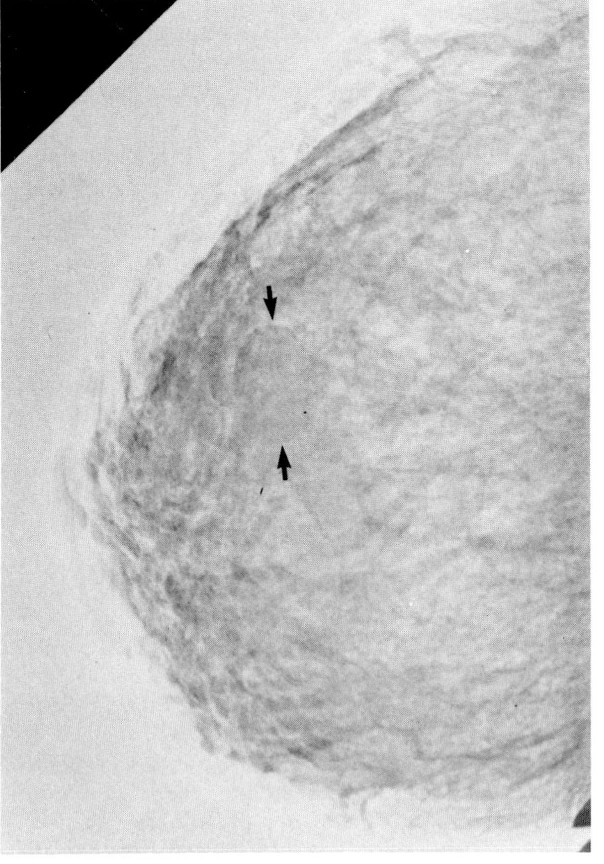

A

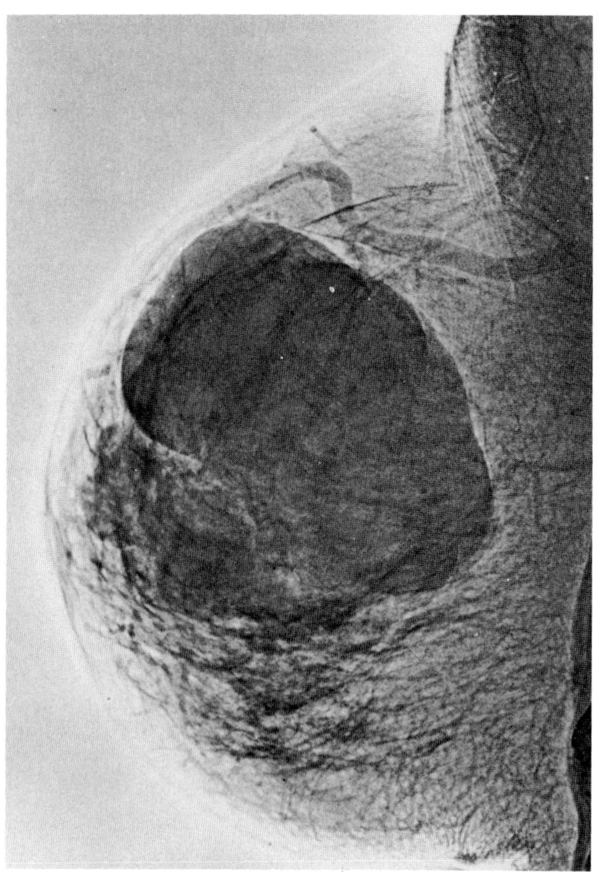

B

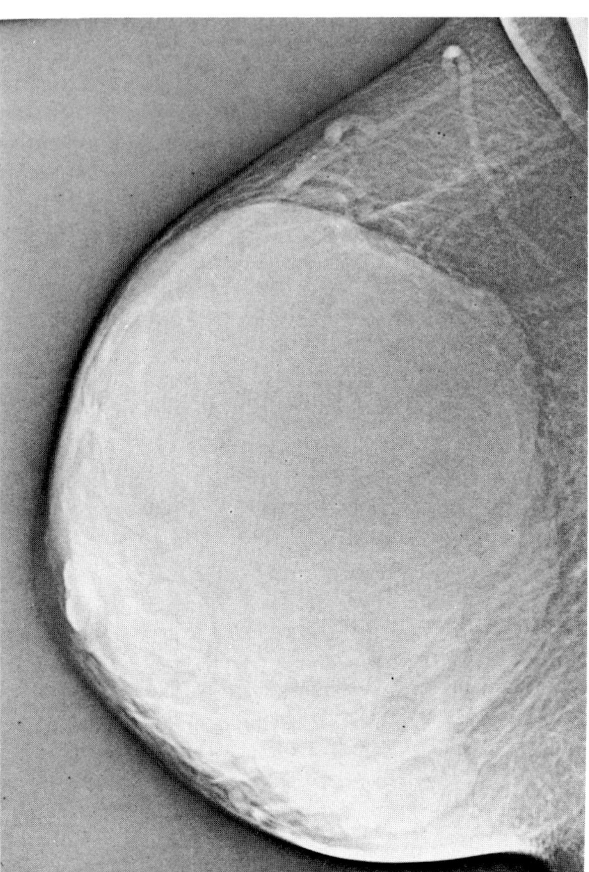

C

Figure 1-34. Cystosarcoma phylloides. Growth over 7 years. A. The 3-cm smoothly marginated lobulated shadow (arrows) was felt clinically and mammographically to represent fibroadenoma. Patient refused biopsy. B. Four years later, lesion has grown to 8 cm, but still maintains smooth border except inferiorly, where it abuts parenchymal tissue. Diameter of superficial veins has increased to striking extent. Patient again refused surgical intervention. C. Three years later, tumor has filled almost entire breast, but still maintains smooth margination. Patient finally agreed to surgery, which consisted of simple mastectomy because of fixation of tumor to skin. Despite its great size, lesion was nevertheless interpreted pathologically as benign cystosarcoma.

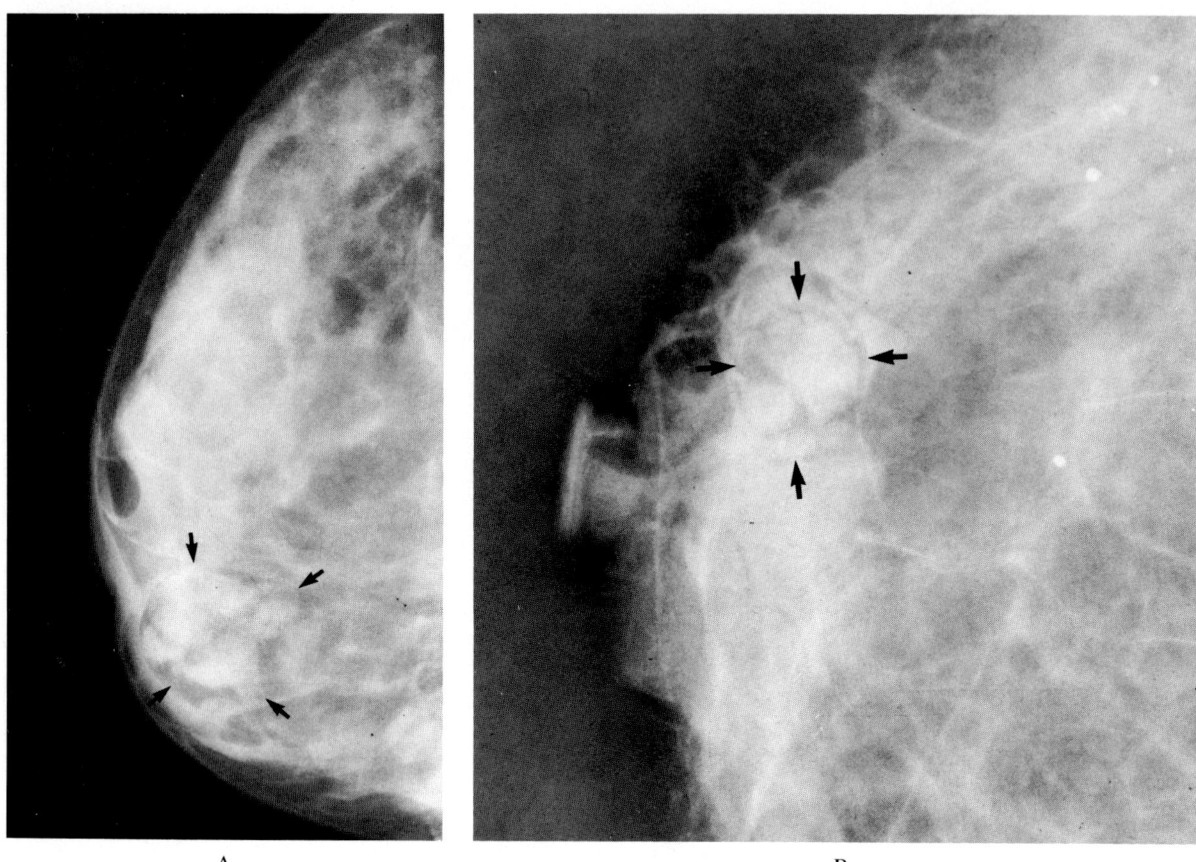

Figure 1-35. Lipofibroadenoma (hamartoma): two cases. A. Lesion (arrows) measures approximately 3 cm in greatest diameter and has pathognomonic features of nonhomogeneous mass containing admixture of fatty and water-density tissue, resulting in cauliflowerlike appearance. Lesion is large enough to cause bulge in breast surface but, because it consisted in large part of fat, was barely palpable. B. Smaller, nonpalpable lipofibroadenoma (arrows) of identical appearance to lesion in A.

size to those found in association with carcinoma, may permeate the lesion, simulating carcinoma calcifications and resulting in the need for a biopsy to exclude malignancy with certainty.

Breast abscesses (Fig. 1-38) may cause diffuse thickening of the skin of the breast, a sign that may be misinterpreted as signifying lymphatic permeation by a carcinoma.[13] Although carcinoma must always be suspected first among the causes of diffuse skin thickening, breast abscess frequently can be excluded only by biopsy. The abscess may be surrounded by intense edema, creating a mammographic and clinical appearance simulating lymphatic carcinomatosis or inflammatory carcinoma. Mammographic calcifications are not a feature of breast abscess.

Traumatic fat necrosis (Fig. 1-39) is a nonsuppurative inframammary process that may result in a variety of mammographic appearances, many of which may be confused with carcinoma. It can also mimic mammary carcinoma on clinical examination.[1,3,14,31] Branching, rodlike, or angular microcalcifications identical to those of carcinoma may be seen (Fig. 1-39F). Other mammographic features may include a spiculated density indistinguishable from carcinoma, associated localized thickening and deformity of the skin that may further raise suspicion of carcinoma, and single or multiple benign-appearing, lipid-filled cavities with or without calcified walls.[4] A location close to the skin or areola is a clue that the lesion may have resulted from blunt or surgical trauma.

Plasma cell mastitis is another disorder that may simulate carcinoma clinically and mammographically.[11,14,15] Clues to diagnosis include a tendency to subareolar location and to bilaterality. The desmoplastic reaction accompanying plasma cell mastitis may resemble that accompanying infiltrating carcinoma and may result in fixation and retraction of the overlying skin and nipple.

SKIN THICKENING: DIFFERENTIAL DIAGNOSIS

The thickness of the skin of normal breasts seldom exceeds 1.5 mm. The exception to this rule is the normally thicker skin of the crease. The inframammary

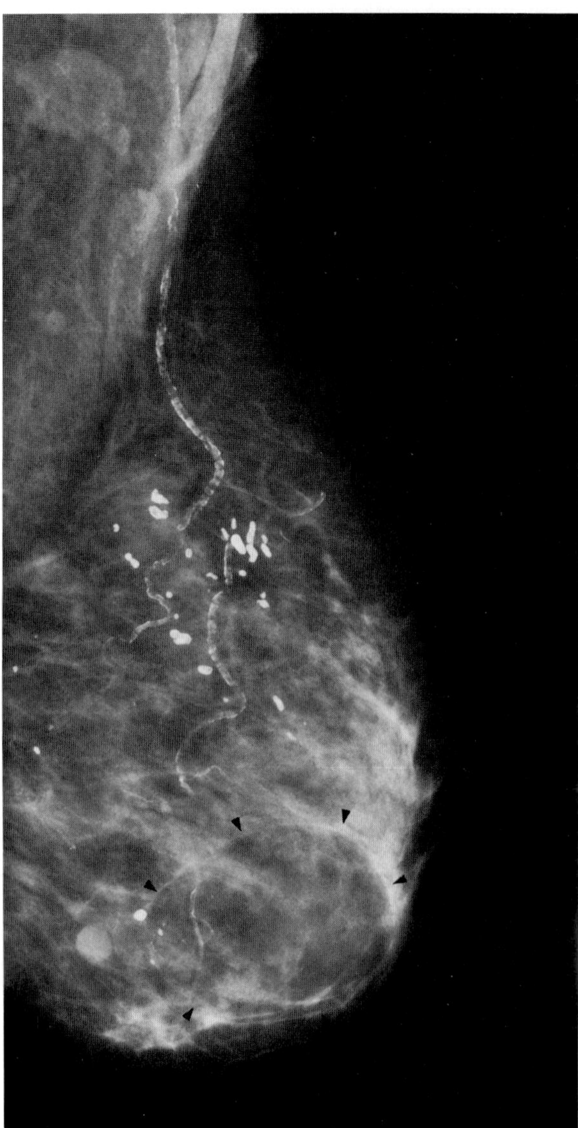

Figure 1-36. Lipoma surrounded by thin wall (arrowheads), difficult to perceive because adjacent parenchyma is composed primarily of fat.

skin of small, firm breasts may appear thickened in mammograms because of the difficulty in achieving optimal compression of these breasts; since the skin tangential to the x-rays is less closely apposed to the film than the skin of larger, flabby, easily compressible breasts, the end result is roentgenographic magnification and, hence, apparent thickening of skin.

Diffuse thickening of the skin suggests lymphatic permeation by the metastases of an underlying primary carcinoma. Although carcinoma must always be considered first, other causes, benign and malignant, are possible:[13] abscess, fat necrosis, radiation therapy,[25] subcutaneous extravasation of pleural fluid after thoracentesis, progressive systemic sclerosis, obstruction of the superior vena cava, pemphigus, nephrotic syndrome, lymphoma, and lymphatic extension from contralateral breast carcinoma. In a bedridden woman, congestive heart failure may lead to edematous skin of a dependent breast.

RADIOGRAPHY OF THE MALE BREAST

Because it consists predominantly of fat and contains few secretory ducts, the normal male breast (Fig. 1-40A) is homogeneously radiolucent, with few if any strands of ductal or interlobar connective tissue and without suspensory ligaments of Cooper. Gynecomastia (Figs. 1-40B and C) is an abnormal increase in both stromal and ductal components. Breast enlargement that results from excessive fat, such as accompanies obesity, is not true gynecomastia. Gynecomastia and adiposity, although not always distinguishable by palpation, are easily differentiated by mammography.

Gynecomastia has been characterized as the male analog of female fibrocystic changes. Enlargement of the breast in gynecomastia is due primarily to the proliferation of stroma in which hypervascularity, fibroblasts, and hyalinization are prominent features, and in which true acinar lobules are usually absent. Two patterns of gynecomastia may be observed: (1) a florid triangular pattern, seen in association with breast enlargement of recent onset; and (2) a dendritic pattern, seen in association with breast enlargement of 6 months or more.[29]

Nonhormonal drugs that may induce gynecomastia include digitalis, reserpine, ergotamine, diphenylhydantoin, phenothiazine, spironolactone, and thiazide diuretics. Other causes of gynecomastia include exogenous estrogen administration, embryonal cell carcinoma or choriocarcinoma of the testis, Klinefelter's syndrome, adrenal carcinoma, marijuana use (Figs. 1-40B and C), cirrhosis of the liver, and chronic renal dialysis.

Carcinoma of the male breast (Figs. 1-40D, E, and F) is rare (fewer than 1.0 percent of all combined male and female breast carcinomas and fewer than 1.5 percent of all cancers in men). The radiographic detection of breast cancer in the male with gynecomastia is subject to the same pitfalls that pertain to the detection of breast cancer in the female with fibrocystic changes. The diffuse increase in radiographic density accompanying florid gynecomastia may mask the underlying carcinoma. The mammographic criteria for carcinoma of the male breast are the same as for the female. Although gynecomastia is not always readily distinguished from carcinoma, the latter tends toward an eccentric location relative to the nipple, spiculation, and in some cases calcifications or involvement of the skin and nipple.[8,29]

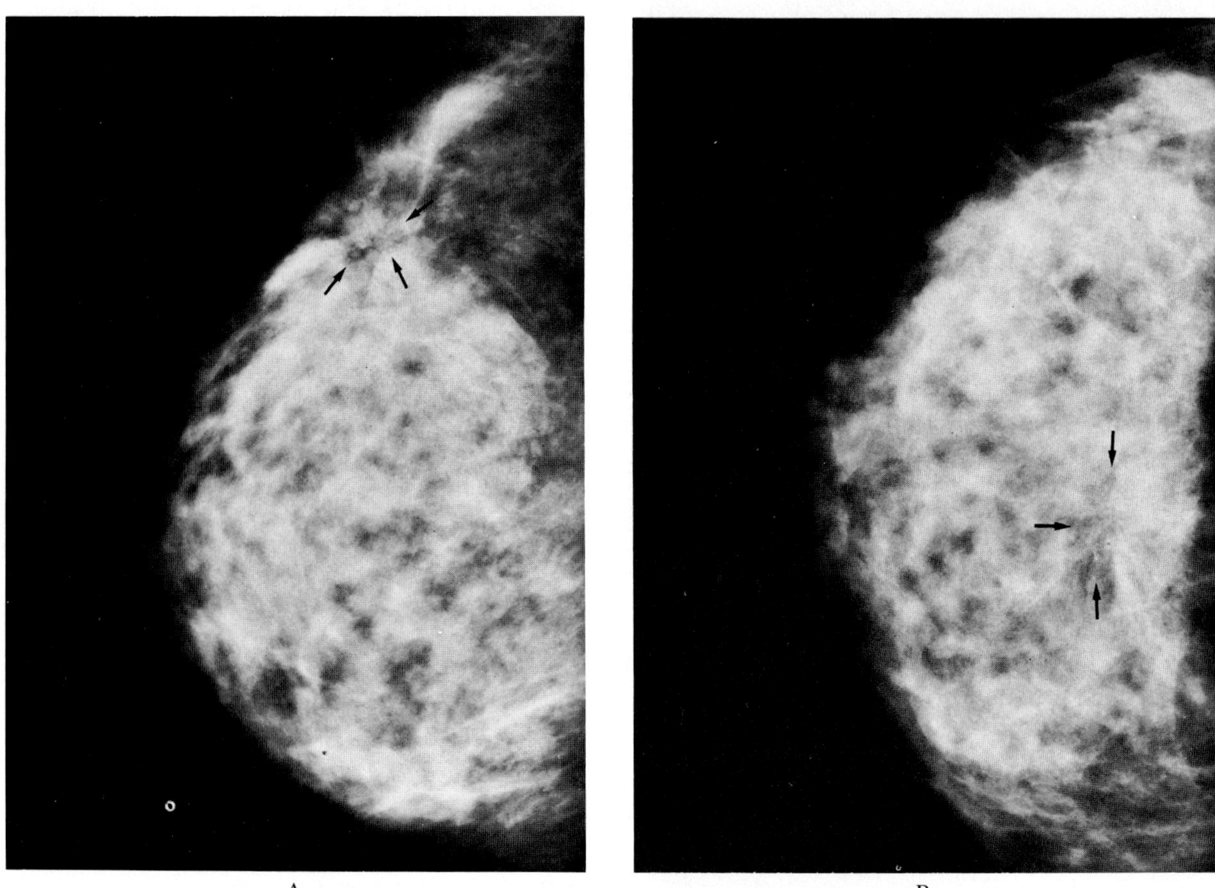

A B

Figure 1-37. Sclerosing adenosis (arrows). A. Mediolateral view. B. Cephalocaudal view. C. Close-up of lesion in B. Diffuse, mottled, and nodular densities throughout breast are characteristic of fibrocystic changes. Arrows encompass spiculated shadow containing faint microcalcifications, combination characteristic of scirrhous carcinoma. Biopsy, however, yielded only fibrocystic changes with sclerosing adenosis. D. Histologic section reveals distortion, compression, and separation of lobular constituents by dense fibrous connective tissue (hematoxylin and eosin stain, original ×160). E. Another focus of sclerosing adenosis at same magnification. Process features chronic inflammatory cells, calcification (arrow), and, in center of field, epithelial proliferation of terminal ductule within remnant of lobule. Entire process is encircled by fibroblasts.

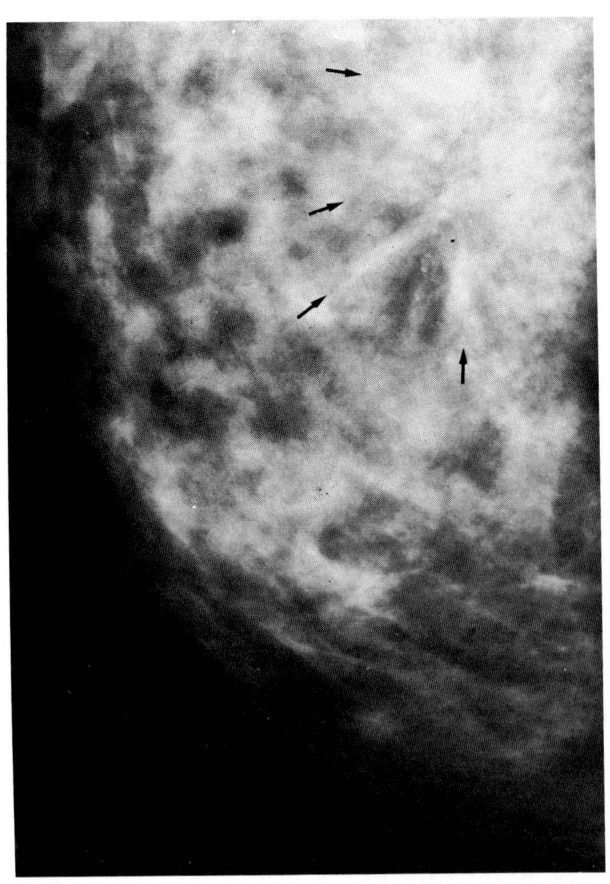
C

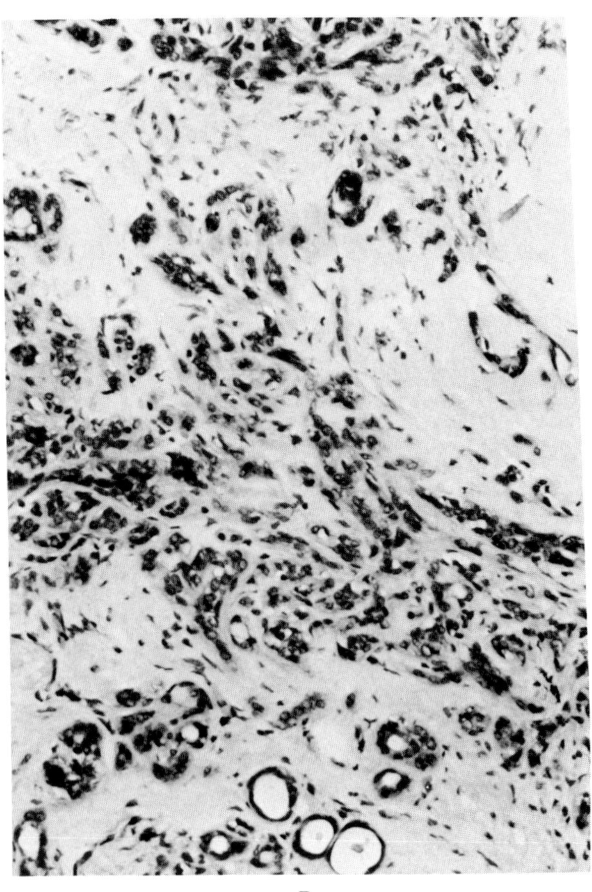
D

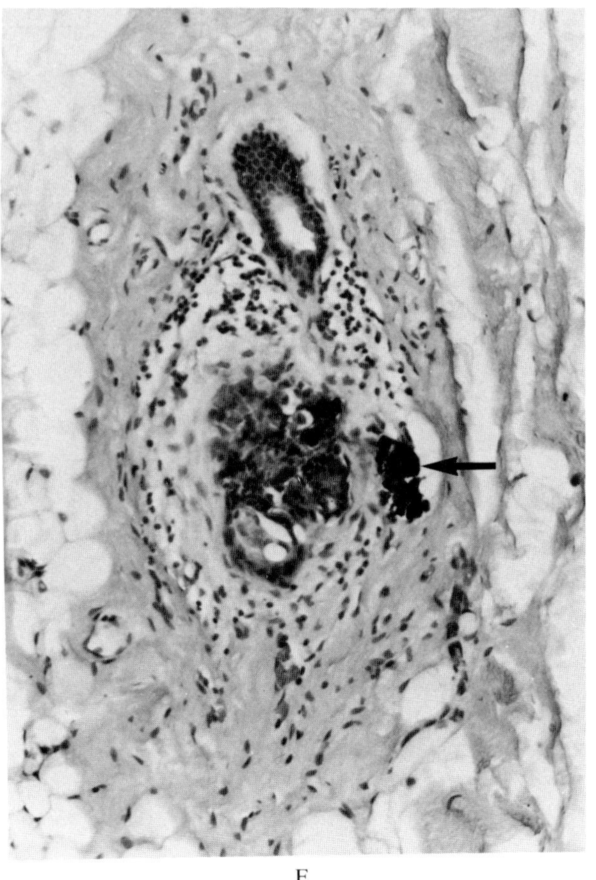
E

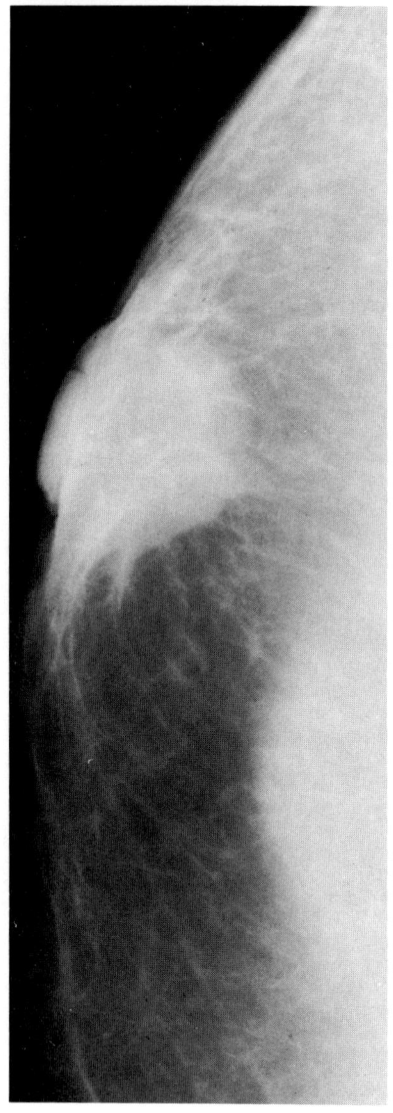

A

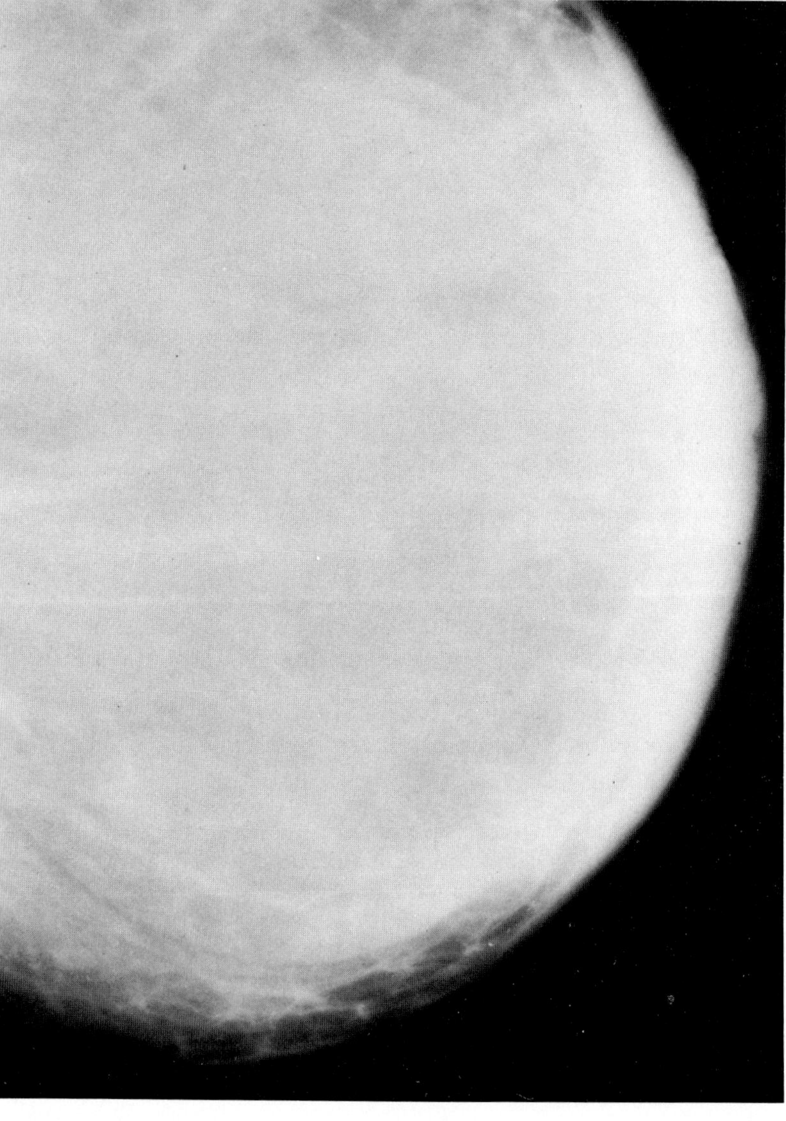

B

Figure 1-38. Breast abscesses. A. Retroareolar abscess in male breast. Edema surrounding abscess has resulted in slightly indistinct margin that suggests infiltrating carcinoma. B. Abscess characterized by diffuse skin thickening and extensive edema. Key differential diagnosis is between abscess and carcinoma with lymphangitic spread. As shown here, abscess (or carcinoma) may be completely obscured by intense surrounding edema.

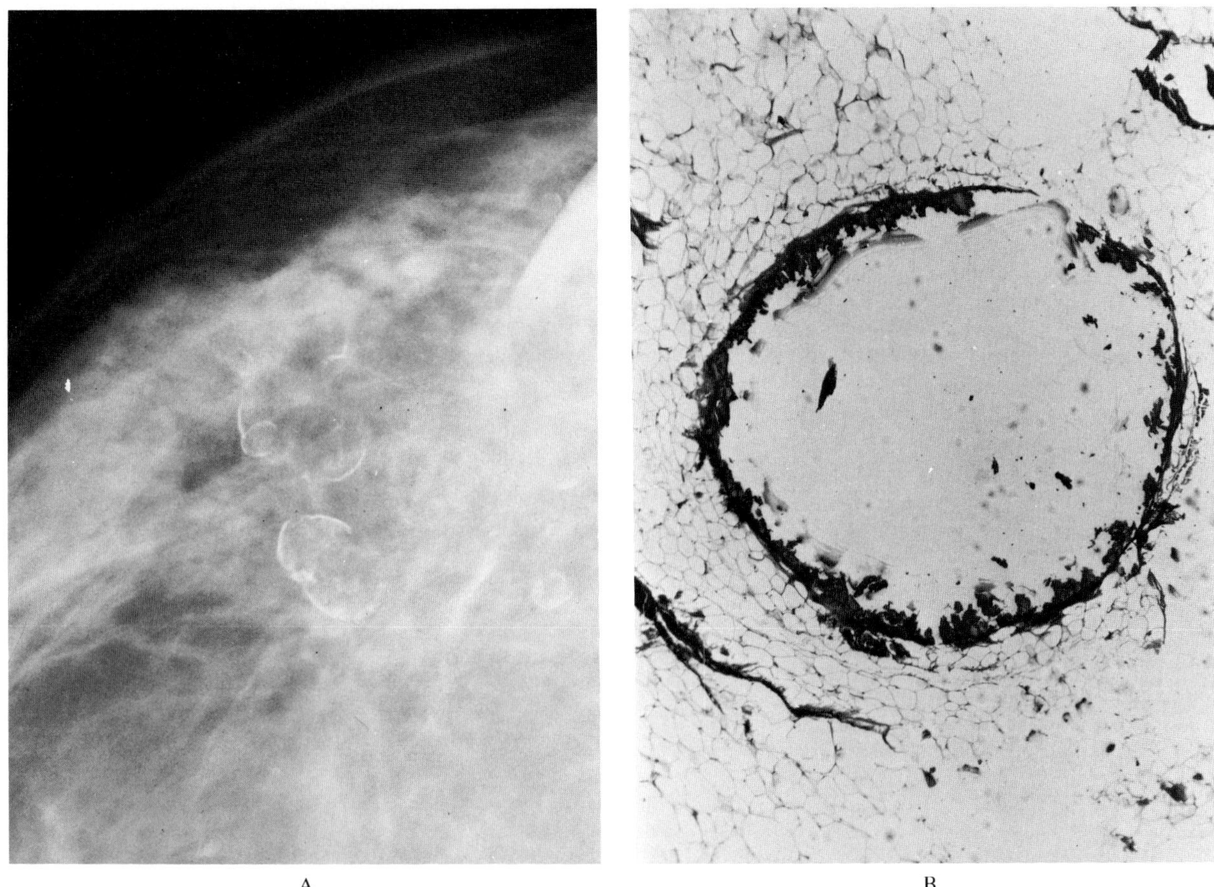

A B

Figure 1-39. Mammographic spectrum of traumatic fat necrosis. A. Close-up of calcification in walls of fat-density cystlike lesions. B. Histologic correlation with A. Calcification is present along inner margin of intact fibrous ring (hematoxylin and eosin stain, original ×25). C. Extensively calcified lipid-filled cavity with calcified wall. Scattered calcifications nearby and focus of skin retraction behind nipple are additional changes of fat necrosis. D. Spiculated shadow and overlying skin thickening and retraction raise specter of carcinoma, but biopsy revealed only focus of fat necrosis resulting from previous biopsy. E. Histologic appearance of fat necrosis. Process is characterized by aggregates of chronic inflammatory cells, dense, irregularly infiltrative fibrosis, and foreign-body reaction to necrotic fat. Fingerlike extension of fibrosis (arrow) extends into adjacent fat, mimicking scirrhous carcinoma (hematoxylin and eosin stain, original ×25). F. Fat necrosis with branching calcifications and skin thickening mimicking carcinoma. This 53-year-old woman complained of slowly enlarging mass for 2 years. Two biopsies had revealed only chronic inflammation. Physical examination disclosed 5 × 6-cm fixed nontender mass and diffuse orange-peel-like skin. Because of deformity, patient requested mastectomy, well aware that lesion might not be malignant. Due to bizarre nature of case, entire mastectomy specimen was extensively evaluated by many pathologists. Pathologic diagnosis: fat necrosis with foci of calcifications within ducts; no evidence of carcinoma. This case, with mammographic appearance indistinguishable from comedocarcinoma, leads us to conclude that carcinoma, while in some cases manifesting characteristic features, exhibits no features that can be called truly pathognomonic.

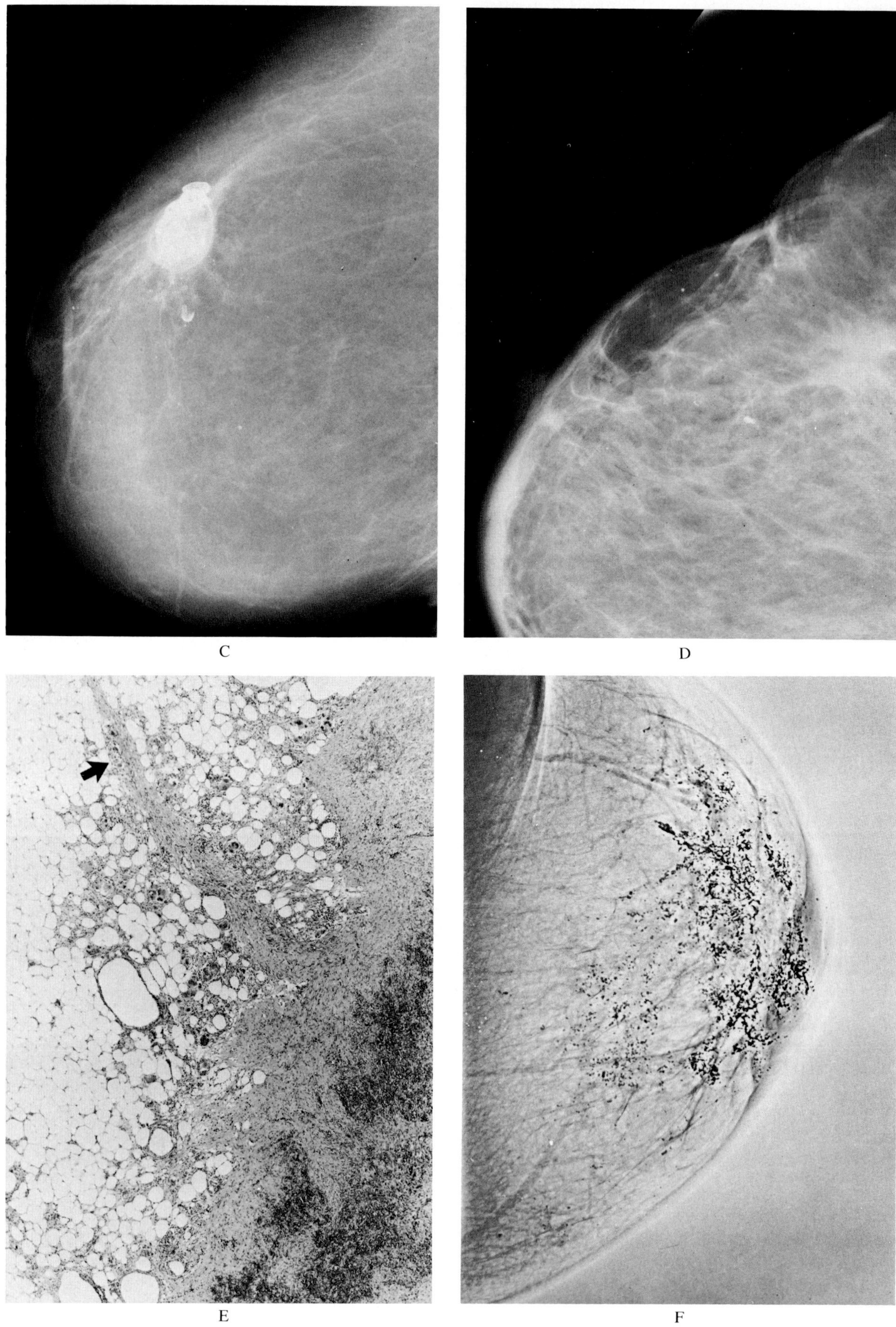
C
D
E
F

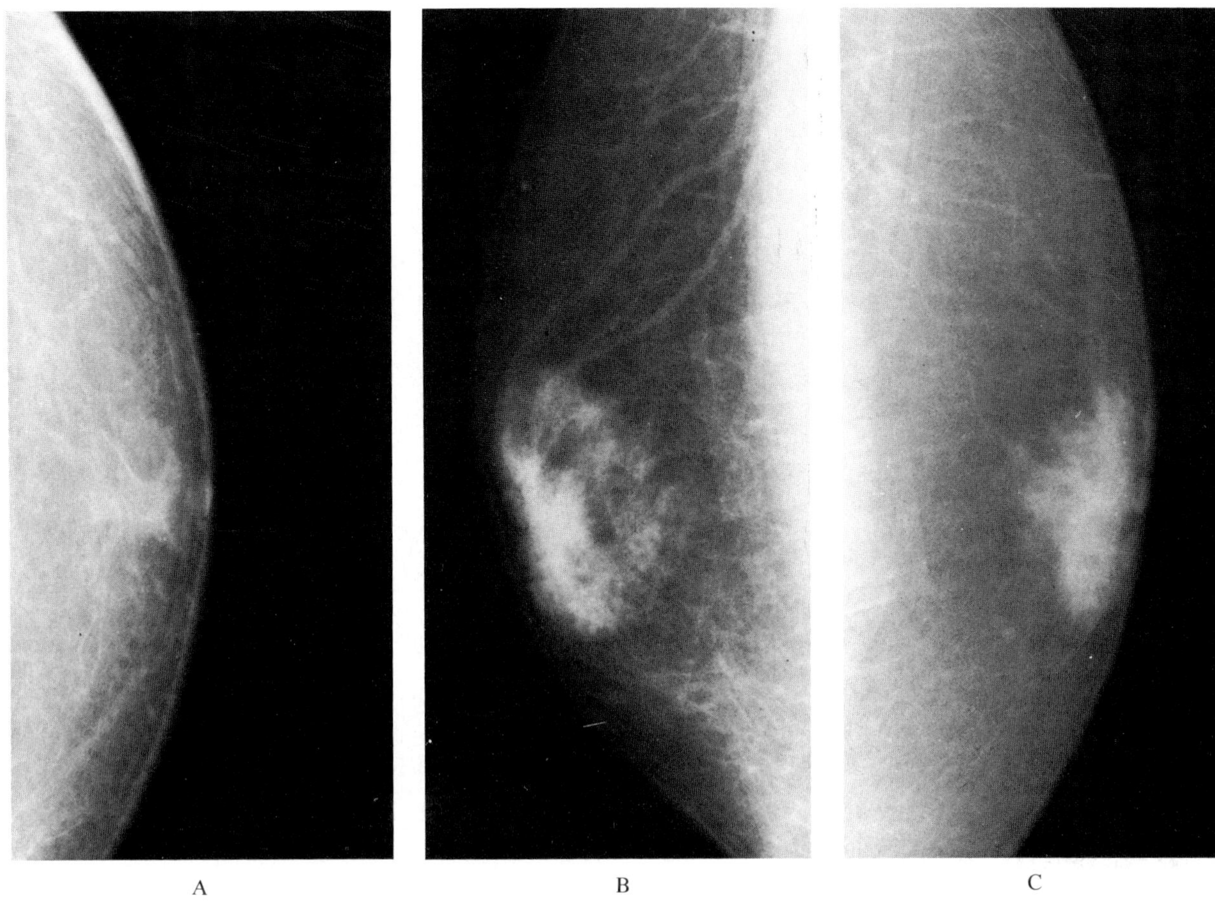

A B C

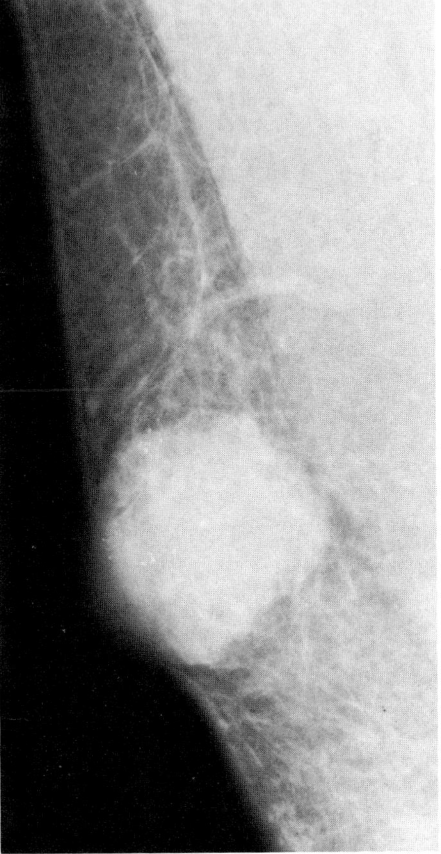

D

Figure 1-40. Radiography of male breast. A. Normal male breast. Because it consists predominantly of fat and contains few secretory ducts, normal male breast is homogeneously radiolucent, with few if any strands of ductal or intralobular connective tissue and without suspensory ligaments of Cooper. B. Gynecomastia resulting from heavy use of marijuana. Right breast. C. Left breast of man whose right breast was shown in B. Gynecomastia is less severe on left. D. Carcinoma. Although this 4-cm tumor is well circumscribed, its margin is indistinct. Lesion, because of its central retroareolar location, would have been difficult to distinguish mammographically from gynecomastia had it not contained numerous microcalcifications of varying size and irregular shape, typical of carcinoma. (Courtesy of Edward A. Sickles, M.D.). E. Well-circumscribed carcinoma. Although this 2-cm lesion is even more smoothly outlined than carcinoma in D, its asymmetry in relationship to nipple and prominent duct between it and nipple are characteristic of carcinoma of male breast. F. Close-up view. Border of carcinoma is not perfectly smooth, as would befit benign mass, but is slightly irregular. Prominent duct results from proliferation of fibrous connective tissue and is highly suggestive of malignancy.

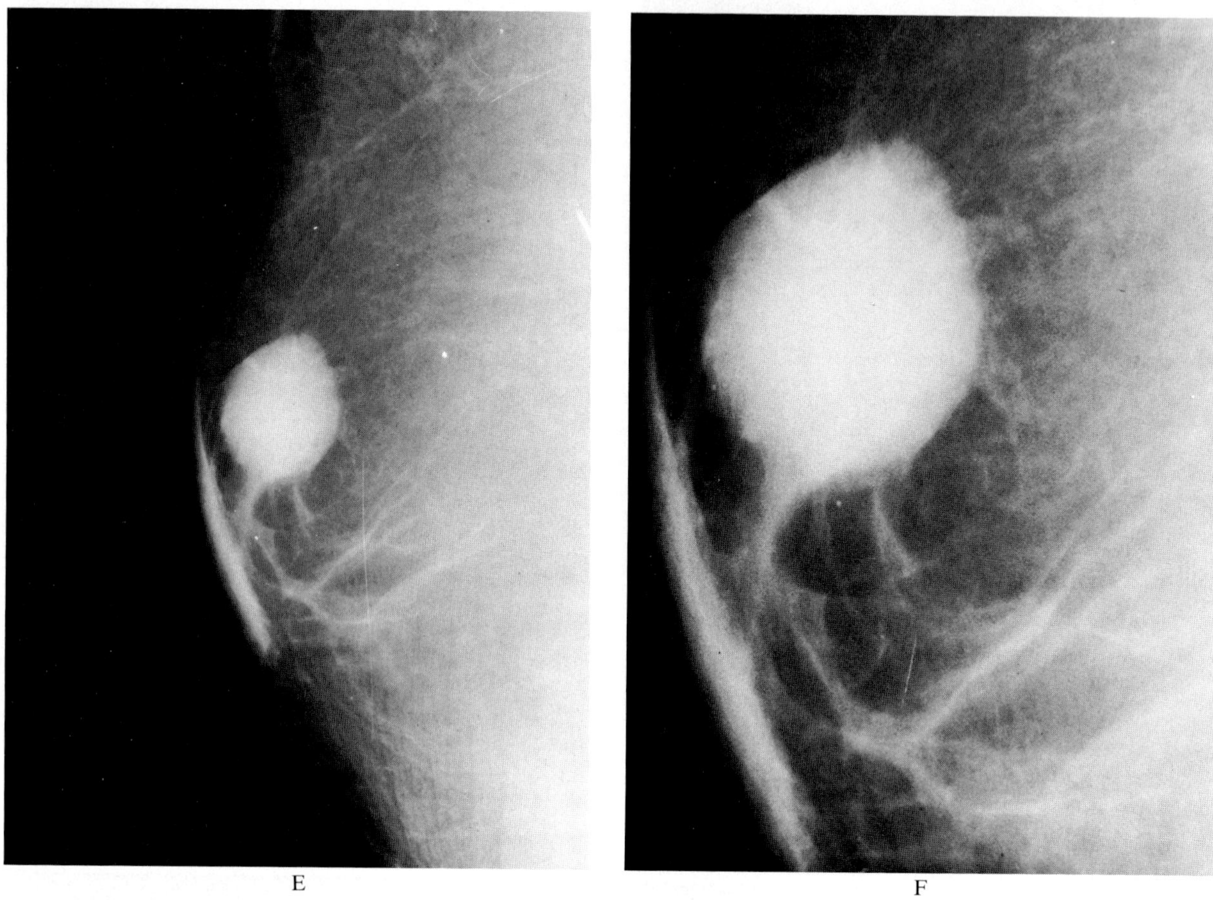

Figure 1-41. Parenchymal patterns as risk markers for breast cancer, according to Wolfe.[41] A. N1, lowest risk—parenchyma is composed entirely of fat with, at most, small amounts of fibrocystic changes and no visible ducts. B. P1, low risk—parenchyma is primarily fat, with prominent ducts in anterior portion of breast and occupying up to one-fourth of the breast volume; alternatively, this pattern may be reflected by thin band of ducts extending into one quadrant. C. P2, highest risk—severe duct prominence occupies more than one-fourth of breast volume. D. DY, high risk—severe fibrocystic changes which, in most severe form, appears homogeneous and may obscure underlying prominent duct pattern.

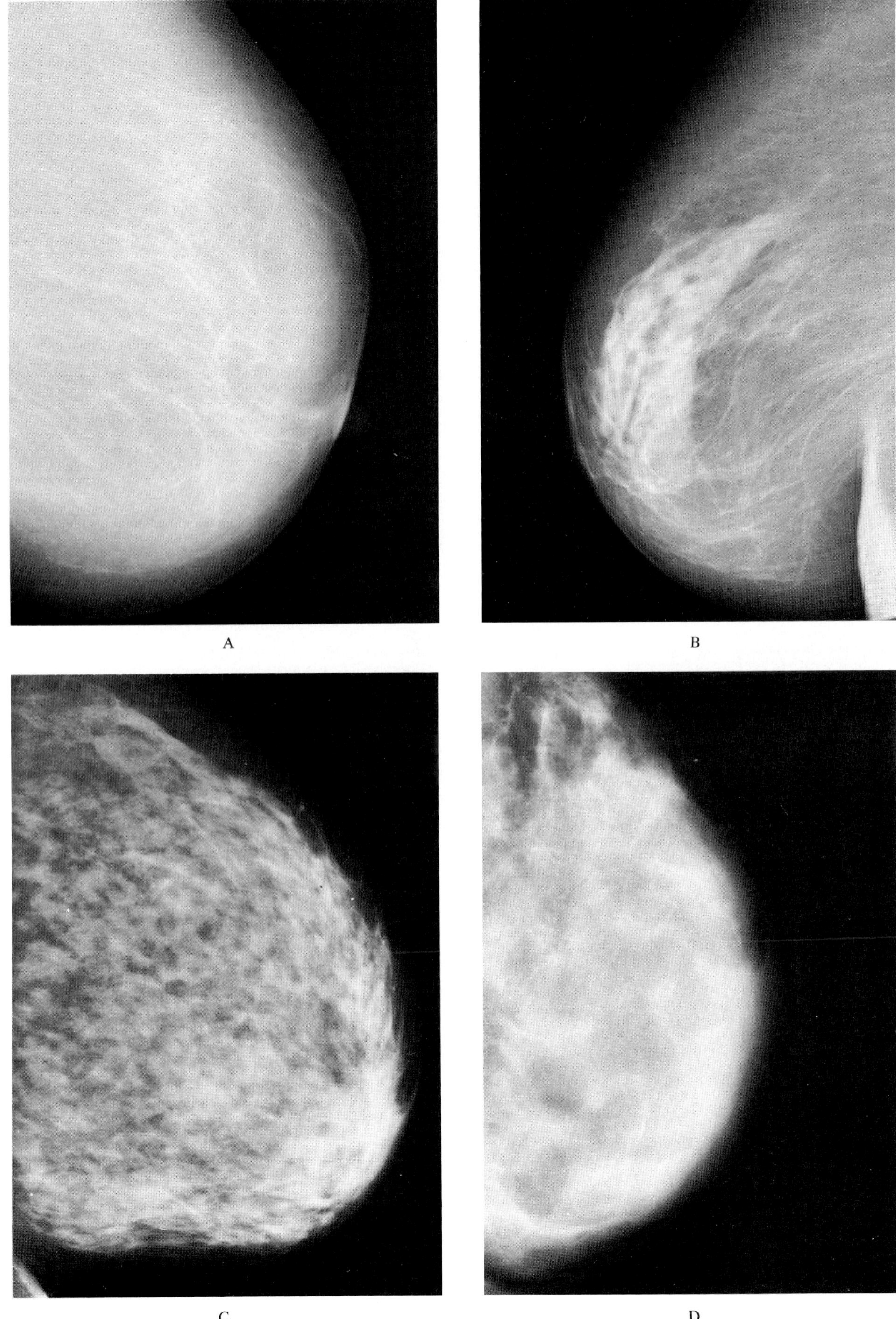
A B C D

PARENCHYMAL PATTERNS AS RISK MARKERS FOR BREAST CANCER

According to Wolfe, it is possible to predict which women are more likely to develop breast cancer solely on the basis of their parenchymal patterns as disclosed by mammography.[6,41] This hypothesis is controversial and is not endorsed by all authorities. The 4 patterns are as follows:

1. N1, lowest risk (Fig. 1-41A): The parenchyma is composed almost entirely of fat with, at most, small amounts of fibrocystic changes and no visible ducts.
2. P1, low risk (Fig. 1-41B): The parenchyma is primarily fat, with prominent ducts in the anterior portion of the breast and occupying up to one-fourth of the breast volume; alternatively, this pattern may be reflected by a thin band of ducts extending into one quadrant.
3. P2, highest risk (Fig. 1-41C): There is severe duct prominence occupying more than one-fourth of the breast volume.
4. DY, high risk (Fig. 1-41D): There is severe fibrocystic change (dysplasia), which, in its most severe form, appears homogeneous and may obscure an underlying prominent duct pattern.

N1 and P1 may broadly be considered as *low*-risk patterns, whereas P2 and DY may be considered as *high*-risk patterns. In an analysis of 332 incident breast carcinomas, Wolfe found that most cancers occurred in the P2 breast, a smaller number in the DY, and only 12 percent in the combined N1–P1 types. Wolfe also found a significant diminution in the proportion of cases falling into the DY category after age 50, and less so for the P2 category.[42]

The mammographic appearance of the parenchymal patterns has been correlated with histology. [40] N1 breasts show normal stroma, ducts, and lobules. P1 breasts have mild to moderate periductal and perilobular fibrosis with some atypical lobules. DY breasts are generally similar to P2 breasts but with more high-gradc atypical lobules and extensive, confluent fibrosis. The highest grades of histologically precancerous lesions are in P2 breasts and are rarely seen in N1 breasts. Wolfe's mammographic risk patterns thus correlate with established histological risk-grading patterns.

REFERENCES

1. Adair FE, Munzer JT: Fat necrosis of the female breast: Report of 110 cases. Am J Surg 74:117–128, 1947
2. Bassett LW, Gold RH: Breast radiography using the oblique projection. Radiology 149:585–587, 1983
3. Bassett LW, Gold RH, Cove HC: Mammographic spectrum of traumatic fat necrosis: The fallibility of "pathognomonic" signs of carcinoma. AJR 130:119–122, 1978
4. Bassett LW, Gold RH, Mirra JM: Non-neoplastic breast calcifications in lipid cysts: Development after excision and primary irradiation. AJR 138:335–338, 1982
5. Bohman LG, Bassett LW, Gold RH, et al: Breast metastases from extramammary malignancies. Radiology 144:309–312, 1982
6. Carlile T, Kopecky KJ, Thompson DJ, et al: Breast cancer prediction and the Wolfe classification of mammograms. JAMA 254:1050–1053, 1985
7. Deos PH, Norris HJ: Well-differentiated (tubular) carcinoma of the breast: A clinico-pathologic study of 145 pure and mixed cases. Am J Clin Pathol 78:1–7, 1982
8. Dershaw DD: Male mammography. AJR 146:127–131, 1986
9. Feig SA, Shaber GS, Patchefsky A, et al: Analysis of clinically occult and mammographically occult breast tumors. AJR 128:404–408, 1977
10. Feig SA, Shaber GS, Patchefsky AS, et al: Tubular carcinoma of the breast: Mammographic apearance and pathologic correlation. Radiology 129:311–314, 1978
11. Gershon-Cohen J, Ingleby H: Secretory disease and plasma-cell mastitis in female breast: Roentgenologic and pathologic studies. Surg Gynecol Obstet 95:497–504, 1952
12. Gershon-Cohen J, Ingleby H, Hermel MB: Calcification and secretory disease of the breast. AJR 76:132–135, 1956
13. Gold RH, Montgomery CK, Minagi H, et al: The significance of mammary skin thickening in disorders other than primary carcinoma: Roentgenologic-pathologic correlation. AJR 112:613–621, 1971
14. Gold RH, Montgomery CK, Rambo ON: Significance of margination of benign and malignant infiltrative mammary lesions: Roentgenologic-pathologic correlation. AJR 118:881–894, 1973
15. Haagensen CD: Mammary-duct ectasia: Disease that may simulate carcinoma. Cancer 4:749–761, 1951
16. Hessler C, Schnyder P, Ozzello L: Hamartoma of the breast: Diagnostic observation of 16 cases. Radiology 126:95–98, 1978
17. Hutter RVP, Albores-Saaveda J, Anderson E, et al: Is fibrocystic disease of the breast precancerous? Consensus Meeting, Oct. 3–5, 1985, New York. Convened by the Cancer Committee of the College of American Pathologists. Supported by a grant from the American Cancer Society. Arch Pathol Lab Med 110:171–173, 1986
18. Hutter RVP: Goodbye to "fibrocystic disease." N Engl J Med 312:179–181, 1985
19. Jensen SR, Mackey JK: Xeromammography after augmentation mammoplasty. AJR 144:629–633, 1985
20. Kalisher L: Factors influencing false negative rates in xeromammography. Radiology 133:297–301, 1979
21. Kalisher L, Chu AM, Peyster RG: Clinicopathological correlation of xeroradiography in determining involvement of metastatic axillary nodes in female breast cancer. Radiology 121:333–335, 1976
22. Kopans DB, Meyer JE, Homer MJ, et al: Dermal deposits mistaken for breast calcifications. Radiology 149:592–594, 1983
23. Kopans DB, Meyer JE, Murphy GF: Benign lymph nodes associated with dermatitis presenting as breast masses. Radiology 137:15–19, 1980

24. Libshitz HI, Montague ED, Paulus DD: Calcifications and the therapeutically irradiated breast. AJR 128:1021–1025, 1977
25. Libshitz HI, Montague ED, Paulus DD: Skin thickness in the therapeutically irradiated breast. AJR 130:345–347, 1978
26. Martin JE, Moskowitz NM, Milbrath JR: Breast carcinoma missed by mammography. AJR 132:737–739, 1979
27. McDivitt RW, Farrow JH, Stewart FW: Breast carcinoma arising in solitary fibroadenomas. Surg Gynecol Obstet 125:572–576, 1967
28. McDivitt RW, Stewart FW, Berg JW: Tumors of the Breast. Armed Forces Institute of Pathology, 1968
29. Michels LG, Gold RH, Arndt R-D: Radiography of gynecomastia and other disorders of the male breast. Radiology 122:117–122, 1977
30. Millis RR, Davis R, Stacey AJ: The detection and significance of calcifications in the breast: A radiological and pathological study. Br J Radiol 49:12–26, 1976
31. Minagi H, Youker JE: Roentgen appearance of fat necrosis in the breast. Radiology 90:62–65, 1968
32. Minagi H, Youker JE, Knudson HW: Roentgen appearance of injected silicone in the breast. Radiology 90:57–61, 1968
33. Moskowitz M: Screening is not diagnosis. Radiology 133:265–268, 1979
34. Sickles EA: Further experience with microfocal spot magnification mammography in the assessment of clustered breast microcalcifications. Radiology 137:9–14, 1980
35. Sickles EA: Mammographic features of 300 consecutive nonpalpable breast cancers. AJR 146:661–663, 1986
36. Sickles EA, Abele JS: Milk of calcium within tiny benign breast cysts. Radiology 141:655–658, 1981
37. Sickles EA, Herzog KA: Intramammary scar tissue: A mimic of the mammographic appearance of carcinoma. AJR 135:349–352, 1980
38. Tabár L, Pentek Z, Dean PB: The diagnostic and therapeutic value of breast cyst puncture and pneumocystography. Radiology 141:659–663, 1981
39. Urban JA, Adair FE: Sclerosing adenosis. Cancer 2:625–634, 1949
40. Wellings SR, Wolfe JN: Correlative studies of the histological and radiographic appearance of the breast parenchyma. Radiology 129:299–306, 1978
41. Wolfe JN: Breast patterns as an index of risk for developing breast cancer. AJR 126:1130–1139, 1976
42. Wolfe JN, Albert S, Belle S, et al: Breast parenchymal patterns: Analysis of 332 incident breast carcinomas. AJR 138:113–118, 1982

Lester Kalisher, M.D.
Robert V. P. Hutter, M.D.

2

The Team Approach to Diagnosis: Preoperative Localization and Specimen Radiography

Until the advent of clinically acceptable mammography, breast cancer detection and localization was done exclusively by palpation. The lesion was most often discovered by the patient, the palpable mass was confirmed by the physician, and the appropriate management was planned. The role of the pathologist was to examine the mass grossly and microscopically to establish a diagnosis. The radiologist's role was nonexistent. Even relatively small, palpable cancers had a significant rate of axillary metastasis.

In the past 20 years, great improvements have been made in mammographic techniques. In the late 1950s and 1960s the work of Gershon-Cohen, Egan, Wolfe, and others pioneered modern-day mammography. High-resolution, low-dose systems utilizing film or xeroradiographic imaging methods are now available. Highly skilled technicians carry out examinations with equipment dedicated to the mammographic procedure. These technical advances have drastically changed the working relationships between primary physicians, surgeons, pathologists, and radiologists. Radiologists now routinely diagnose clinically unsuspected lesions in mammograms of asymptomatic women, recommend surgery for nonpalpable lesions, and find their recommendations accepted.

The 20-year actuarial survival rate of patients with minimal breast cancers has been reported as high as 93 percent.[11] However, the radiological detection of these highly favorable lesions has created potential problems. After the identification of the suspicious area in the mammogram, how does the surgeon localize and excise it, and how does the pathologist confirm that the surgical specimen contains the lesion in question?

PREOPERATIVE LOCALIZATION

Background and Methodology

Many terms are used to describe the unsuspected breast cancer that is discovered by mammography. In order to avoid confusion, specific definitions must be applied. *Clinically occult carcinoma* is any nonpalpable carcinoma, regardless of size. For example, a 4-cm cancer may be hidden in a large, fatty breast; even though nonpalpable, it would manifest the same prognosis as

We wish to acknowledge Mrs. Barbara Friedman for her assistance.

BREAST CANCER DETECTION
ISBN 0-8089-1842-7

any palpable carcinoma of similar size, location, and histology. A clinically occult carcinoma is therefore not necessarily an early one. *Minimal carcinoma* is defined as noninfiltrating ductal or lobular carcinoma, or focally invasive infiltrating carcinoma less than 5 mm in diameter.[20]

The oldest method of directing the surgeon to the location of a nonpalpable lesion was by written or verbal description alone. A suspicious area was described by its quadrant, the distance from the nipple, or its locus on a clockface.[1,2,28] These landmarks were located while the patient was sitting or lying in a decubitus position at the time of radiographic imaging. At surgery, with the patient supine, the lesion invariably shifted in its relation to the described landmarks, making the surgical localization very difficult. Quadrantectomies were often undertaken, and the specimen was then incised in numerous planes in search of the lesion before being sent to the pathologist. Radiographic interpretation of the specimen was difficult because of the distortions introduced by random sectioning.

Four basic approaches have evolved for localization of nonpalpable lesions: surface localization, spot techniques, hard-needle systems, and needle/wire systems. Each approach has distinct advantages and disadvantages.

1. *Surface localization*. This noninvasive technique, as described above, provides the surgeon with a map demonstrating the relative position of the suspicious area within the breast. Specific measurements related to the transverse and vertical midnipple lines may also be obtained. The advantage of this method is its simplicity. No special equipment is needed, it is quick and painless, and there are no risks to the patient. It is also the most inaccurate method, since any errors in transposition will result in missing the lesion and, more importantly, the lesion will shift in position with respect to the original mammogram when the patient lies supine for surgery. Frankl and Rosenfeld[10] attempted to overcome this shortcoming by taping to the skin of the breast radiopaque letters and numbers in vertical and horizontal orientations, respectively, allowing coordinates to be taken directly from the mammogram. There was, however, still considerable change in location of the lesion with respect to the markers when the patient was placed in the supine position.
2. *Spot method*.[4,7,15,22] A dye, sometimes mixed with an oily or water-soluble radiopaque contrast agent, is injected into the breast in or near the nonpalpable lesion. Simon et al.[25] recommended a mixture of Evans blue and pantopaque, while others preferred various alternative vital dyes and contrast agents. The dye/contrast mixture is injected through a small-gauge needle after the skin has been locally anesthetized. Some mammographers prefer not to use local anesthesia because of the relative pain insensitivity of breast tissue and the danger of an allergic reaction. Needles are repositioned as needed until repeated mammograms reveal that the needle tip is in or near the lesion. A tiny bolus (0.1 cc) of dye/contrast mixture is injected, and a trail of the mixture is made to the skin surface as the needle is withdrawn. The major advantage of this sytem is the ease with which the lesion is located at biopsy, provided that the biopsy is performed within 4 hours of injection. If the biopsy is prolonged beyond this time, the vital dye may become excessively diffused or may even disappear. Oily contrast material may obscure microcalcifications or small lesions on the specimen radiograph. Since the patient must be able to cooperate during the procedure, premedication for surgery should await the completion of localization.
3. *Needle localization*. Numerous techniques for placing needles into the area of suspicion have been developed. Most use a single hypodermic needle of appropriate length placed into the breast parallel to the chest wall from either the horizontal or vertical approach.[19] If the needle is misplaced, it can be repositioned. Dodd et al.[5] suggested using two needles at right angles, but Threatt et al.[29] found this unnecessary for accurate localization. Debnam et al.[3] place a second needle in the breast if the first needle is inaccurately positioned, permitting the first needle to serve as a guide. The needle hub is often difficult to secure since the hub can act as a lever and become displaced. Drucker[6] placed a Teflon sheath over the needle and then placed the combination into the breast, after which the needle was removed and the sheath that was left behind in the breast was sutured in place. Kalisher and Peyster,[17,21] recognizing the difficulty of anchoring conventional needles, developed flat-hub needles of various lengths that can be placed in the breast after the site of entrance is determined from the mammograms. The needles are secured by radially placed Steri-Strips.

   A word of caution about needle placement: although a horizontal anterior approach allows mammographic compression, this approach increases the danger of passing the needle into the chest wall or pleural space, with possible resultant pneumothorax or, rarely, tumor contamination of the pleural cavity.

   One variation of the needle-localization technique consists of using a Plexiglas compression plate containing multiple holes that is attached directly to the mammographic unit. After the mammogram is obtained, the specific hole overlying the lesion is identified, and a needle is passed through it and into the breast. The diameter of the hole should be larger than that of the hub of the needle. Needle-localization methods are tedious, since the measurements must be exact, and it may be difficult to compress the breast properly during confirmatory mammography after the needle is in place.

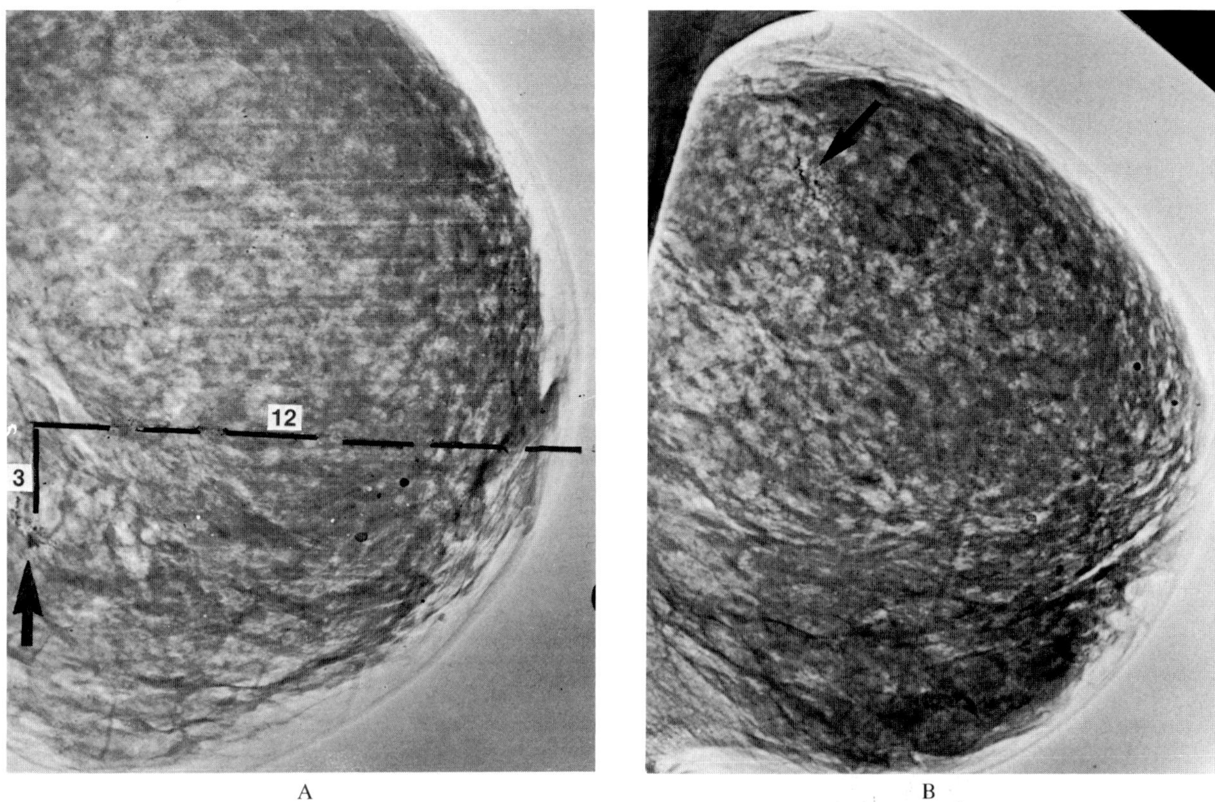

Figure 2-1. Cephalocaudal and lateral xeromammograms. A. Cephalocaudal view shows clustered microcalcifications (arrow) near chest wall. Line extends from nipple perpendicular to chest wall. Second line is drawn from lesion perpendicular to first line. First axis measures 12 cm, second axis, 3 cm. B. Lateral view shows microcalcifications (arrow) superiorly, near chest wall.

Regarding local anesthesia prior to needle localization, although minor discomfort may occur when the localizing needle is inserted, the needle dispensing the local anesthetic is usually no less discomforting. Some radiologists, therefore, prefer not to use local anesthesia. Because the patient must sit and be able to cooperate during the localization procedure, premedication for the biopsy should be withheld until localization has been completed.

4. *Needle/wire localization.*[12,15,16] Stiff needles may shift in the fatty breast, especially when compression is used. However, a malleable wire with a barbed hook at its tip will remain in place when introduced into the breast. Frank et al.[9] used a 25-gauge wire hooked at its end and "preloaded" into a 25-gauge needle. This assembly was introduced through a small skin incision along a line perpendicular to the chest wall at a location and depth estimated from the initial mammograms.[14] Kopans and de Luca[18] used an overbent spring hook to hold the wire in place, and Stephenson[27] used a Chiba needle to introduce the wire. Once the wire is in place, it is secure and can be compressed without fear of dislodgement during mammography performed to confirm accurate placement.

   A few disadvantages have been reported with this approach. Wires have been sheared by the cutting edge of the needle and, rarely, have migrated into the soft tissues of the upper limb. Since the wire, once inserted, cannot be easily removed, initial placement must be accurate. Finally, the wire may be difficult for the surgeon to palpate and could be subjected to accidental electrocautery or transection. Homer[14] devised a retractable wire with a curved end that may be withdrawn through the needle for improved ease of positioning. If xeroradiographic technique is utilized to image needles, radiopaque contrast agent, or wires, use of the negative mode will minimize the obscuration of the lesion by "toner robbing," a major disadvantage of the positive mode.

We have found the following simple method to be useful in the localization of nonpalpable lesions of the breast.[21] The cephalocaudal mammogram from the initial examination is used to estimate the position of the lesion. On the image, a line is drawn from the nipple perpendicular to and extending to the chest wall. A second line is drawn through the lesion perpendicular to the first line (Fig. 2-1). The distances along these two

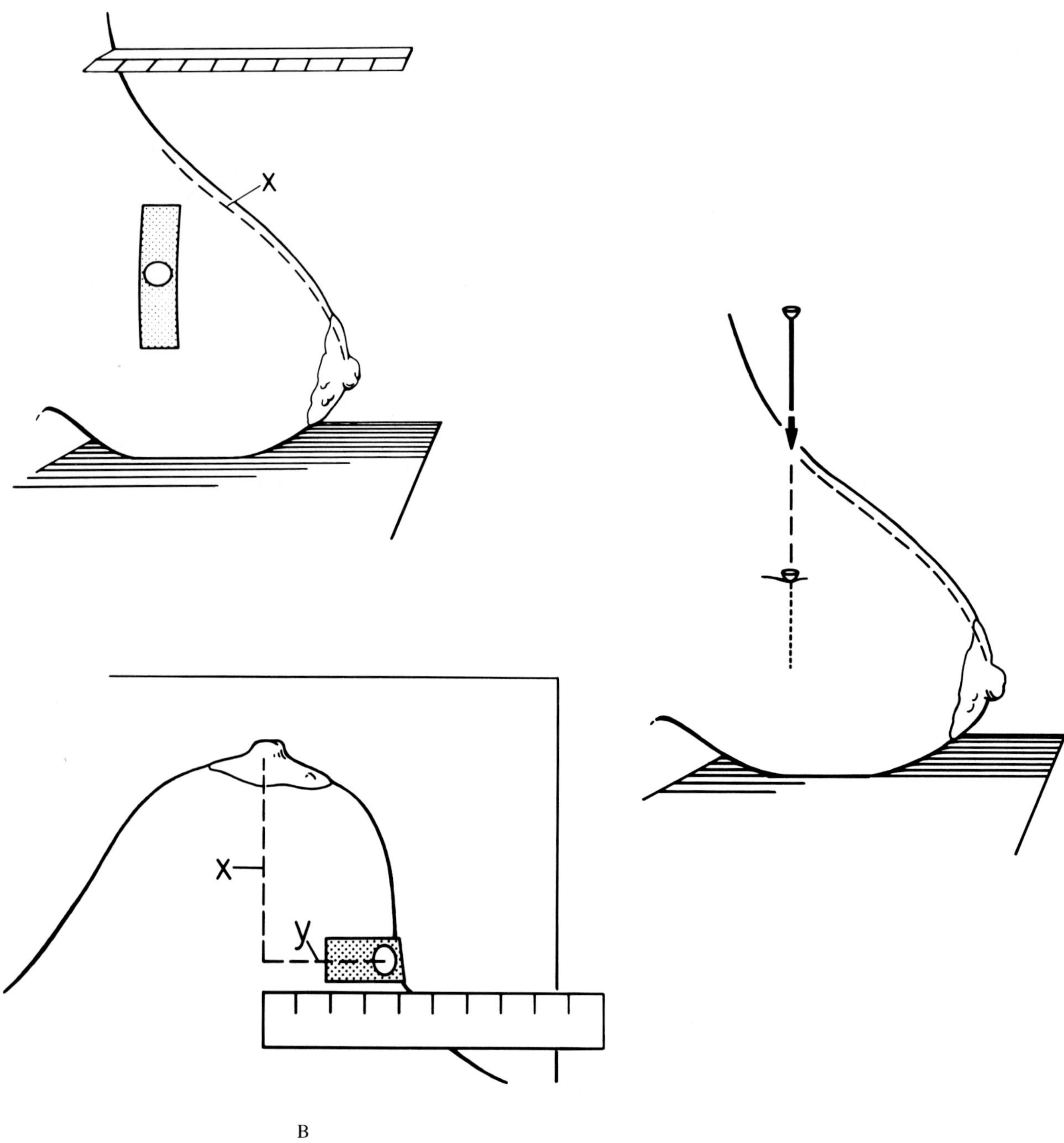

Figure 2-2. Breast as viewed by operator during localization procedure. A. (from side) and B (from above). Metallic marker is taped over site in breast corresponding to measurements along two axes described in Figure 2-1A. Needle is inserted, directed inferiorly, parallel to chest wall. C. Needle is embedded all the way to its hub.

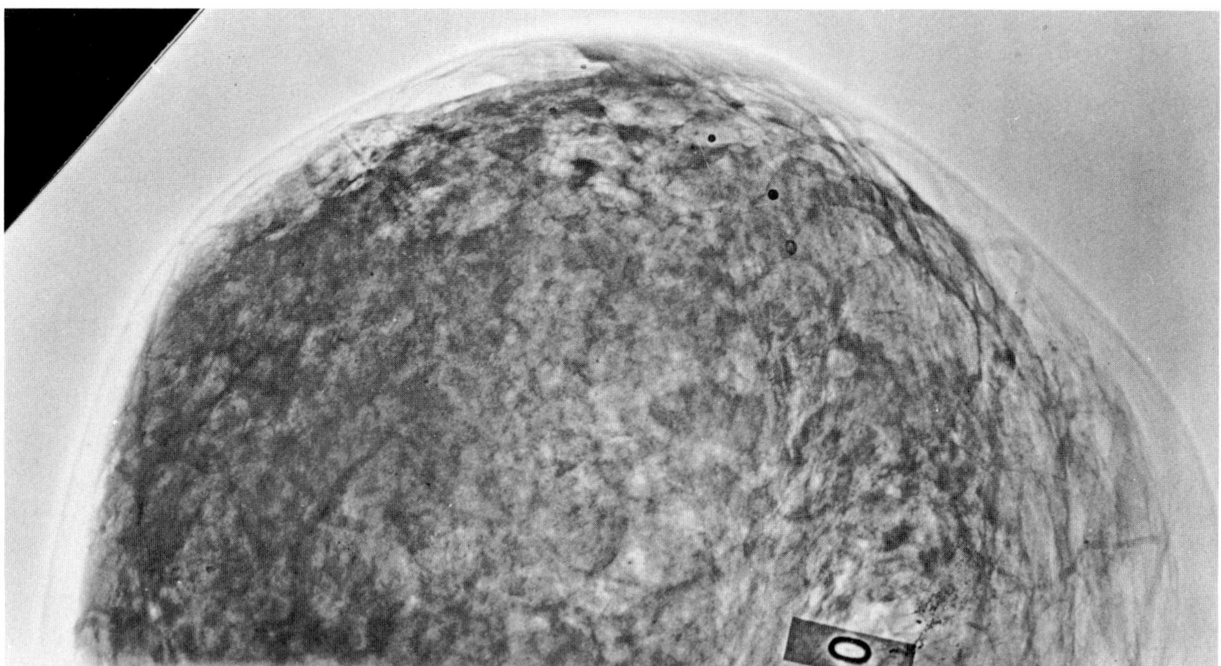

Figure 2-3. Cephalocaudal mammogram demonstrates metallic marker just lateral to microcalcifications. Appropriate adjustment is made when applying india-ink mark.

axes are measured. The patient is seated in a chair, and the breast is placed upon an x-ray receptor so that it lies in the same plane as during the original mammogram. The previously measured axes are plotted on the breast as they were on the mammogram, and a metallic marker is placed over the expected site of the lesion (Fig. 2-2A and B). A cephalocaudal projection is then taken (Fig. 2-3). In most patients, the marker will be projected over the lesion. If not, the appropriate adjustment is made. A mark is made with india ink at the site of the marker, and the marker is removed.

The region of the breast around and including the ink mark is prepared with Betadine (povidone-iodine) and alcohol, and an aseptic technique is maintained throughout. The operator stands behind the patient and directs the patient to look to the side opposite the breast being stüdied. The appropriate-length 22-gauge flat-headed needle* is selected on the basis of the size of the breast and the depth of the lesion. If flat-headed needles are not available, a conventional 22-gauge hypodermic needle can be substituted, provided that the hub of the embedded needle is well secured to the skin by sterile paper tape or Steri-Strips. No premedication or local anesthesia is used, since the burning sensation caused by the local anesthesia exceeds the minimal discomfort associated with needle placement.

The operator places the needle tip at the ink mark and directs it inferiorly, parallel to the chest wall and perpendicular to the x-ray receptor (Figs. 2-2B and C). If the needle is inserted in this manner, there is no possibility of creating a pneumothorax or propelling tumor cells into the chest wall. The needle should transfix the lesion.

Mediolateral and cephalocaudal projections are then taken to evaluate the position of the needle relative to the lesion (Figs. 2-4A and B)., In all patients in our series, the needle either transfixed the lesion or was sufficiently close to it to guide the surgeon effectively. The needle is taped in position by radial Steri-Strips, and the patient is sent to the operating room. The films are reviewed with the surgeon, who is then able to excise a small specimen at the appropriate place along the needle course. The specimen is then sent to the mammography clinic or pathology department, where x-rays are taken and compared with the original mammograms to ascertain that the suspicious lesion has been removed (Fig. 2-5). The specimen is then prepared for histological examination. If any doubt remains as to the correct area being excised, follow-up mammograms are recommended.

A needle wire assembly is a simple, useful means of localizing a nonpalpable lesion. A frontal approach is safe and effective provided that care is taken to use a needle of appropriate length. Moreover, a mechanical stop attached to the needle prevents the needle tip from passing into the chest wall. Using this method, the needle position can be altered until the tip is in the lesion. Then, as the needle is removed, the hook wire is retained in the breast. Mammograms confirm the position of the tip of the wire in the lesion (Fig. 2-6)

* *Popper & Sons, Inc., New Hyde Park, NY 11040*

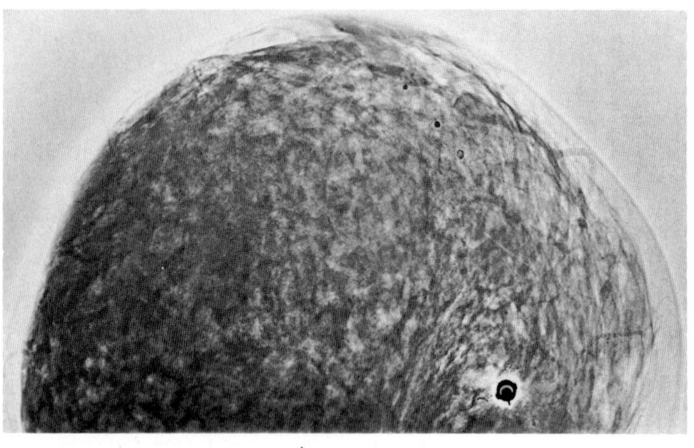

A

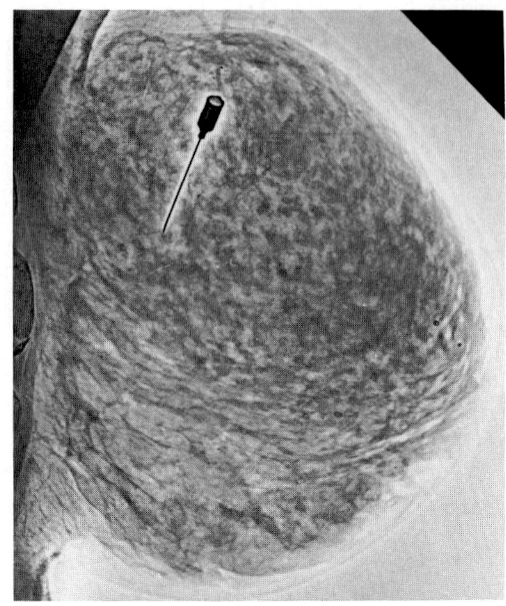

B

Figure 2-4. Cephalocaudal and mediolateral views, positive xeroradiographic mode, showing relationship of needle to lesion. A. Cephalocaudal view reveals needle projected directly on microcalcifications. B. Mediolateral view shows tip of needle slightly inferior to microcalcifications. (Use of negative mode would have diminished calcium obscuration caused by "toner robbing.")

SURGICAL APPROACHES

Two possible approaches may be taken by the surgeon. One is to use an elliptical incision overlying the needle or wire, cutting down to the lesion. The second is to make a circumareolar incision extending posteriorly toward the chest wall, feeling for the needle or wire along the way. Although the latter approach usually results in a less-prominent scar, it may also make it more difficult to feel the wire or needle. The surgeon, after removing the localized lesion and sending it to be radiographed, awaits notification by the radiologist and pathologist that the correct area has been removed.

SPECIMEN RADIOGRAPHY

Once the specimen is obtained from the operating room, it is first examined radiologically to confirm the presence of the lesion. In this endeavor, the radiologist and pathologist work hand in hand. A radiograph of the intact specimen may be performed with the mammography X-ray unit in the radiology department, using either film or xeroradiographic technique. An alternate method is to use a small x-ray unit (Hewlitt-Packard Faxitron) dedicated to the radiography of pathologic specimens.[26] The Faxitron is simple to use and provides an image of consistently high quality. It does not require a radiographic room, and waiting patients need not be exposed to the sight of surgical specimens. Xeroradiographic, industrial-film, or mammographic screen-film receptors are all suitable for use with the Faxitron.

After the specimen radiograph has been compared with the original mammograms and the presence of the lesion has been confirmed, the specimen is sequentially sliced into sections 3–5 mm thick; each section is labeled with radiopaque markers, and the specimen is then reradiographed. Appropriate samples for microscopic examination are then taken from the areas that are roentgenographically the most suspicious. Rarely, it may be necessary to radiograph the subsequent paraffin blocks to ascertain whether microcalcifications are present.[23,24,27]

If the lesion is not seen in the specimen radiograph, the surgeon is informed, and further exploration is carried out. Should only one or two calcifications of a more extensive cluster be noted in the specimen, they may be used to help orient the surgeon toward a more

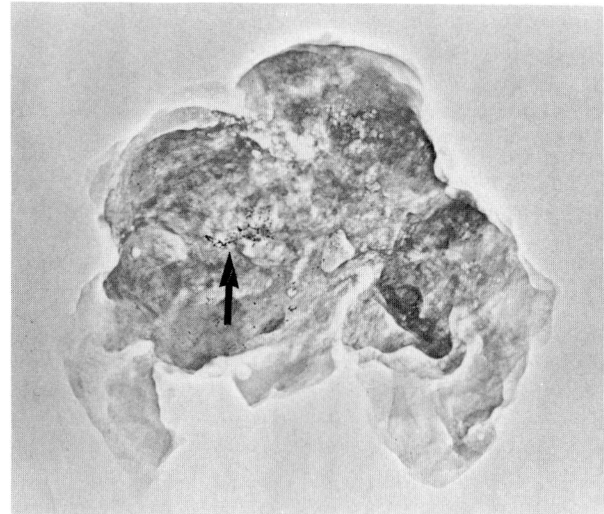

Figure 2-5. Specimen xeroradiograph revealing microcalcifications.

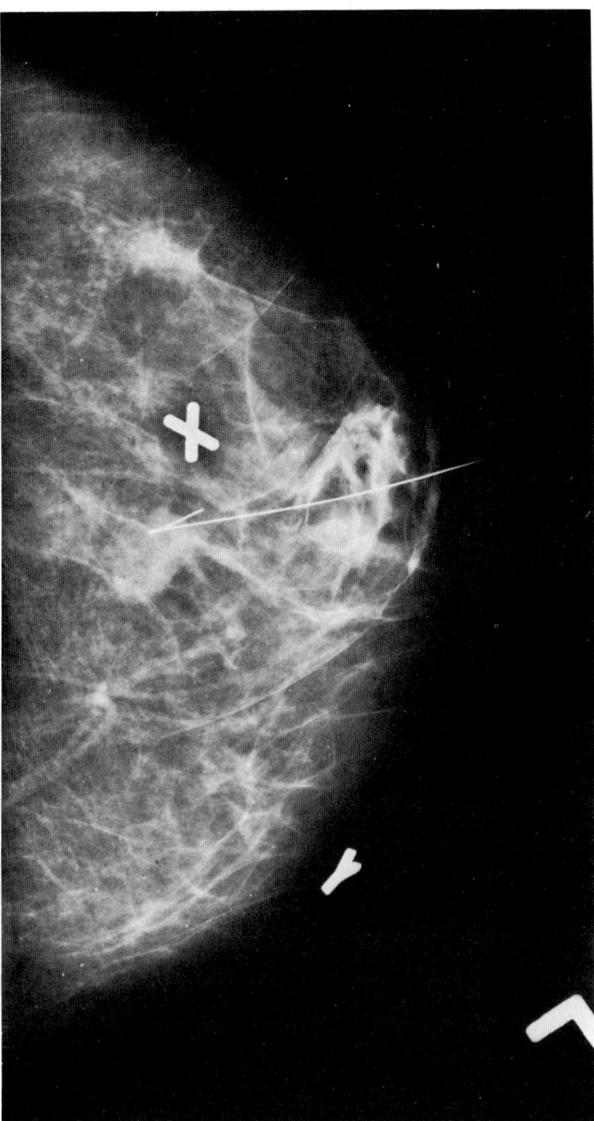

Figure 2-6. Hookwire at site of nonpalpable mass. Overlying "X" and "Y" skin markers guided placement of needle-wire assembly.

productive site for a second biopsy specimen. If benign cysts are inadvertently incised, this information should be transmitted to the pathologist and radiologist.

CONSIDERATIONS FOR THE FUTURE

Although needle and wire systems for localization of nonpalpable lesions are presently the most commonly used, no ideal system is available. The success rate depends on the experience and expertise of the radiologist. A real-time fluoroscopic or ultrasonic system in which the lesion is identified in two planes while a marker is placed directly into the suspicious area would be ideal. Such a system, possibly with computer enhancement, may be on the horizon. In the meantime, tools now are available that permit reliable localization of nonpalpable lesions. Rapid communication between radiologist, pathologist, and surgeon is necessary, and communication systems are now available that transmit to the operating room video images of specimen radiographs and gross and microscopic sections of the specimen.

In conclusion, the importance of cooperation between surgeon, radiologist, and pathologist cannot be overemphasized. By working together as a team, these physicians enable the discovery of the nonpalpable lesion and facilitate its localization and removal. If the lesion is benign, the patient loses only a small amount of breast tissue, with little, if any resultant deformity. If the lesion is malignant, a proper, unhurried approach to the treatment of the lesions is undertaken. Egan[8] stated that the word *team* is defined as "a group on one side in a match with a desire to win . . . with each team member contributing and willing to learn from and share with his team members."

REFERENCES

1. Berger SM, Curcio BM, Gershon-Cohen J, et al: Mammographic localization of unsuspected breast cancer. AJR 96:1046–1052, 1966
2. Curcio BM: Technique for radiographic localization of nonpalpable breast tumors. Radiol Technol 42:155–160, 1970
3. Debnam JW, deSevilla E, Staple TW: Preoperative localization of occult breast lesions: A new technic. South Med J 70:204–235, 1977
4. Dietler OC, Wineland RE, Matolo NM: Localization of nonpalpable breast lesions detected by xeromammography. Am Surg 42:810–811, 1976
5. Dodd GD, Frey K, Delaney W: Preoperative localization of nonpalpable lesions. Conference on Detection and Treatment of Early Breast Cancer, Buena Vista, FL, March 1974. HS Gallager (ed), New York, Wiley, 1974, pp 151–153
6. Drucker L: Localization of nonpalpable carcinoma of the breast utilizing xeromammography-technique B. Breast 2:28–29, 1976
7. Egan JF, Sayler CB, Goodman MJ: A technique for localizing occult breast lesions. CA 26:32–37, 1976
8. Egan RL: Evolution of the team approach in breast cancer. Cancer 36:1815–1822, 1975
9. Frank HA, Hall FM, Steer ML: Postoperative localization of nonpalpable breast lesions demonstrated by mammography. N Engl J Med 295:259–260, 1976
10. Frankl G, Rosenfeld D: Xeroradiographic detection of occult breast cancer. Cancer 35:542–548, 1975
11. Frazier T: Prognosis and treatment in minimal breast cancer. Am J Surg 133:697–701, 1977
12. Funderbush WV, Flax RL: Localization of nonpalpable carcinoma of the breast utilizing xeromammography-technique A. Breast 2:28–29, 1976
13. Homer MJ: Nonpalpable breast lesion localization using a curved-end retractable wire. Radiology 157:259–260, 1985

14. Homer MJ: Percutaneous localization of breast lesions: Experience with the Frank Breast Biopsy Guide. J Can Assoc Radiol 30:238–241, 1979
15. Horns JW, Arndt RD: Percutaneous spot localization of nonpalpable breast lesions. AJR 127:253–256, 1976
16. Jensen SR, Luttenegger TJ: Wire localization of nonpalpable breast lesions. Radiology 132:484–485, 1979
17. Kalisher L: An improved needle for localization of nonpalpable breast lesions. Radiology 128:815–817, 1978
18. Kopans DB, de Luca S: A modified needle-hookwire technique to simplify preoperative localization of occult breast lesions. Radiology 134:781, 1980
19. Libshitz HE, Feig SA, Fetouh S: Needle localization of nonpalpable breast lesions. Radiology 121:557–560, 1976
20. Martin JE, Gallager HS: Mammographic diagnosis of minimal breast cancer. Cancer 28:1519–1526, 1971
21. Peyster RG, Kalisher L: Needle localization of nonpalpable lesions of the breast. Surg Gynecol Obstet 148:703–706, 1979
22. Raininko R, Linna ME, Rasanen O: Preoperative localization of nonpalpable breast tumours. Acta Chir Scand 142:575–578, 1976
23. Rosen PP, Snyder RE: Nonpalpable breast lesions detected by mammography and confirmed by specimen radiography: Recent experience. Breast 3:13–16, 1977
24. Rosen PP, Snyder RE, Robbins G: Specimen radiography for nonpalpable breast lesions found by mammography: Procedures and results. Cancer 36:1815–1822, 1975
25. Simon N, Lesnick GJ, Lerer WN, et al: Roentgenographic localization of small lesions of the breast by the spot method. Surg Gynecol Obstet 134:527–574, 1972
26. Snyder RE, Rosen P: Radiography of breast specimens. Cancer 28:1608–1611, 1971
27. Stephenson TF: Chiba needle-barbed wire technique for breast biopsy localization. AJR 135:184–185, 1980
28. Stevens GM, Jamplis RW: Mammographically directed biopsy of nonpalpable breast lesions. Arch Surg 102:292–295, 1971
29. Threatt B, Appleman H, Dow R, et al: Percutaneous needle localization of clustered mammary microcalcifications prior to biopsy. AJR 121:839–842, 1974

Section 3
Performing the Examination

Wende W. Logan, M.D.
Joyce A. Janus, M.D.

1

Screen-Film Mammography

In the late 1960s and early 1970s, concern about the relatively high x-ray exposure required for industrial-film mammography led to the development of screen-film detector systems capable of producing detailed breast images at low x-ray doses.[14,15,18] A calcium tungstate intensifying-screen-single-emulsion film combination kept in intimate contact by a vacuum yielded a mammographic image of diagnostic quality and with even better resolution than that obtained with the same screen and double-emulsion film.[15,18] Another advantage of the new film was its suitability for rapid and automatic processing. It is fortunate that the developmental work had already been accomplished by 1975, prior to the onset of widespread negative publicity concerning the high x-ray dosage required for conventional nonscreen, industrial-film mammography.

Although additional screen-film systems were subsequently developed,[3,17] the DuPont Lo-Dose II calcium tungstate system and the Eastman Kodak Min-R rare-earth system became the ones in widest use in the United States. The average glandular dose with these screen-film combinations is only 200–300 mrads per two-view examination.[12] Fear of radiation-induced breast carcinoma by physicians and the public was the major factor causing many mammographers to convert from xeromammography and conventional nonscreen film mammography to screen-film combinations.

Although the inherent resolution of these combinations is less than that of industrial nonscreen hand-processed film, the increased speed of screen-film systems, in combination with breast compression and low peak-kilovoltage (kvp) technique, compensates for the decreased resolution by providing higher image contrast. Diminished exposure times result in less object motion and reduced motion unsharpness. The smaller focal spots and longer target-to-image distances featured by the newest dedicated units have further improved the resolution of screen-film combinations. Indeed, when performed with state-of-the-art dedicated mammography equipment, screen-film images are equal or superior to those of reduced-dose xeromammography and far superior to nonscreen film mammograms.

TECHNICAL CONSIDERATIONS

Screen-film X-ray Equipment

Unlike xeromammography or conventional film mammography, optimum screen-film mammograms require the use of specially designed x-ray units. The first dedicated mammography unit was introduced by Dr. Charles Gros in France in the mid-1960s.[5] Its molybdenum target provided the "soft" x-ray beam required for enhanced contrast between low-density breast structures. The unit also housed a device capable of providing vigorous breast compression to reduce scattered

BREAST CANCER DETECTION
ISBN 0-8089-1842-7

radiation. These two components made it possible to visualize minute microcalcifications and the contrasting density of masses.

The relatively homogeneous x-ray spectrum produced by the molybdenum target could increase the contrast between low-density structures by enhancing the photoelectric effect. For this purpose, a technique of 25–28 kvp and a molybdenum filter with an equivalent half-value layer no greater than 0.3 mm of aluminum proved to be ideal. (The substitution of aluminum for molybdenum filters is detrimental and is reserved for use with grids and for magnification.) The resulting low-energy x-ray spectrum greatly enhances the contrast between calcifications, masses, and surrounding breast tissues. The increased speed of screen-film image receptors allowed the use of the lower-energy x-ray beam while still permitting exposure times far more rapid than those required by xeromammographic and nonscreen film techniques. It cannot be overly stressed that the use of conventional tungsten targets results in a "hard" beam that degrades the screen-film image by severely impairing contrast and, hence, the detection of both microcalcifications and masses (Fig. 1-1).

Vigorous compression of the breast during the x-ray exposure is mandatory in screen-film examinations for the following reasons:

1. It minimizes geometric unsharpness by bringing the entire breast as close as possible to the image receptor.[6]
2. It increases image contrast by diminishing scattered radiation.[1]
3. It decreases motion unsharpness by preventing patient movement during the exposures.
4. It allows a reduction in average dose by decreasing breast thickness.
5. It results in a nearly uniform thickness of the anterior and posterior parts of the breast, allowing nearly equal penetration by the x-ray beam.
6. It allows a more accurate assessment of the true density of masses, an important factor distinguishing benign masses of low density, such as cysts, from carcinomas, which are characterized by high, uneven density.
7. It separates the breast structures, allowing optimal evaluation of lesional borders that might otherwise be obscured by overlying tissue.

The average breast can be compressed to approximately 4 cm in thickness. In order to obtain the full cooperation of the patient, the value of compression should be carefully explained before it is applied. Moreover, the compression, although it must be vigorously applied, is benign; in over 20,000 patients, I have yet to personally encounter an injury due to compression of the breasts.

The optimal compressing surface for screen-film mammography should be perfectly parallel to the film surface and not sloped at its posterior edge. Sloping of the posterior edge of a compression device, as in the one commonly used in xeromammography, hinders compression of the base of the breast and leads to underpenetration by the x-ray beam (Figs. 1-2A and C). Ideally, the posterior part of the compressing plane should be bent sharply upward to a height of 2 in (Fig. 1-2B). This alteration displaces the axillary fold, which overlies the posterolateral aspect of the breast on the cephalocaudal view. The sharply raised edge also strengthens the device by buttressing it. In addition, the sharp posterior angle allows the device to grip the posterior aspect of the breast tissue as it compresses it, rather than allowing it to slide out from underneath. The result of vigorous compression with a properly engineered device is optimal visualization of the posterior aspect of the breast (Fig. 1-2D). If the compression device on a screen-film dedicated unit does not fulfill

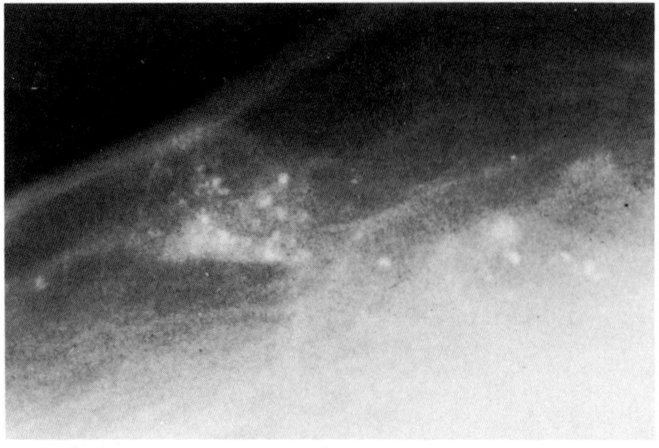

A

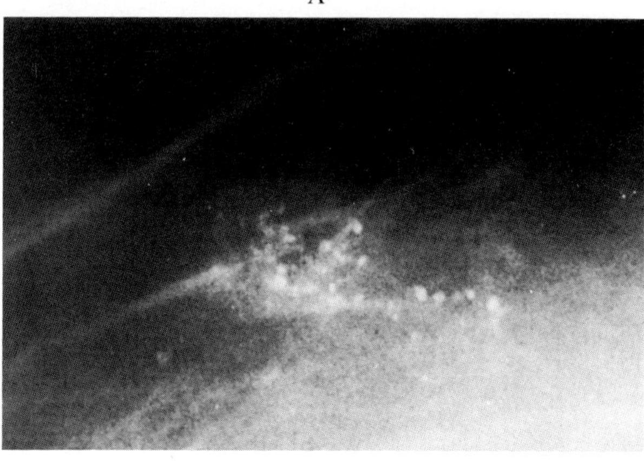

B

Figure 1-1. Detection of microcalcifications impaired by use of excessively "hard" x-ray beam (above 28 kvp). A. First mammogram was performed at 29 kvp with Min-R screen-film system on GE MMX unit. B. Second mammogram was performed with same factors except exposure was performed at 25 kvp at slight increase in exposure time. Calcifications are more readily detected and additional calcifications are now seen because of improved contrast. From Logan WW, Muntz EP (eds): Reduced Dose Mammography. New York, Masson USA, 1979, p 425. With permission.

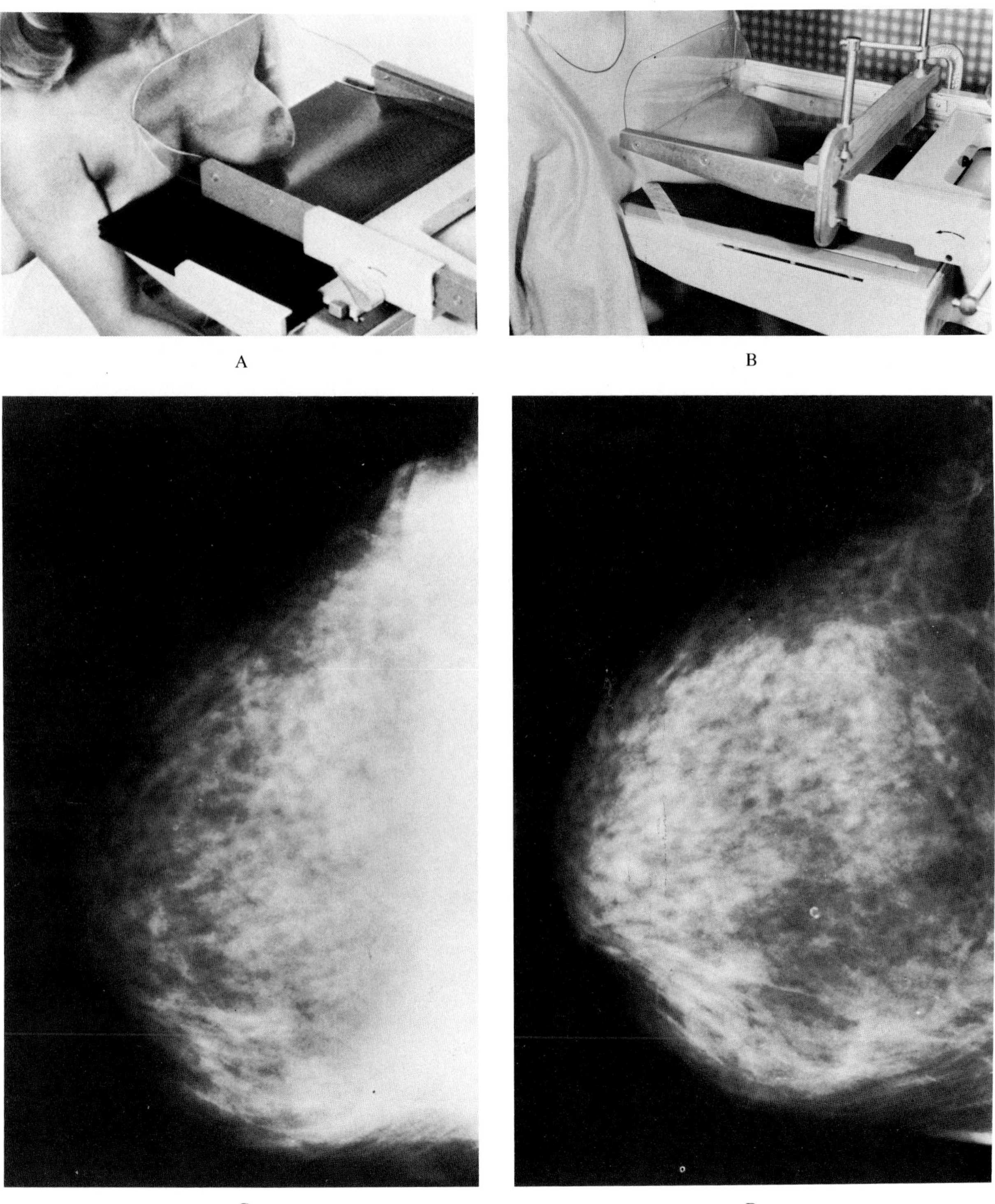

Figure 1-2. A. Two types of compression device. Gently sloping posterior edge of this compression device (GE MMX) results in geometric unsharpness and underpenetration of posterior breast tissues. B. Optimal compression devices have posterior surface bent sharply upward. C. Mediolateral mammogram performed with gradually sloping compression device reveals underpenetration of posterior aspect of breast (25 kvp at 1 second, Min-R screen—Min-R single-emulsion film vacuum-packaged in Picker polyethylene bag). D. Mediolateral mammogram performed 1 year later with redesigned (GE) compression device shows improved compression of posterior aspect of breast (25 kvp at 0.25 second, Min-R screen—Kodak NMB film vacuum-packaged in Picker polyethylene bag). Proper posterior compression of breast enables use of slightly faster and more contrasty film, which also aids in dose reduction. From Logan WW, Muntz EP (eds): Reduced Dose Mammography. New York, Masson USA, 1979, p 423. With permission.

these criteria, it can be replace with a 1-mm thick Lexan shield (not a fire-retardant form) that has been bent at a sharp 85° angle posteriorly. A suitably rigid compression device is now a feature of the Elscint microfocal-spot tungsten-target unit employed for magnification mammography (Fig. 1-3).[8,9]

Choice of a Screen-film Combination

The Kodak Min-R and DuPont Lo-Dose II systems are currently most popular. Only film with emulsion on one side is suitable for screen-film mammography. The reason is that film with emulsion on both sides will suffer excessive diffusion of the light produced by the intensifying-screen phosphor crystals on the emulsion coating farthest from the screen. This "crossover" effect degrades the mammographic image.

When screen-film combinations have equivalent spatial resolution and system speed, the one that produces the most contrast per given half-value layer is to be preferred. I use Kodak OM-1 film, which possesses slightly more contrast and speed than Kodak Min-R film, in combination with a Kodak Min-R rare-earth screen. If this system produces an image with a graininess or noise level that is unacceptable, the DuPont Lo-Dose II system, which has less contrast, is recommended.

Prior to mammographic exposure, intimate contact must be obtained between screen and film. This contact is best achieved by placing the screen-film combination in a Picker or DuPont polyethylene bag that is air-evacuated and sealed in a Picker or DuPont vacuum sealer.[14] With these methods, the mammographer will gain the least attenuation of the x-ray beam by image receptor, permitting the lowest-possible x-ray exposure and the highest-possible image contrast (Figs. 1-4C and D). The EZ-EM polyvinyl chloride vac-bag is an unacceptable vacuum system because it absorbs and "hardens" the x-ray beam exiting from the breast to too great an extent (Fig. 1-4A). An acceptable alternative to the vacuum-sealing device is the Kodak screen-film vacuum cassette (Fig. 1-4B)

Screens should be cleaned daily with Kodak screen-cleaning solution. The Picker or DuPont polyethylene bags can be reused approximately five times. In order to prevent static marks on the film, the inside of each bag should be sprayed before its initial use with an antistatic spray.* Screens and films should not be exposed to these sprays, which may leave an elevated residue.

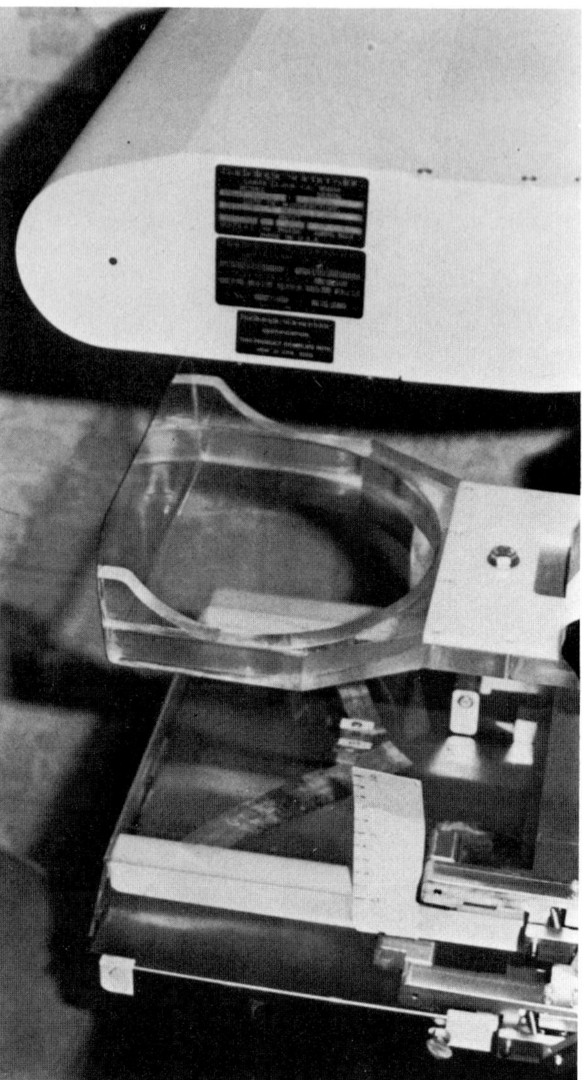

Figure 1-3. Compression device designed for Radiologic Sciences, Inc. magnification mammography unit (now marketed by Elscint, Inc.). Plastic material is angled 90° superiorly at breast base in order to push axillary fold tissue posteriorly, so that it will not be superimposed over glandular tissue. Sharp angle is preferable because (1) it enables last few millimeters of posterior glandular tissue to be well penetrated by x-ray beam and (2) it grips compressed breast better so that breast cannot slide out from underneath when compression is applied. From Logan WW, Muntz EP (eds): Reduced Dose Mammography. New York, Masson USA, 1979, p 424. With permission.

Patient Positioning

Most screen-film mammographers employ a mediolateral and a cephalocaudal view performed with vigorous compression for routine examinations. A routine lateromedial projection is not recommended, since 70 percent of all breast carinomas are in the lateral hemisphere and the lateromedial projection would result in unnecessary geometric unsharpness and scattered radiation in the area of most interest. Exaggerated medial and lateral cephalocaudal views are used to localize a deep lesion that is visible only in the mediolateral projection.

* Price Driscoll Corp., Farmingdale, NY

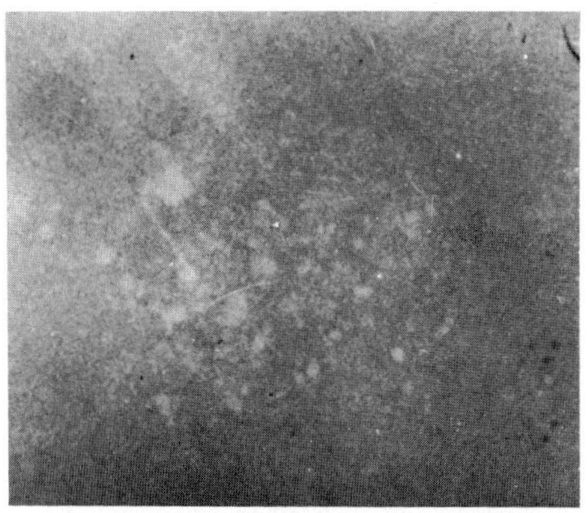

A

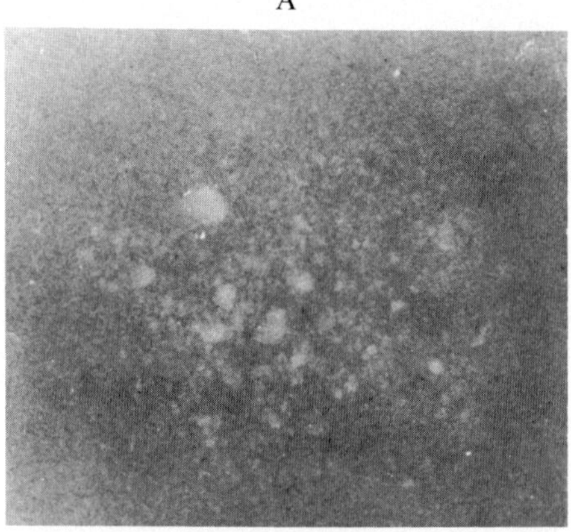

B

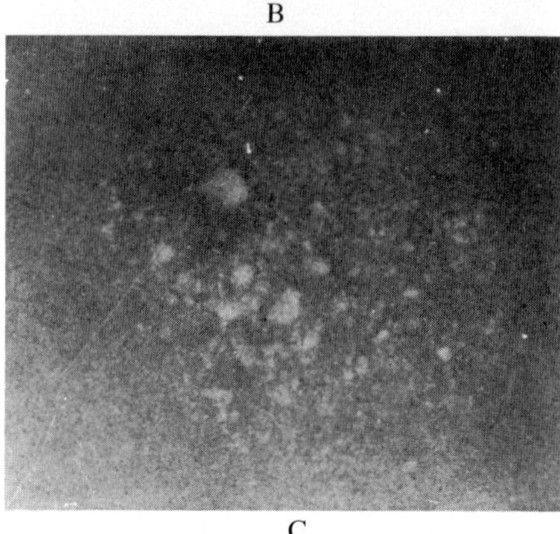

C

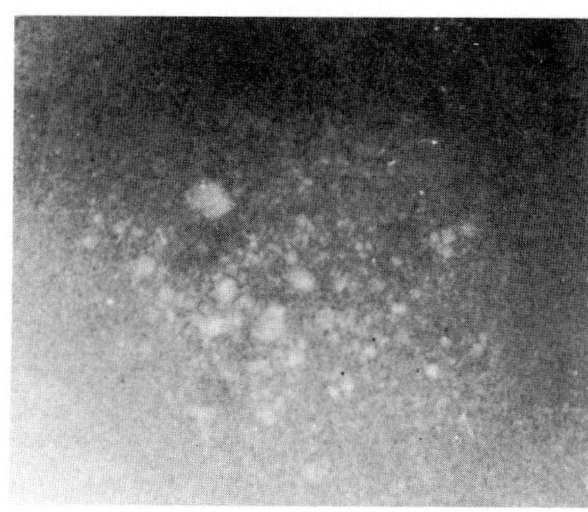

D

Figure 1-4. Radiographic images of Kodak Pathé phantom calcifications (placed on three 1-cm-thick Lucite blocks). A. Kodak Min-R screen—Min-R film within EZ-EM polyvinyl chloride vacuum bag. B. Kodak Min-R screen—Min-R single-emulsion film within Kodak Min-R screen-film vacuum cassette. Slightly improved contrast is observed because Kodak plastic cassette surface attenuates x-ray beam less than EZ-EM bag. C. Min-R screen—Min-R film enclosed in Picker polyethylene vacu-pack. Increased contrast is because Picker polyethylene cover attenuates breast exit beam less than Kodak cassette. D. Min-R screen-Kodak NMB single-emulsion film (slightly faster than Min-R screen-Kodak NMB single emulsion film (slightly faster than Min-R film) enclosed in Picker polyethylene bag. Contrast between calcifications and surrounding Lucite is further improved because of increased film contrast. From Logan WW, Muntz EP (eds): Reduced Dose Mammography. New York, Masson USA, 1979, p 426. With permission.

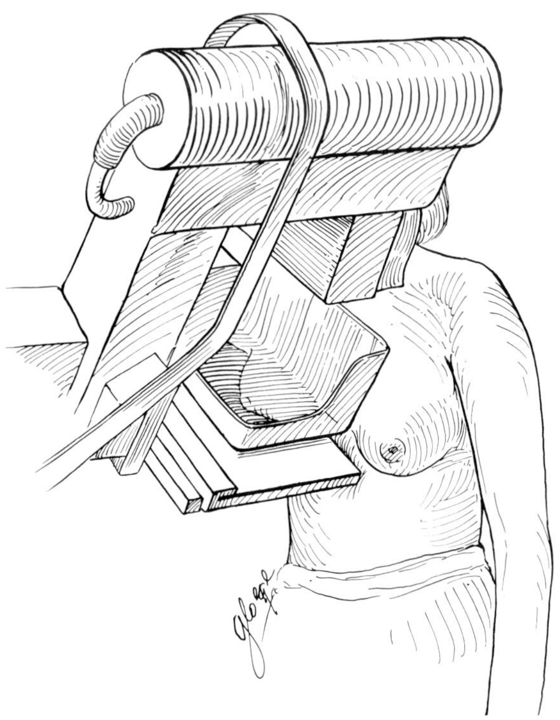

Figure 1-5. Oblique view. The position of the standing patient, in relation to the x-ray tube and compression device, is shown. From Bassett LW, Gold RH: Breast radiography using the oblique projection. Radiology 149:585–587, 1983. With permission.

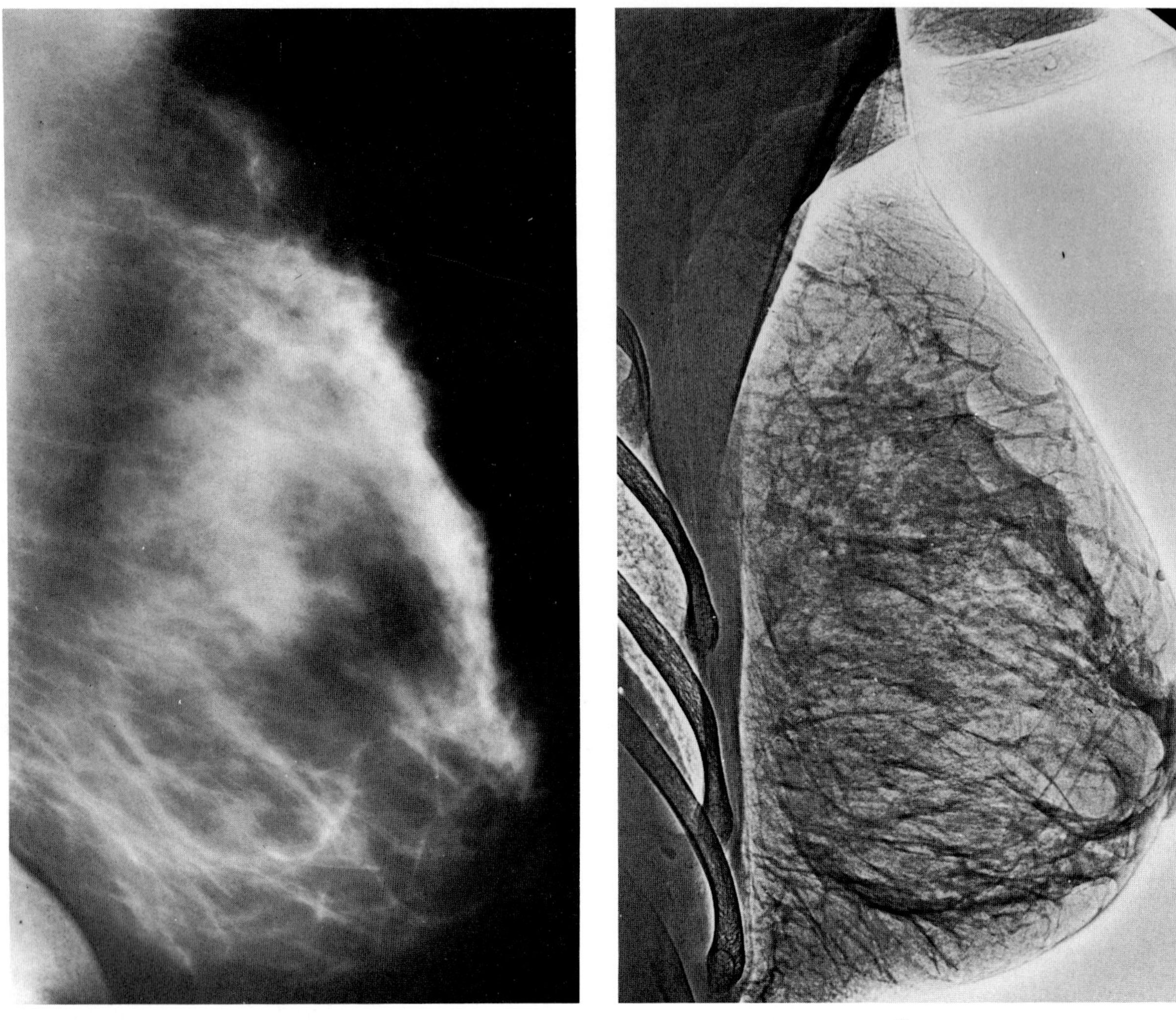

Figure 1-6. A. Properly performed oblique view. Glandular tissue is visualized extending into axillary region. B. Lateral chest wall view xeromammogram, same patient. Note that when proper positioning is performed for oblique screen-film view, glandular tissue can be seen as completely as with xeromammography method, even though ribs are not visualized on screen-film study. From Logan WW, Muntz EP (eds): Reduced Dose Mammography. New York, Masson USA, 1979, p 420. With permission.

I personally prefer an oblique view to the standard mediolateral view for routine examinations (Fig. 1-5). Approximately 5 percent of patients have an auxillary tail of breast tissue that cannot be completely visualized in routine mediolateral and cephalocaudal views. This variation usually occurs in women with relatively small breasts who have had a recent weight gain of 5 pounds or more. Because the skin of the recently enlarged breast has had insufficient time to stretch, difficulty may be encountered in pulling the breast tissue away from the chest wall. Even in a chest wall mediolateral xeromammographic view, it may be possible to see the most posterior segment of glandular tissue. In screen-film mammograms, this problem is recognized when glandular tissue is seen to extend beyond the edge of the film in mediolateral and cephalocaudal views. In contradistinction, the oblique view, performed with the x-ray beam directed from superomedial to inferolateral, usually discloses all of the breast structures, including the posterior segment and the axillary tail, on a single film (Figs. 1-5 through 1-7).[11] Were a single-view mammographic examination ever to be considered acceptable for screening in future years, the oblique view would be the most effective projection for visualizing the entire breast. The primary factor in successfully achieving this view is the compression by the technologist of the underlying pectoral muscles. By compression of these muscles parallel to their longitudinal plane, the breast is displaced anteriorly onto the mammographic image. In contrast, the direction of compres-

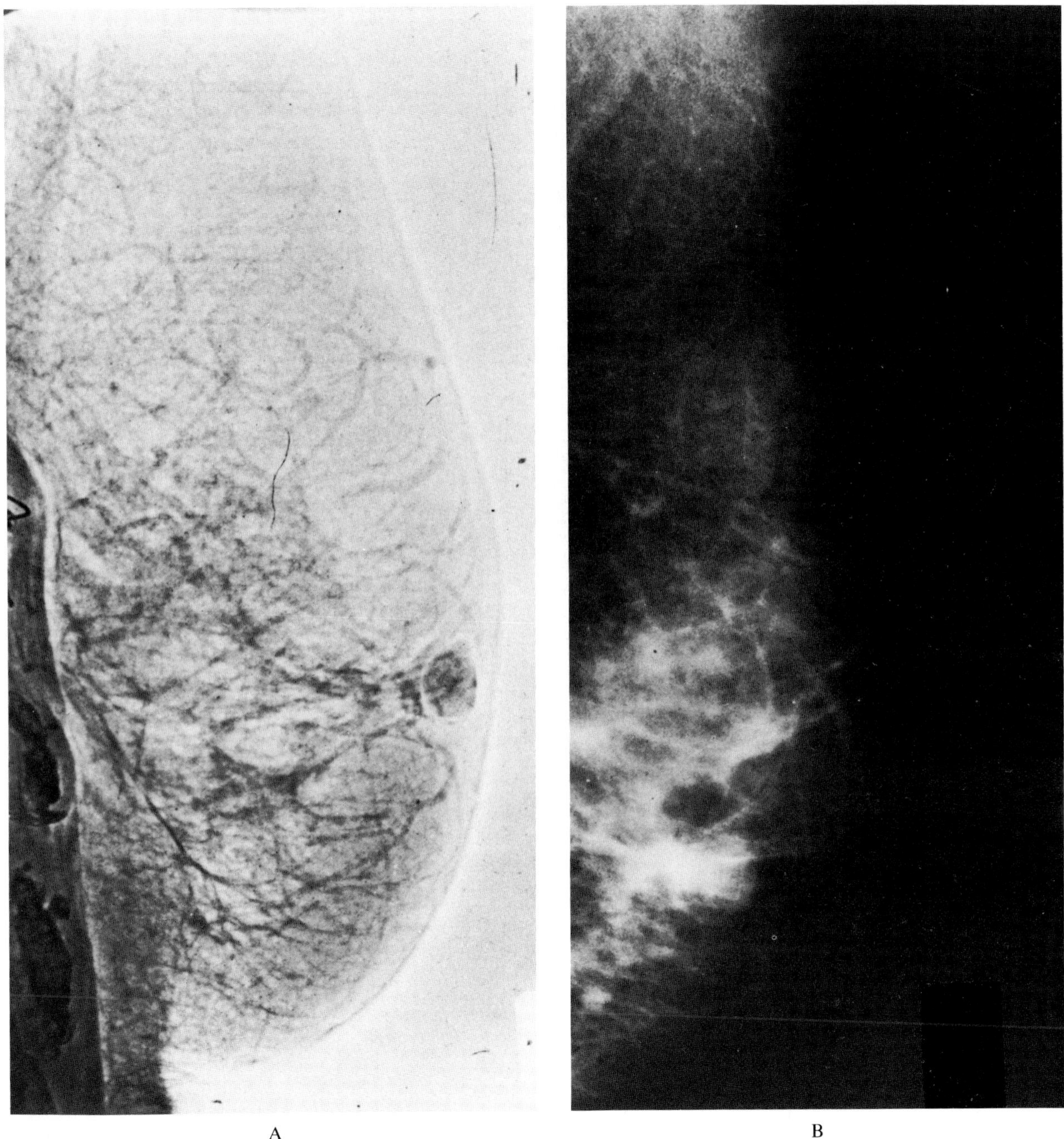

A B

Figure 1-7. Mammograms of patient with 20-pound weight gain over a 5-year period, resulting in breast enlargement and skin tightening. Lateral chest wall xeromammogram (A) and mediolateral screen-film mammogram (B) reveal no abnormalities. Cephalocaudal xeromammogram (C) and screen-film mammogram (D) reveal glandular tissue extending from subareolar region to posterolateral breast. E. A 45° oblique view (x-ray beam directed from superomedial to inferolateral). Large, soft, nonpalpable lobulated carcinoma is now visualized.

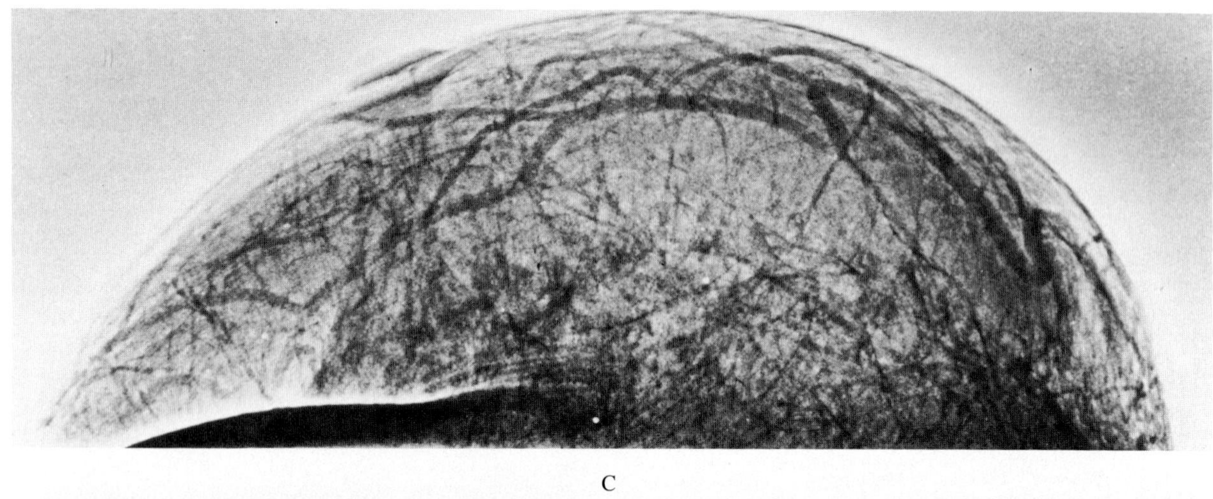

C

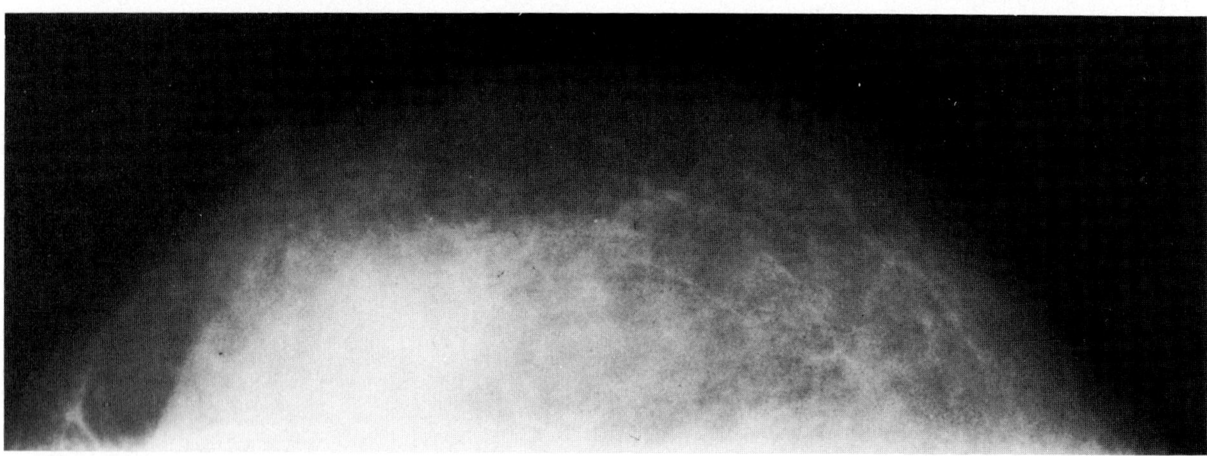

D

E

Figure 1-7 (cont.)

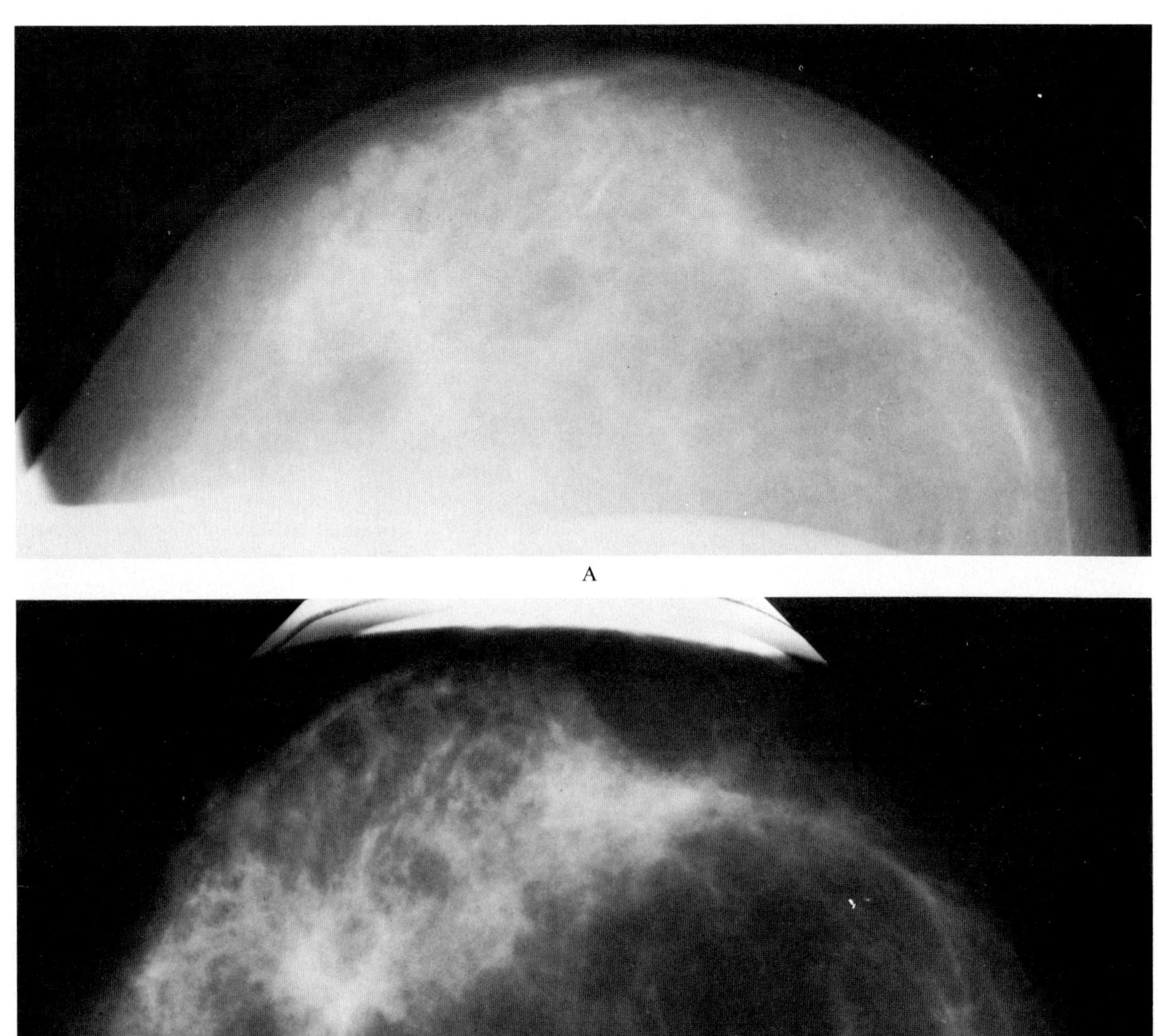

Figure 1-8. Mammograms of patient with large palpable "soft" mass in left upper outer quadrant. A. Cephalocaudal mammogram (Min-R screen-Min-R film, in Kodak Min-R screen cassette) performed with nondedicated x-ray unit with tungsten target shows poor contrast between soft tissue and fatty tissue. B. Cephalocaudal screen-film mammogram (Min-R screen-Kodak NMB film) performed on dedicated GE MNX unit shows high contrast between breast tissues. Stellate mass is now visualized. Increased contrast is due to combined effects of soft molybdenum x-ray beam and vigorous compression obtained with dedicated mammography compression device.

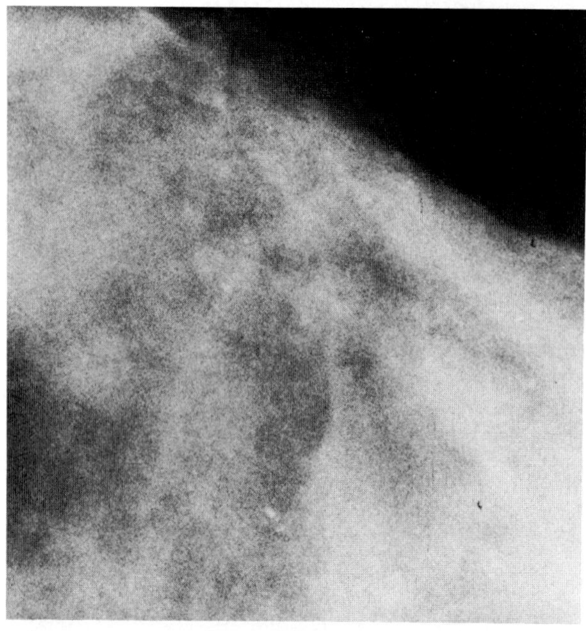

A

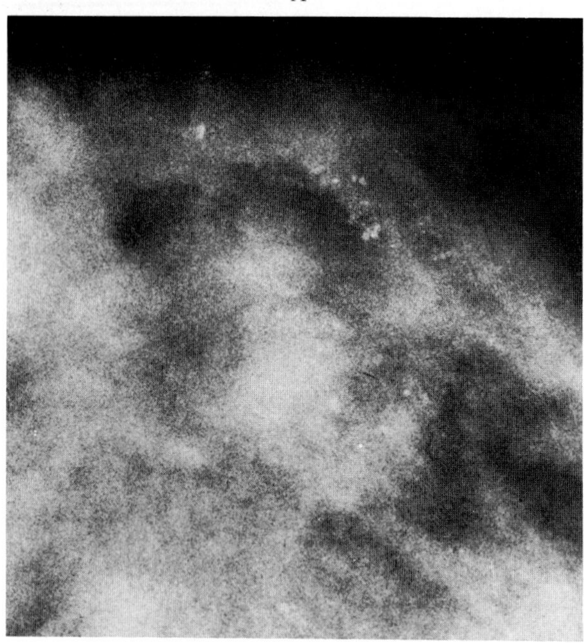

B

Figure 1-9. Magnification screen-film mammography. A. Screen-film mammogram film reveals dense glandular tissue and poorly defined fine calcifications. B. A 1.5 × magnification view was performed with 150μ tungsten focal spot (Radiologic Sciences, Inc.—now marketed by Elscint, Inc.). Magnification view shows greater detail of calcifications as well as many more. (Image has been reduced to size of contact mammogram to facilitate comparison.) From Logan WW, Muntz EP (eds): Reduced Dose Mammography. New York, Masson USA, 1979, p 427. With permission.

sion for the standard mediolateral view is antagonistic to the true longitudinal alignment of the pectoral muscles, resulting in suboptimal displacement of the breast from the underlying rib cage. This problem is compounded in the cephalocaudal view, in which the compression is almost directly counter to the alignment of the pectoral muscles. This problem in positioning can be appreciated by pinching the skin in front of one's biceps muscle from medial to lateral (the equivalent to the mediolateral and cephalocaudal views). When one discovers how much more tissue can be displaced away from the muscle in a true medial-to-lateral pinch, the value of the oblique view becomes clear. As the direction of the pectoral muscles differs from one patient to another, the angle of the oblique view must vary from 40° to 50°, but is usually 45°. When the oblique view is used, it is important to compress both breasts at identical angles. Labeling each radiograph with the angle of obliquity used during the oblique view facilitates the localization of lesions.

In my office, a routine mammographic examination consists of cephalocaudal and oblique views. Whenever a nonpalpable lesion is discovered, a supplemental mediolateral view is performed in order to correctly localize the lesion in three dimensions.

CONVERSION FROM XEROMAMMOGRAPHY OR NONSCREEN FILM MAMMOGRAPHY TO SCREEN-FILM MAMMOGRAPHY

Unless xeromammography has been performed with a dedicated mammography unit, conversion to the screen-film method should not be attempted until specialized x-ray equipment has been obtained. Even large carcinomas may go undetected when screen-film techniques are attempted without a dedicated unit (Fig. 1-8). The considerable recording latitude of xeromammography enables the denser regions, such as the most posterior breast structures and the ribs, to be visualized as adequately as the nipple and skin in a single xeromammographic chest wall view. This latitude, however, is obtained with the sacrifice of broad area contrast, the lack of which leads to difficulty in assessing the density of lesions. Contrast is further sacrificed by the added aluminum filtration required for reduced-dose xeromammography. The comparatively minimal recording latitude of screen-film combinations will not allow adequate simultaneous visualization of the peripheral thinner breast structures and the thicker and denser chest wall structures. Therefore, the "soft" x-ray beam required for screen-film mammography cannot adequately image both the rib cage and superficial structures. While severe beam "hardening" will allow rib penetration in screen-film studies, the resultant diminution in contrast of the breast is unacceptable. Many xeromammographers contend that rib visualization is necessary to ensure that the entire posterior part of the

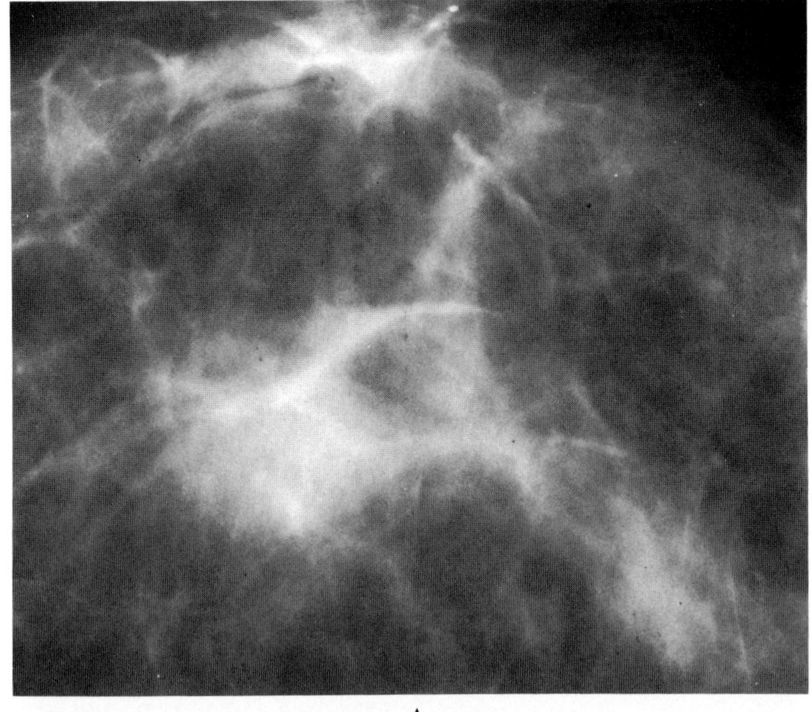

A

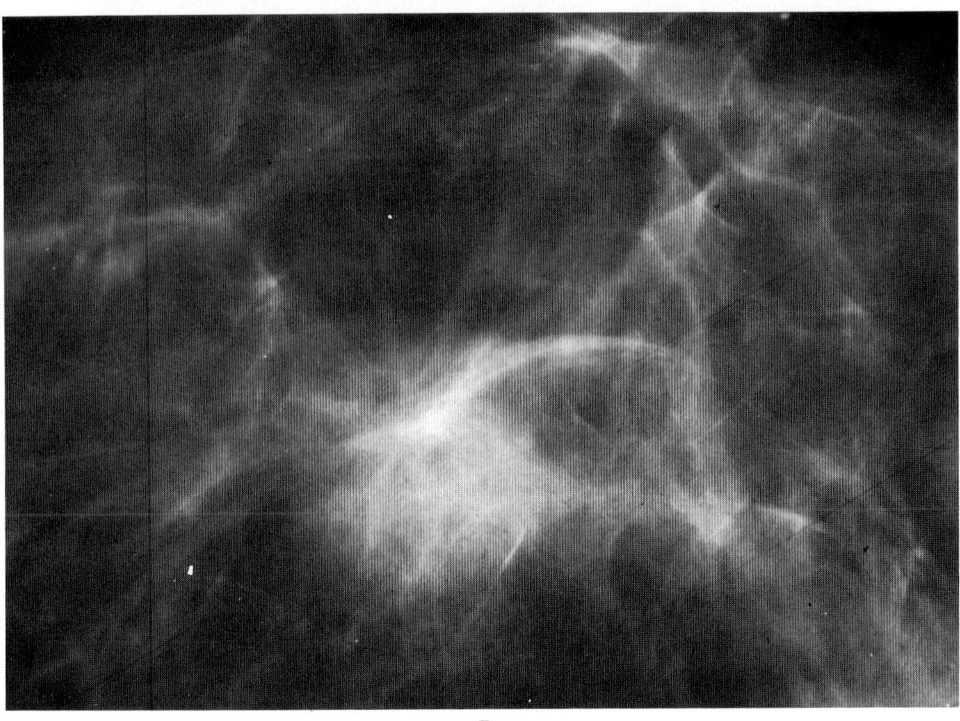

B

Figure 1-10. Magnification and grids in screen-film mammography. A. Screen-film mammogram obtained with molybdenum target. Contrast is excellent, enabling good visualization of border of carcinoma. However, some geometric unsharpness is present because focal spot is 1 mm in diameter. B. Magnification (Elscint microfocus unit) and grid screen-film mammograms, same patient. Because of spectral distribution of tungsten target, there would be less contrast between outline of carcinoma and surrounding fatty tissue. However, grid was utilized to absorb scattered radiation, so that resulting image contains excellent contrast and virtually no geometric unsharpness. Border of the carcinoma is more clearly defined, showing irregularity superiorly. As faster film could be utilized for grid-microfocus unit study, resulting average glandular x-ray dose to patient's breast was the same in both studies.

breast has been imaged. This contention is not only debatable, but the inclusion of the chest wall has in some cases been shown to be detrimental.[2] If the technologist adequately pulls the breast away from the chest wall as the breast is positioned on the dedicated-unit film holder, the breast will usually be completely imaged. The patient's arm should be elevated to 90° but kept as close as possible to the breast. Pulling the arm back or elevating it excessively results in tightening of the skin of the breast, making it difficult for the technologist to adequately pull the breast away from the chest wall and onto the film.

While the latitude of nonscreen film mammograms is not as high as that of xeromammograms, it is nevertheless a relatively high-latitude technique. Many of the problems encountered in converting from nonscreen film (conventional) mammography to screen-film mammography are similar to those encountered with xeromammography. A change from obsolete nonscreen to modern screen-film mammography also requires a change from a conventional tungsten target to a state-of-the-art dedicated mammography unit with molybdenum target and breast compression. The changeover, however, will bear great dividends in the increased number of cancers detected and in the added confidence of the mammographer in the examination.

ADVANCES IN DEDICATED SCREEN-FILM MAMMOGRAPHY EQUIPMENT

The earliest dedicated units had relatively large focal spots and short target-to-film distances, factors favoring geometric unsharpness. This unsharpness was partially offset by application of vigorous compression. The images produced by these units will benefit by conversion to a longer compression cone, such as the one designed by Haus, which lengthens the target-to-film distance to 66 cm, considerably reducing geometric unsharpness.[6] Most commercially available American and European units dedicated to screen-film mammography produced in the last 3 or 4 years have the capacity for focal spot-to-film distances of 50 cm or greater.

A microfocal spot allows considerable versatility when suspicious findings are detected in routine mammograms. Magnification views of these areas provide greater resolution, while background noise remains unchanged (Fig. 1-9 and 1-10).[7–9,16] Magnification mammography requires a focal spot no greater than 300 μ in measured diameter.[13] When investigating a unit for magnification, knowledge of the *actual* measured focal spot, not the nominal size, is essential. (Magnification mammography is discussed in detail in Section 3, Chapter 3.)

An improvement in image quality occurred with the addition of a moving grid to dedicated units. The grid permits dense glandular and dysplastic tissues to be evaluated as effectively as with xeromammography.[10] To avoid an increase in dose, the grid must be used with a fast screen-film combination. For use with older dedicated systems without a built-in grid, an ultrahigh-strip-density, stationary, focused grid that fits inside a standard mammographic cassette is available.[4]

ADVANCES IN SCREEN-FILM COMBINATIONS

In an attempt to further reduce doses, some radiologists have advocated screen-film combinations even faster than those in current use. Newer screen-film systems are continually being evaluated. Eastman Kodak OM-1 film and DuPont MRF-31 film are 50 percent faster than Kodak NMB film and twice as fast as Min-R film; of the two, the Kodak yields the most contrast but, consequently, the most noise.

Actually, the average breast dose obtained with the "soft" x-ray beam utilized for current screen-film mammography has recently been determined to be less than originally proposed. The midplane breast dose is only 5–10 percent of the surface exposure, rather than the 25 percent originally assumed. Therefore, the use of faster screen-film combinations is unjustified when advances in speed take place at the expense of image resolution. The use of faster combinations is feasible only when microfocal spot magnification techniques and/or grids are employed to offset the diminished resolution.

SUMMARY

The development of screen-film mammography has resulted in the re-emergence of confidence, rather than fear, in mammography. When screen-film mammography is performed with state-of-the-art dedicated equipment utilizing vigorous breast compression and a "soft" x-ray beam for improved contrast, screen-film images are equivalent or superior to those of reduced-dose xeromammography and superior to those of nonscreen film mammography. Technological aids for conversion from xeromammographic or nonscreen film mammographic techniques to screen-film techniques have been described. Screen-film mammography should not be attempted until dedicated equipment has been obtained and the importance of vigorous compression has been understood.

REFERENCES

1. Barnes GT, Brezovich IA: Contrast: Effect of scattered radiation. In Logan WW (ed): Breast Carcinoma: The Radiologist's Expanded Role, New York, Wiley, 1977, pp 73–82.
2. Bassett LW, Pagani JJ, Gold RH: Pitfalls in mammography. Radiology 136:641–645, 1980
3. Chang CH, Sibala JL, Martin NL, et al: Film mam-

mography: New low radiation technology. Radiology 121:215–217, 1976

4. Dershaw DD, Masterson ME, Malik S, et al: Mammography using an ultrahigh-strip-density, stationary, focused grid. Radiology 156:541–544, 1985
5. Gros CM: Méthodologie. Symposium sur le sein. J Radiol Electr 48:638–655, 1967
6. Haus AG: The effect of geometric unsharpness in mammography and xeroradiography. In Logan WW: Breast Carcinoma, pp 93–108.
7. Kubo Kanji, MD: Enlargement mammography for early diagnosis of breast cancer. Third International Symposium on Detection and Prevention of Cancer, New York City, April 28, 1976
8. Logan WW: Closing remarks, In Logan WW, Muntz EP (eds): Reduced Dose Mammography. New York, Masson USA, 1979, pp 543–550
9. Logan WW: Overview of the radiologist's role in breast cancer detection. In Logan WW: Breast Carcinoma, pp 344–352
10. Logan WW, Stanton L: Grid versus magnification use in clinical mammography. In Logan WW, Muntz EP (eds): Reduced Dose Mammography. New York, Masson USA, 1979, pp 265–279
11. Lundgren B: The oblique view at mammography. Br J Radiol 50:626–628, 1976
12. Muntz EP: Average, mid-plane entrance and other hybrid doses in mammography. In Logan WW, Muntz EP (eds): Reduced Dose Mammography. New York, Masson USA, 1979, pp 57–60
13. Muntz EP, Logan WW: Focal spot size and scatter suppression in magnification mammography. AJR 133:453–459, 1979
14. Ostrum BJ, Becker W, Isard H: Low-dose mammography. Radiology 109:323–326, 1973
15. Price JL, Butler PD: The reduction of radiation and exposure time in mammography. Br J Radiol 43:251–255, 1970
16. Sickles EA, Doi K, Genant HK: Magnification film mammography: Image quality and clinical studies. Radiology 125:69–76, 1977
17. Skucas J, Logan WW, Gorski J, et al: Improved mammography system, NY State Med J 76:1992–1993, 1976
18. Weiss JP, Wayrynen RE: Imaging system for low-dose mammography. J Appl Photogr Engr 2:7–10, 1976

Stephen A. Feig, M.D.

2

Xeromammography

In xeroradiography, a selenium-coated aluminum plate is the counterpart of the x-ray film. Semiconductors such as selenium normally inhibit the passage of electrons, but become good conductors under the influence of light, heat, electricity, or x-rays. A latent image in the form of a pattern of electrical changes is produced on a uniformly charged selenium plate after exposure to x-rays. Since the process by which this latent image is developed into a visible image does not necessitate the wet chemicals required for photography, it has come to be known as xeroradiography, from the Greek word xeros, meaning "dry."

THE XERORADIOGRAPHIC PROCESS

The xeroradiographic process[34] begins before x-ray exposure, when the plate is charged in the Xerox conditioning unit (Figs. 2-1 and 2-2). The charged plate now contains positive charges within the selenium layer and an equal number of negative charges (electrons) that have been attracted to the aluminum surface adjacent to the selenium layer. A light-tight, electrically insulated cassette is then inserted into the conditioner to receive the charged plate. The cassette with its enclosed charged plate is removed from the conditioner by the technologist and positioned under the breast so that x-rays passing through the breast selectively discharge the plate in inverse proportion to the radiographic density of the overlying tissue, i.e., the discharge is greatest below fatty tissue and least below calcifications. A high-resolution latent image of the breast in the form of a nonuniformly distributed electron charge is thus formed on the selenium-coated plate (Fig. 2-3).

After x-ray exposure, the cassette is inserted into the Xerox processing unit so that the pattern of electrical charges on the plate can be transcribed into a visible image (Fig. 2-2). Within the processor, the plate is automatically extracted from the cassette and sprayed with ionized blue toner particles, which are attracted to the plate according to the regional plate charge. The blue powder cloud is blown into the development chamber with blasts of air (toner "bursts"), which then become charged in the chamber. Since regions on the plate corresponding to denser breast tissues have retained higher proportions of the positive charges, they attract a higher concentration of negatively charged blue toner particles during positive-mode development. Next, a sheet of plastic-coated paper is transported to make contact with the powder-bearing surface of the plate. The paper is then charged electrostatically so that, upon separation from the plate, the toner adheres to the paper. After the paper is heated and cooled, the toner particles are encapsulated into its plastic surface. The xeromammogram is then ready for interpretation.

In the processing unit, any residual toner particles are loosened from the plate by an ion-generating device

BREAST CANCER DETECTION
ISBN 0-8089-1842-7

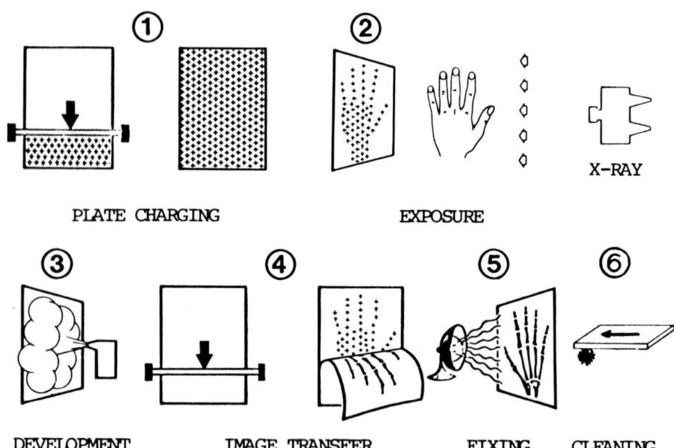

Figure 2-1. Simplified version of xeroradiographic process. From: The Principles of the Xeroradiographic Process. Pasadena, CA, Xerox Corporation, 1975, p 3. With permission.

and removed by a rotating brush. The cleaned plates are then manually transported from the processor back to the conditioner, where they are briefly heated and cooled to remove any remnants of the previous image. This process of "relaxation" prepares the plate for re-use.[3,6,34,37]

126 System

The new Xerox 126 System (Fig. 2-4) allows better efficiency and quality control than does the previous 125 model. By means of lighted digital display messages, the 126 conditioner keeps the technologist aware of its operating status. (*ready, please wait, plate transfer box empty*), plates (number available), and plate charge (*high* for mammography, *low* for thicker body parts). Similarly, the 126 processor alerts the technologist as to its status (*replace box, add paper, warm-up*) and the type of examination (negative- or positive-mode mammography, negative- or positive-mode special for thick body parts, or general for thinner body parts). If its normal operation is interrupted, the system senses eight jam conditions, e.g., jams at the elevator, at the transfer station, at the paper-feeder, etc., which are then indicated on the display panel. Printed instructions and illustrations on the undersurface of the hood direct the operator to the location of the problem and explain how to clear it so as to minimize down-time.

The push-button control panel on the front of the 126 processor allows the technologist to easily increase or decrease the number of toner bursts in order to adjust image density, and to increase or decrease the development (back bias) voltage in order to adjust image contrast. In the positive mode, lowering the back bias voltage will increase contrast and edge enhancement. Increasing the back-bias voltage will decrease contrast and edge enhancement and improve skin line visibility. In the negative mode, back bias is automatically set.

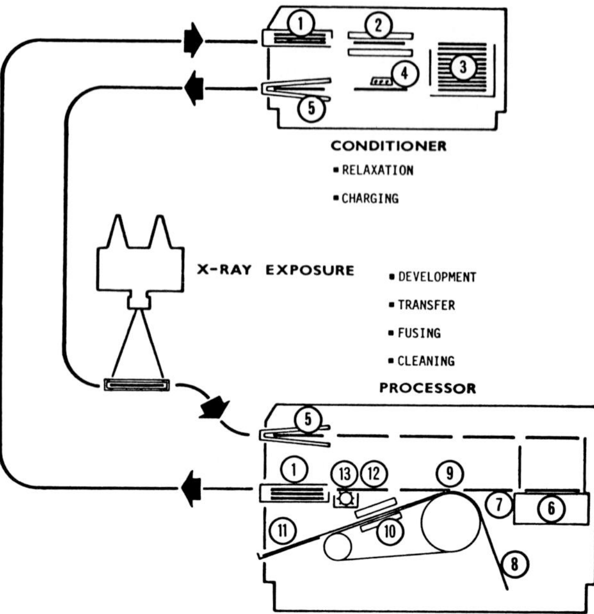

Figure 2-2. Flow diagram of Xerox conditioner and processor. In conditioner: Storage box station (1) receives loaded cassette, plate of which is then removed and heated in relaxation oven (2), where any remaining charges are removed. Plate is stored (3) and recharged (4). Empty cassette is inserted into cassette station (5), where it receives another charged plate. Cassette and enclosed charged plate are ready for x-ray exposure. In processor: Following x-ray exposure, cassette with exposed plate is inserted into cassette station (5), where plate is removed. Plate is then transported to development chamber (6), where it is sprayed with charged toner particles. Pre-transfer ion-charging device (7) loosens particles for transfer to paper arriving from paper feeder (8). Ion-transfer charging device (9) attracts powder to paper. Paths of plate and paper now diverge. Within fusing oven (10), powder image is annealed to paper. Finished xeroradiograph is released via output tray (11). Toner particles remaining on plate are loosened by pre-cleaning ion-generating device (12) and removed by rotating brush (13). Cleaned plates are deposited in processor storage box (1), which, when filled to capacity, is automatically released from processor and manually transfered to storage box in conditioner. From: The Principles of the Xeroradiographic Process. Pasadena, CA, Xerox Corporation, 1975, p 8. With permission.

Positive and Negative Modes

Xeroradiographic images may be developed in either a positive or a negative mode (Fig. 2-5). The photoelectric charges placed on the selenium plate are identical for both modes. The powder cloud produced in the development chamber contains equal numbers of positively

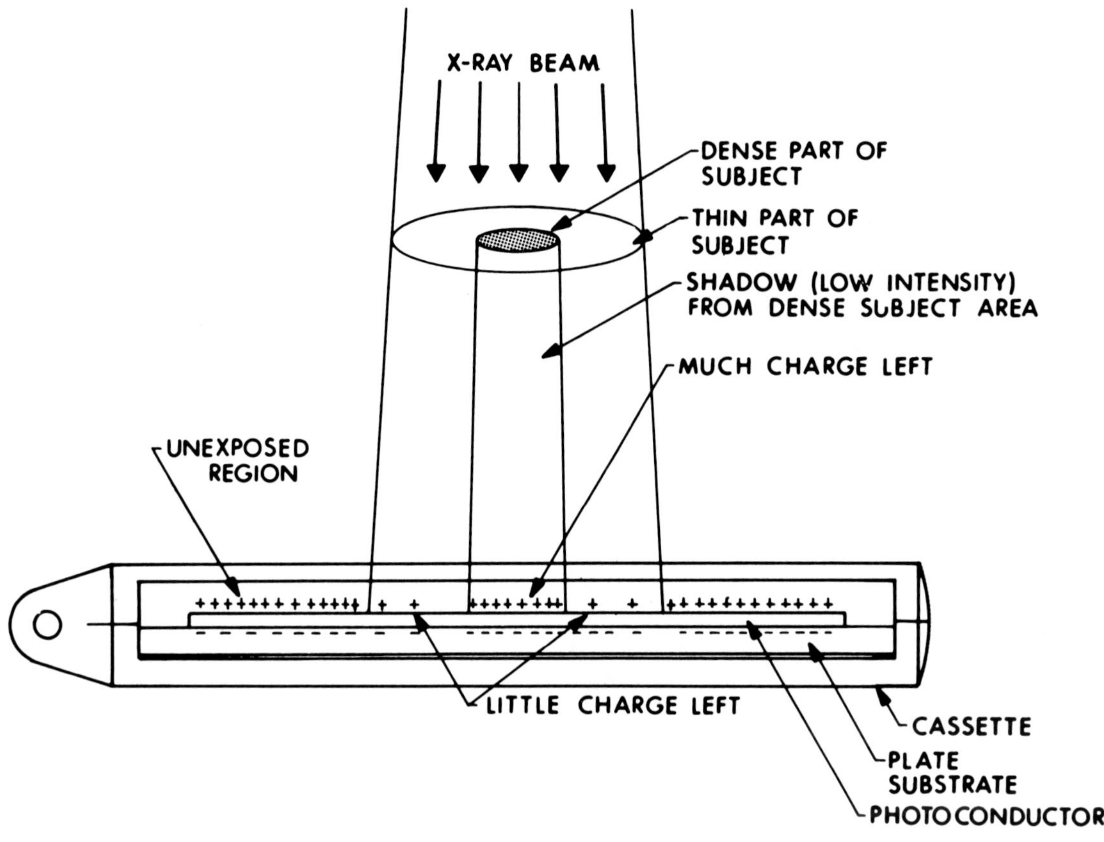

Figure 2-3. Partially discharged xeroradiographic plate, enclosed within cassette, following x-ray exposure. Amount of regional discharge is inversely proportional to density of overlying tissue. From: The Principles of the Xeroradiographic Process. Pasadena, CA, Xerox Corporation, 1975, p 4. With permission.

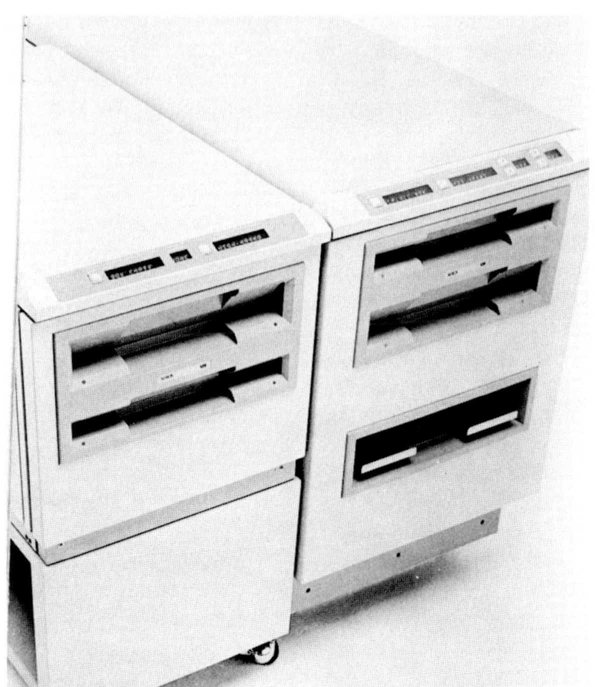

Figure 2-4. Xerox 126 conditioner and processor (courtesy of the Xerox Corporation).

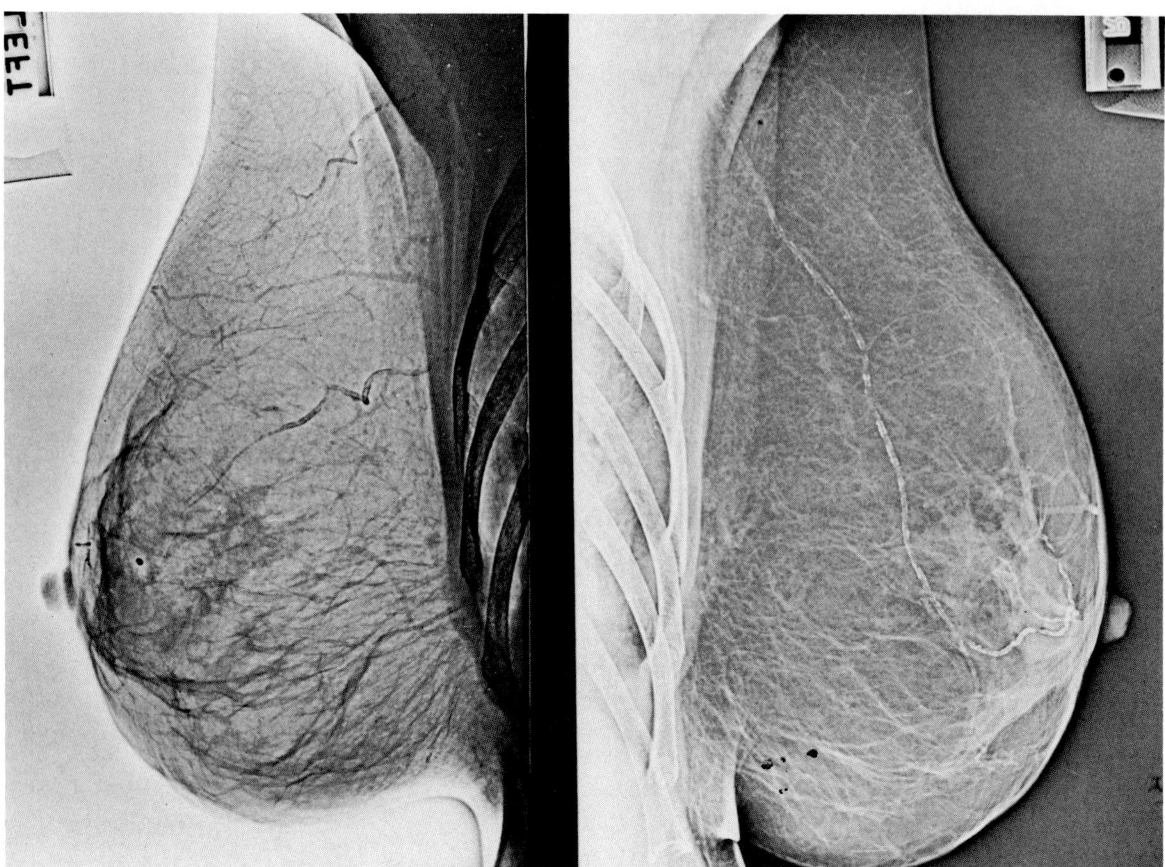

Figure 2-5. Tonal relationships of positive- and negative-mode xeromammograms. Actual xeromammographic images are in varying shades of blue to white, but are presented as degrees of black to white in these illustrations. Densest structures, such as ribs and calcifications, are dark blue (black) in positive mode (A), but white in negative mode (B). Tissues of intermediate radiographic density, such as those in subareolar region, are medium-blue in positive mode and light blue in negative mode. Fatty tissue is light blue in positive mode and medium blue in negative mode. Exposed background is white to light blue in positive mode, but medium to dark blue in negative mode.

and negatively charged toner particles regardless of development mode. In the positive mode, a positive-bias voltage is applied to the back of the plate (back bias), and negatively charged blue toner particles are attracted toward the least-discharged regions on the plate surface. These regions correspond to foci of high radiographic density, such as calcifications. In the negative mode, a negative-bias voltage is applied to the back of the plate, and the positively charged blue toner particles are attracted toward the most heavily discharged regions of the plate surface. In the negative mode, these heavily discharged areas correspond to regions of low radiographic density, such as fatty tissue.[41] A greater amount of toner is required for the negative mode than for the positive mode.

The positive mode is currently the one most preferred by xeromammographers. This choice can be explained by a physiologic principle of vision: it is easier for the human eye to perceive subtle differences between darker hues than between lighter hues. Xeromammograms containing extremely dense objects, such as silicone implants or biopsy localization needles, are better developed in the negative than in the positive mode, because the latter produces a "toner robbing" phenomenon in the tissues adjacent to these objects.

IMAGE CHARACTERISTICS

Xeroradiographic and film images differ in several important aspects. Xeromammograms possess two unique characteristics that affect the visualization of breast pathology: wide recording latitude and edge enhancement.

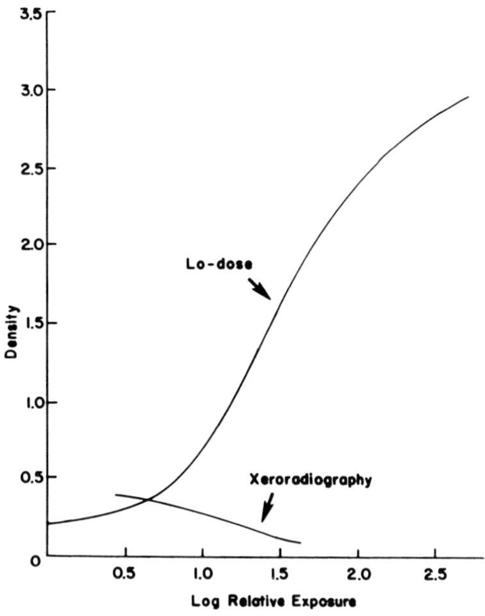

Figure 2-6. Characteristic curves for DuPont Lo-dose I screen-film system and xeroradiography. From Haus AG, Doi K, Metz EE, et al: Image quality in mammography. Radiology 125:83, 1977. With permission.

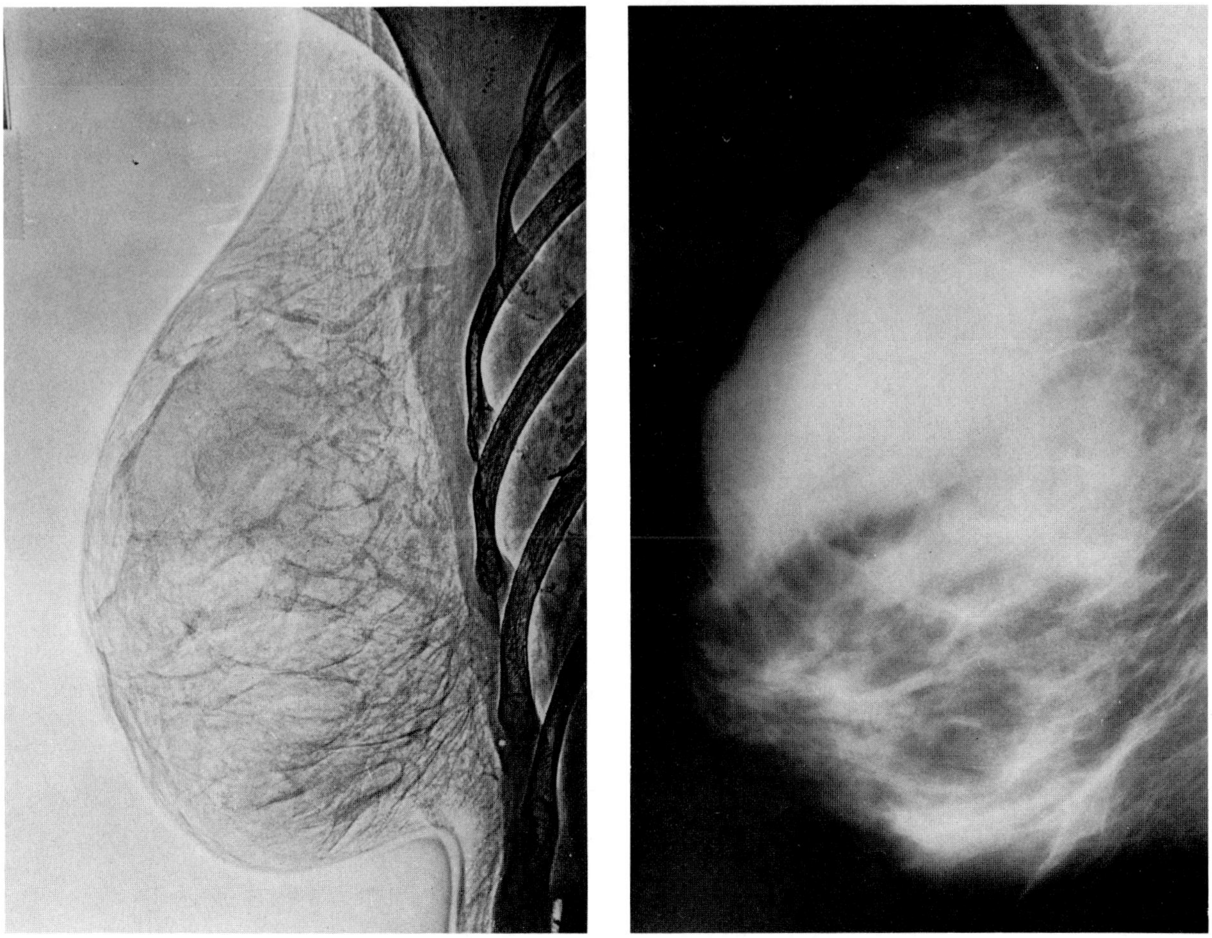

A

B

Figure 2-7. Broad-area contrast is less with xeromammography (A) than with screen-film mammography (B). Hence, overall density differences among soft tissue structures are less apparent on xeromammography.

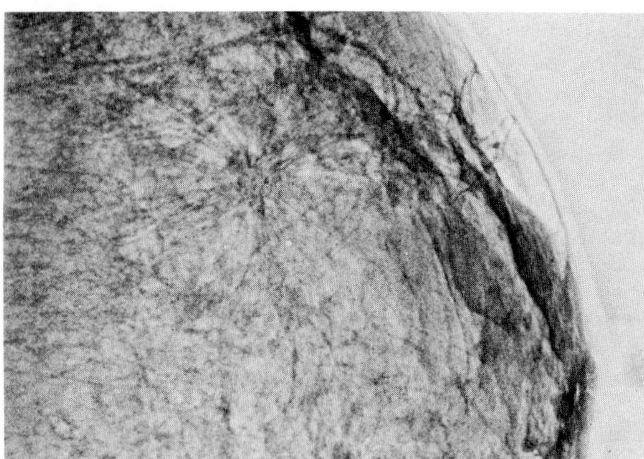

Figure 2-8. Relatively high kV used in xeromammography allows penetration of dense fibroglandular tissue to demonstrate this carcinoma. Edge enhancement aids in visualization of spiculations. However, relatively low broad-area contrast of xeromammography will reduce contrast between mass and surrounding tissue.

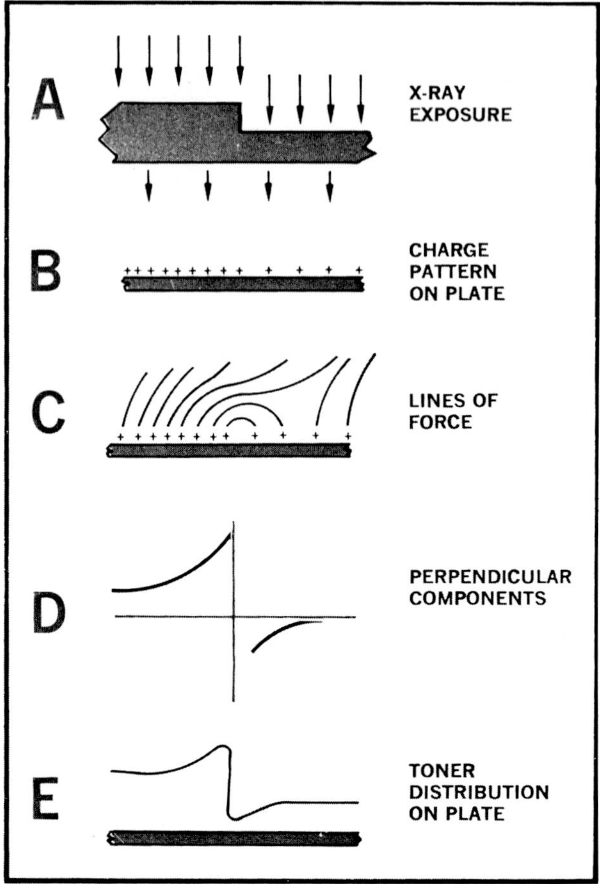

Figure 2-9. Edge enhancement in xeroradiographic development. From Xerox Corporation: Technical Application Bulletin 1: What is Edge Enhancement and How Does it Affect the Mammographic Image? Pasadena, CA, Xerox Corporation, 1974, p 2. With permission.

Wide Recording Latitude

Characteristic curves for xeromammography and screen-film mammography determined at equivalent exposure conditions are shown in Figure 2-6. These curves illustrate that for the same differences in exposure, density gradients for xeromammography are much less than in screen-film systems.[9] Because of this wide recording latitude, a single xeromammographic image yields good contrast and detail throughout a wide range of tissue density and thickness. As a result, both the denser chest wall and the thinner peripheral portions of the breast are clearly visualized.

By comparison, the narrower recording latitude (steeper characteristic curve) of screen-film combinations results in areas of overexposure or underexposure if the breast is not compressed to nearly uniform thickness. The chest wall thus cannot be imaged in screen-film mammograms. With xeromammography, however, a high-quality image of the entire breast from the adjacent rib cage to the nipple can be obtained in a single mediolateral chest wall projection.[40] The disadvantage of such a wide recording latitude is that the overall difference in density between a mass and surrounding tissue (broad area contrast) is less in a xeromammogram than in a screen-film mammogram (Fig. 2-7).

Edge Enhancement

On the other hand, xeroradiographic edge enhancement[35] accentuates the visualization of margins of breast masses, spiculations, and calcific particles (Fig. 2-8). The edge-enhancement phenomenon can be explained by lines of electrical force that result from the interaction of the charges on the xerox plate with those applied in the development chamber. Although the actual charge pattern on the plate is not edge enhanced, the toner particle distribution during development results in edge enhancement in the final image. As a result, an area of uniform greater density adjacent to an area of uniform lesser density will create a higher concentration of toner particles at its side of the border than elsewhere. Likewise, the adjacent area of lesser density will have a reduced concentration of toner particles at its side of the border (Fig. 2-9).

Contour density also affects visual perception. Areas within a dark boundary margin appear darker, whereas areas within a light boundary margin appear lighter. This phenomenon, based on neural mechanisms, is known as the Craik-O'Brien effect.[20]

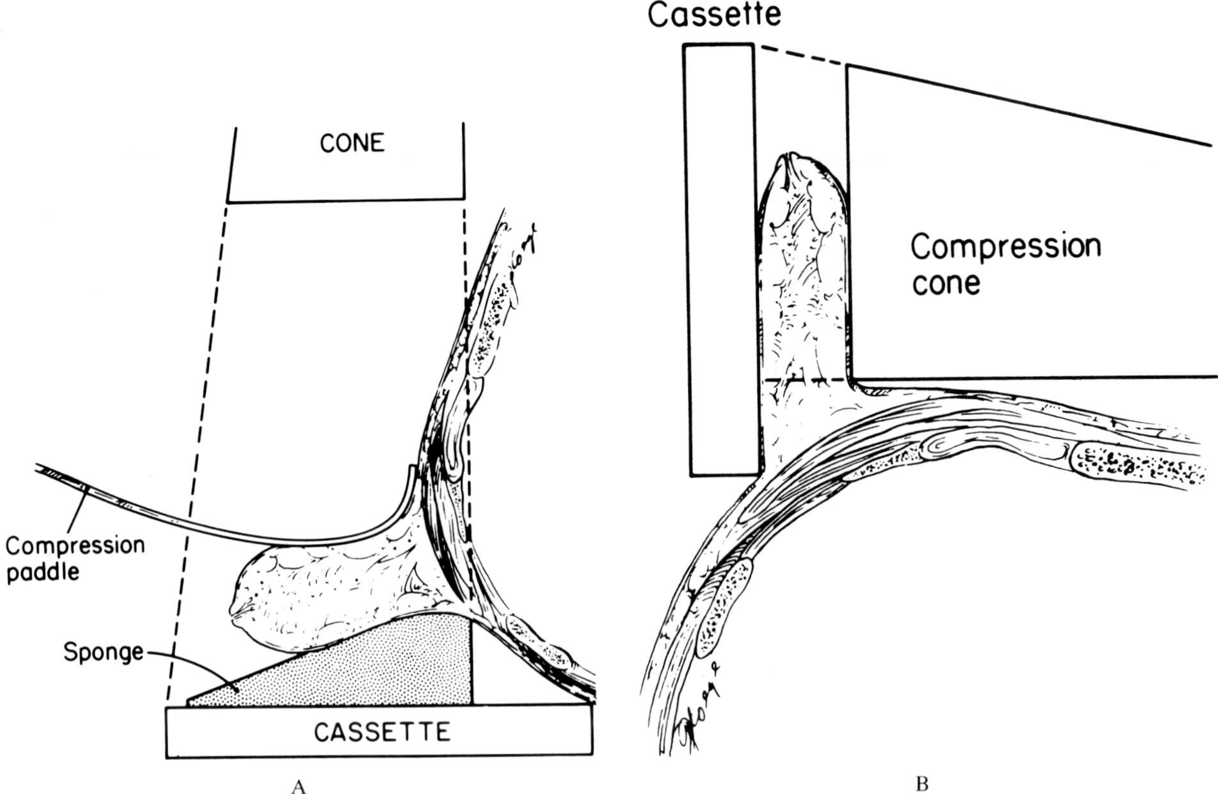

Figure 2-10. Chest wall lateral projection (A) includes more posterior breast tissue than does contact lateral projection (B). The curved compression device and the sponge required for the chest wall lateral view prevent the application of vigorous compression. From Pagani JJ, Bassett LW, Gold RH, et al: Efficacy of combined screen-film/xeromammography: Preliminary report. AJR 135:142, 1980. © Williams and Wilkins Company, 1980. With permission.

RADIOGRAPHIC TECHNIQUE AND EQUIPMENT

Positioning

Two standard projections are used in xeromammography: the cephalocaudal and the chest wall mediolateral. Positioning for the cephalocaudal view is identical to that used for screen-film mammography. The breast is placed on top of the image receptor and compressed, while the x-ray beam passes from the cephalic to the caudal breast surfaces. As in screen-film mammography, exaggerated (rotated) medial or lateral cephalocaudal views can be utilized as supplementary views. The rotated medial cephalocaudal view will visualize more of the medial breast but less of the lateral

Table 2-1
Technical Factors for Xeromammography and Screen-film Mammography

	Xeromammography	Screen-Film
kVp	45–55	26–28 (non-grid) 28–30 (grid)
Filtration	2–3 mm Al	0.03 mm Mo
Target material	Tungsten	Molybdenum

Al = aluminum; Mo = molybdenum

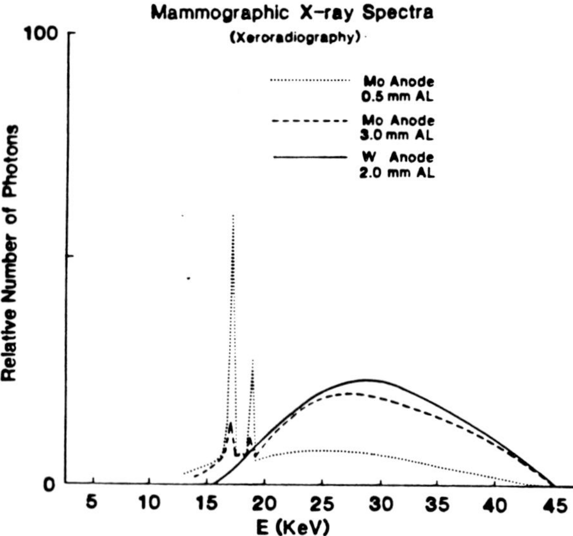

Figure 2-11 X-ray spectra produced at 45 kVp. Tungsten (W) target with 2.0 mm aluminum (AL) filtration results in lowest dose. Molybdenum (Mo) target with 3.0 mm aluminum filtration has only minimally greater contrast, but higher dose due to characteristic radiation spikes at 15–20 keV. These spikes are more pronounced and the dose considerably higher with Mo target and 0.5 mm filtration. From Haus AG: Physical principles and radiation dose in mammography. In Feig SA, McLelland R (eds): Breast Carcinoma: Current Diagnosis and Treatment. New York, Masson USA, 1983, p 103. With permission.

breast than will the routine cephalocaudal view. Similarly, the rotated lateral cephalocaudal view will visualize more of the lateral breast but less of the medial breast than will the standard cephalocaudal projection.

The mediolateral chest wall view includes the chest wall structures immediately posterior to the breast. For this view, the cassette must be separated from the lateral breast surface so as to partially underlie the adjacent rib cage. A radiolucent sponge is therefore interposed between the lateral breast surface and the cassette in order to support the breast and prevent skin folds (Fig. 2-10).

The chest wall lateral view should not be used in screen-film mammography. Since the chest wall is curved and rigid, inclusion of the rib cage in the image can only be accomplished by decreasing the extent of breast compression. In this situation, the thick posterior tissues cannot be sufficiently compressed to allow adequate imaging with the lower kVp technique required for screen-film mammography. On the other hand, the entire breast and chest wall can be visualized in a single mediolateral xeromammogram because:

1. The higher kVp technique of xeromammography requires only moderate compression to obtain adequate penetration of denser structures.
2. The wider recording latitude of xeromammography requires the breast to be compressed to a lesser and nonhomogeneous extent.
3. The higher resolution that results from edge enhancement compensates for the geometric unsharpness that occurs as the image receptor is displaced from the breast by a sponge.

Supplementary views include the contact mediolateral, the lateromedial, and the oblique lateral. For the contact mediolateral, the cassette is placed in direct contact with the breast surface, without an intervening sponge. The contact projection provides less magnification and therefore greater resolution than the noncontact projection with an intervening sponge, but does not include the chest wall.[17] The lateromedial view provides better resolution of medially situated lesions.

Positioning for the oblique lateral projection is similar to that used in screen-film mammography, i.e., the x-ray beam is directed at 45° from superomedial to inferolateral. Since the breast is pulled forward off the chest wall, more of the posterior breast will be visualized than with the contact lateral view. Due to the "dead space" in the xerox cassette, however, approximately 0.7 cm less posterior breast tissue will be seen than with the oblique lateral screen-film view. ("Dead space" in the cassette for the Xerox 175 system, to be available in 1987, will be reduced to only 0.1–0.2 cm.) Because the breast is closer to the image receptor, the oblique lateral projection will provide better resolution than does the chest wall lateral view. Detailed descriptions of xeromammography positioning are available.[31,32]

Compression

As with screen-film mammography, compression is used to reduce overlapping of internal breast structures, increase contrast by reducing scattered radiation, decrease geometric unsharpness, provide uniform tissue thickness, and permit a lower dose. Because of the wider recording latitude and higher kVp of xeromammography, it requires less compression than does screen-film mammography to insure adequate image quality. As with screen-film mammography, however, greater compression will allow a lower dose.[14]

The chest wall lateral projection requires a compression device that is curved to match the contour of the chest wall. It is difficult or impossible to take this projection with a straight compression device. When used for the cephalocaudal projection in xeromammography, curved compression devices will produce moderate rather than vigorous compression and will be more comfortable for the patient. However, utilization of a straight compression device for this projection will enable stronger, more uniform compression with a consequent reduction in dose.

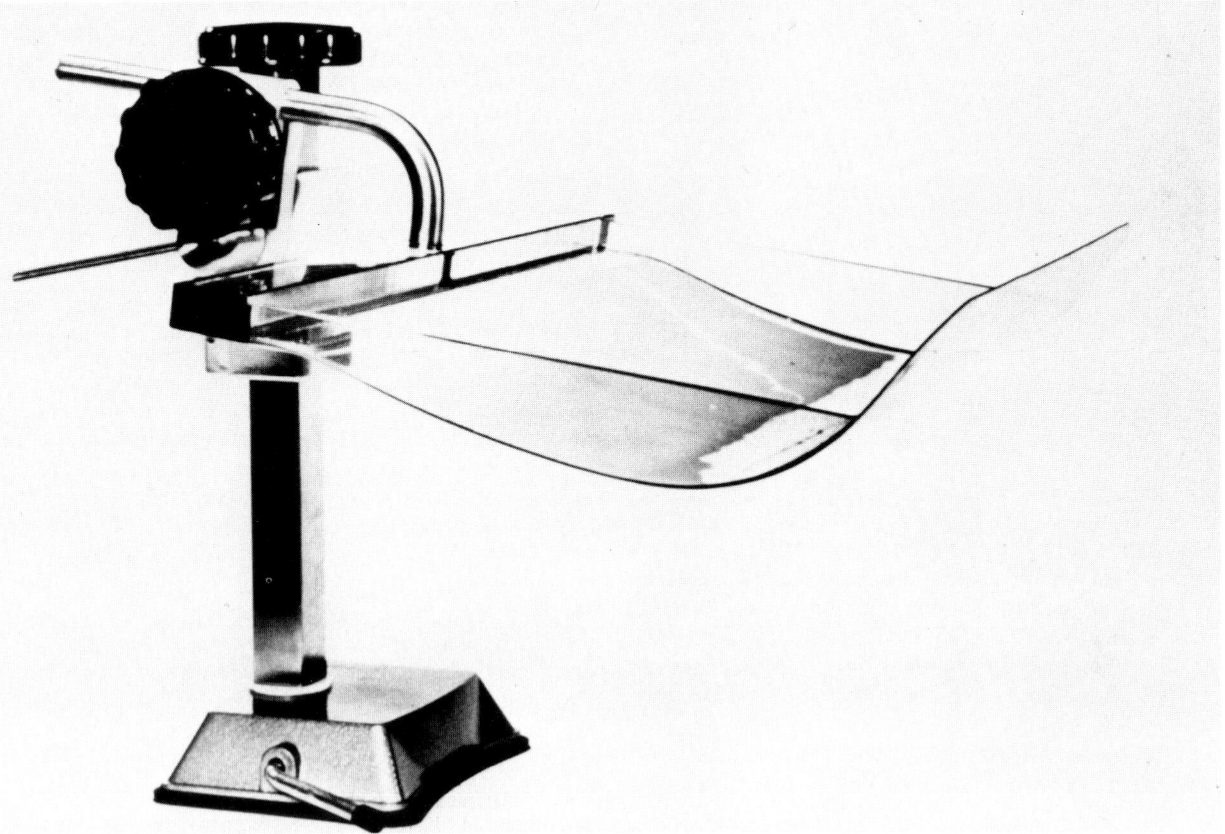

Figure 2-12. The XR mammographic positioner. Its curved shape, designed for the chest wall lateral projection, can also be used for the cephalocaudal xeromammogram. Vacuum base and release lever allow the device to be mounted on and easily detached from table used with a general-purpose radiographic unit. (Courtesy, Xerox Corporation.)

Technique

The differing technical requirements for xeromammography and screen-film mammography are listed in Table 2-1. In order to maintain xeromammography dosage at acceptable limits, higher kVp and greater beam filtration are required than for screen-film mammography. Because of edge enhancement, the higher kVp does not result in an appreciable sacrifice of image quality. In fact, in dense or large breasts, the "harder" beam will yield better penetration.

Mammography Units

While a molybdenum target can produce high-quality xeromammograms, its use for xeromammography should be discouraged because of unacceptably high dose levels. In contrast, at the higher peak kilovoltage and greater filtration levels needed for reduced-dose xeromammography, the "harder" radiation from a tungsten target contributes more to image production and less to dosage (Fig. 2-11).[7,10,15]

Although general-purpose tungsten target x-ray equipment can be used for xeromammography, specialized mammography units with tungsten targets produce higher quality xeromammograms since more vigorous compression can be applied and the geometric factors responsible for high resolution (the smaller focal spot size and/or longer target-film distance) are more favorable.

If a general-purpose unit is used, aluminum filtration must be added to harden the x-ray beam. A compression device may be directly attached to the tube housing, as with a balloon compression device, or may be independent of the tube, usually attached to the x-ray table by a suction apparatus (Fig. 2-12). The cephalocaudal view is obtained with the patient sitting or standing. Since the lateral view must be obtained with the patient lying on her side, examination time will be longer than with a dedicated unit.

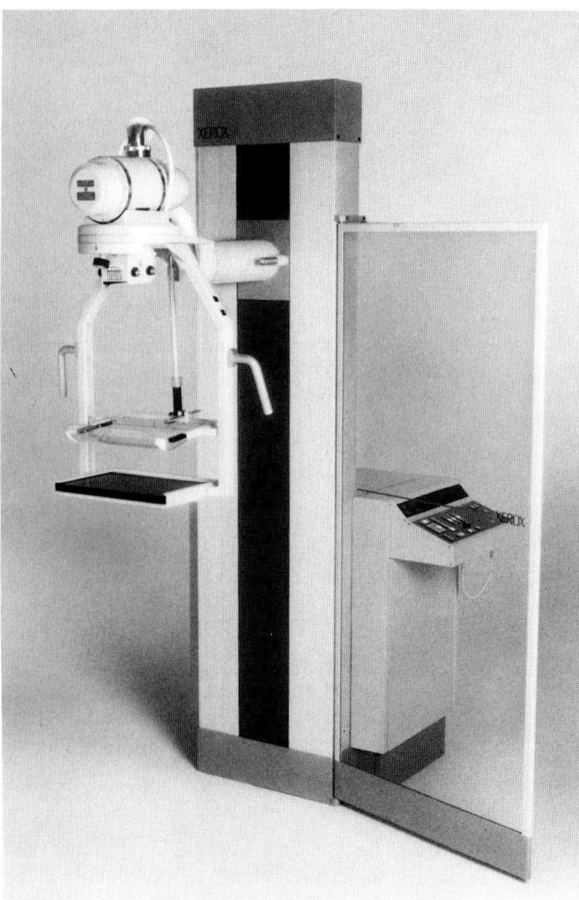

Figure 2-13. The Xerox 120 System, a dedicated mammography unit designed specifically for xeromammography. (Courtesy, Xerox Corporation.)

Although many dedicated mammography units include a tungsten target tube as optional equipment, a system manufactured by Xerox includes features which are optimized for xeromammography, such as a compression and positioning system specifically designed for the chest wall lateral projection (Fig. 2-13).

IMAGE QUALITY

Positioning Technique

Proper positioning is essential. Suboptimal positioning may eventually lead to a cancer being missed. For the cephalocaudal view, the height of the object upon which the breast rests (cassette or table top) should be at the level of the inframammary crease. Thus, the breast will be horizontal rather than dependent. Portions of the breast may be excluded from the image if the breast is higher or lower than this position. The patient should turn her head in the direction opposite the side being radiographed. Skin folds and wrinkles should be eliminated by readjusting the table height and retracting the breast away from the chest wall. The opposite arm should rest on the table and should press the cassette tightly against the chest wall. As compression is applied, the patient should lean forward slightly. The technologist should again pull the breast forward so that the posterior part does not slip out from under the compression device.

The chest wall lateral projection should include the breast, the axilla, and enough of the chest wall to include the retromammary tissues. The nipple should be in profile. The lower edge of the cassette should be located one inch below the inframammary crease. When this projection is taken with the patient supine, the wedge-shaped sponge should be placed with the thick end towards the rib cage. When this view is taken with the patient erect, the thin edge of the sponge should be closest to the rib cage. The breast should be pulled forward and up so that it does not sag. The technologist's hand should be used to smooth out all wrinkles and skin folds between the breast and the sponge as compression is being applied. It is especially important that the technician's hand be placed between the breast and the sponge from behind the patient, and that the technician gently pull the patient's skin back in order to eliminate a long, thick fold that can form parallel to the chest wall.[29,32]

Exposure Characteristics

In xeromammography, the determination of whether an image has been properly exposed can be difficult, especially if previous images of the same breast at different exposure factors are not available for comparison. In most cases, the white halo surrounding the blue skin line in the positive-mode image is an adequate indicator of proper exposure. In the correctly exposed image, the halo will usually have the same width as the skin line: 1–2 mm. Since it is relatively easy to evaluate the width of the skin halo, it has been widely applied as an index of proper exposure. Parenchymal density and overall contrast, though harder to assess, are more direct indices. Indeed, some images with halos too narrow or too wide provide better parenchymal detail than do those with optimal halos.[19] Although the skin-line halo is not present in negative-mode images, the other criteria for judging proper exposure in negative and positive modes are based on similar principles.

Overexposure will "burn out" breast tissues, especially the thinner and less-dense skin and subcutaneous tissues. The overall image will be flat; contrast will be low. In the positive mode, the image will be faint i.e., less blue, and the white halo surrounding the skin will be thinner than is the skin line, usually 1 mm or less (Fig.

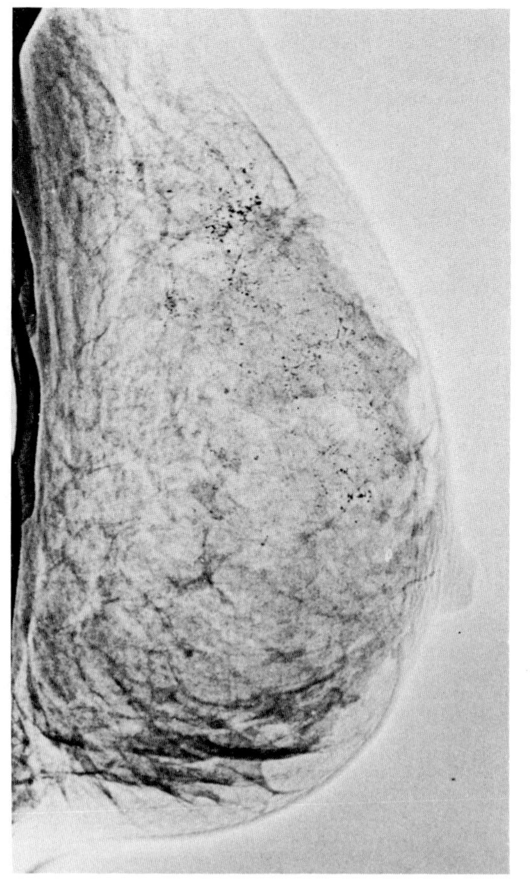

A

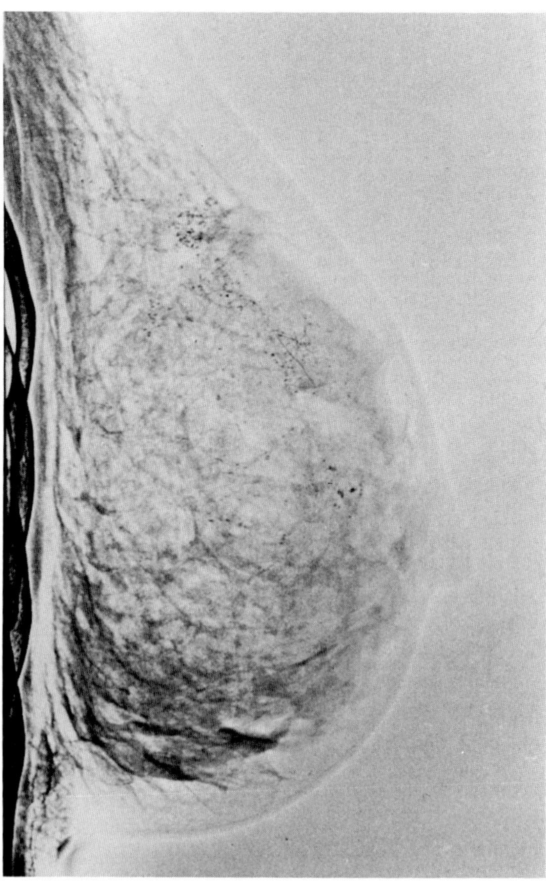

B

Figure 2-14. Evaluating positive-mode image quality. A. Properly exposed xeromammogram. White halo peripheral to skin is approximately the same width as skin itself. Contrast and detail are optimal throughout breast. B. Overexposed image of the same breast. White halo is much narrower than skin line. Overpenetration has resulted in washout of detail of thinner subcutaneous tissues.

2-14). In the negative mode, the image will be too blue (Fig. 2-15).

Conversely, underexposure results in obscuration of abnormalities in the inadequately penetrated denser and thicker areas such as those near the chest wall. In the positive mode, image density will be increased, i.e., too blue. The white halo surrounding the skin will be considerably wider than the skin and may in turn be bounded by a thin, blue, pseudo-skin line. The skin pores may be prominent. Underexposure of a dense breast causes deletion of the skin and subcutaneous tissues because of "toner robbing": imaging the dense parenchymal tissue requires so much toner that there is an insufficient quantity to image the thinner and more fatty structures[30,32,42] (Fig. 2-16). The underexposed negative mode image will be too white and will show excessive contrast, especially in the thin areas of the breast. The skin will appear too white, rather than blue as in the properly exposed negative-mode image. With moderate underexposure, a white line occurs under the skin, resembling a reverse halo (Fig. 2-17).

Artifact Sources

Artifacts interfere with the xeroradiographic image by masking information. When artifacts are present, it is important to identify them, repeat the image if necessary, and promptly initiate corrective action to prevent their recurrence. Numerous illustrations of common and uncommon artifacts are available in the literature.[4,33]

Powder deficiency spots (PDSs) are common artifacts representing areas on the selenium plate where the charge is lost because the selenium has become conductive. Since these areas lack toner deposition, they appear white (PDSs) in the positive mode and blue

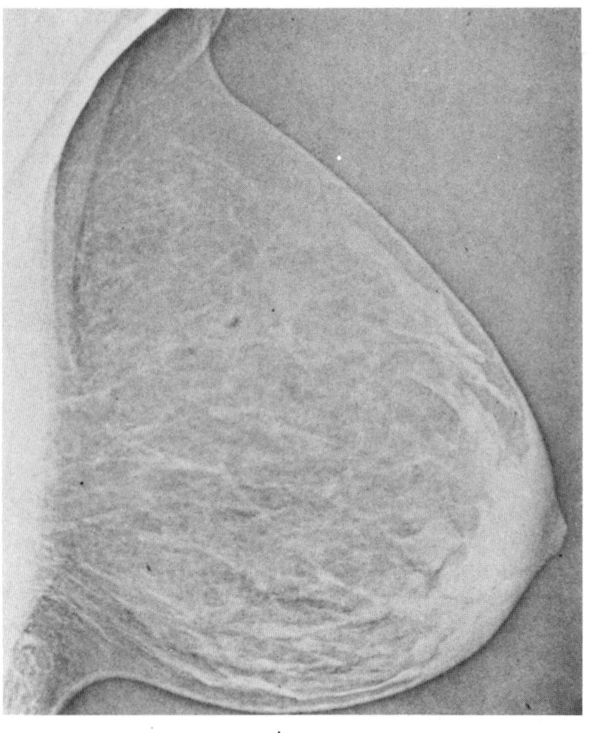

A

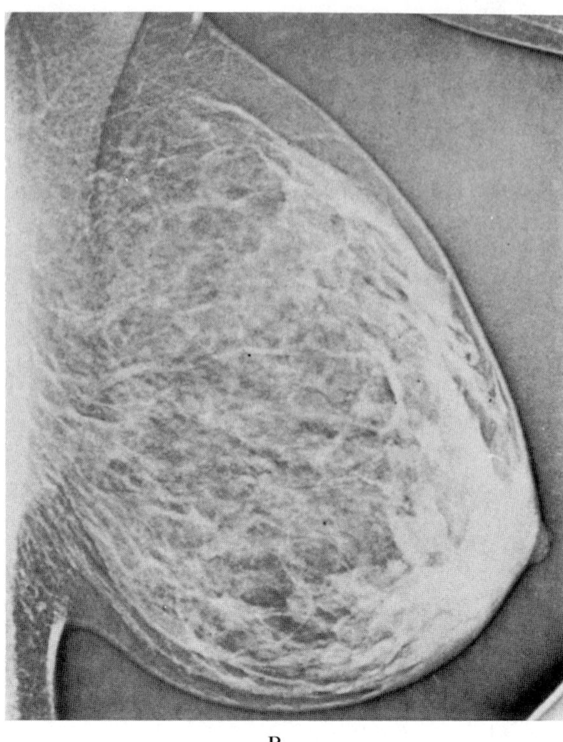

B

Figure 2-15. Evaluating negative-mode image quality. A. Overexposed xeromammogram. Image is too dark and lacks adequate contrast, especially in subcutaneous tissues. B. Properly exposed image of the same breast.

(*PESs or powder excess spots*) in the negative mode. Although PDSs do not mimic microcalcifications (which are blue in the positive mode and white in the negative mode), they may mask them. PDSs may appear as spots ("*Snow*" connotes a large number of PDSs) or lines (Fig. 2-18).

Although a few PDSs may occasionally be seen on a new selenium plate, they generally do not appear in significant numbers until the plate has been used several hundred times.[4] PDSs are the main determinants of plate life. Worn-out plates must be discarded and replaced, since they cannot be repaired.

By means of "dark dusting," PDSs as well as many other artifacts can be readily detected before they interfere with image interpretation. "Dark dusting" means developing a charged plate without exposing it. This quality-assurance test should be performed on all plates periodically, e.g., at weekly intervals. A specific plate can be identified from its serial number, which will appear on the corner of the image.

White lines on an image may also result from scratches on the plate or the paper. A paper scratch can be felt with the tip of the thumbnail as a slight depression in the paper. *Dark lines* on an image are usually due to brush marks that occur when the rotating brush has worn out and is not completely cleaning the selenium plates.

Spots of excess powder, or image "*spatter*," occur when the toner receptacle in the processor is too full or too empty, or when the development chamber requires cleaning. Depletion of toner may also lead to decreased image density of both the breast and background.

Reticulation is a granular appearance of the image due to selenium crystallization on the plate surface (Fig. 2-19). If an image shows a reticulated appearance, the defective plate should be replaced.

Another artifact, "image smear," is characterized by a ground-glass appearance just behind the skin line. This problem can usually be eliminated by cleaning the cassette charging pins.

DOSE REDUCTION

Any discussion of dosage should include a definition of terms.[15,25,26] Skin dose should not be used as a primary index of risk, since virtually no breast cancers arise in the skin or subcutaneous tissues. Skin dose must, however, be used to calculate the mean glandular dose, a more meaningful parameter for estimation of carcinogenic risk, since it represents the average dose to the

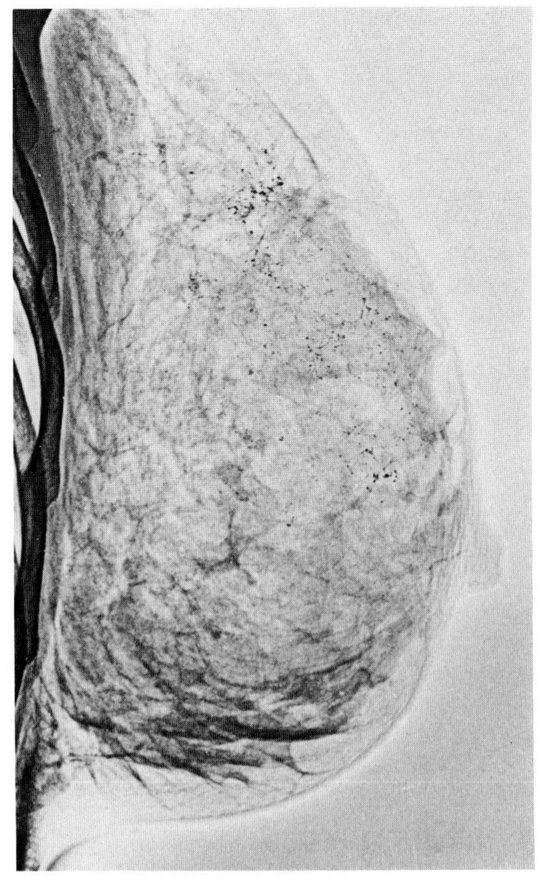

A

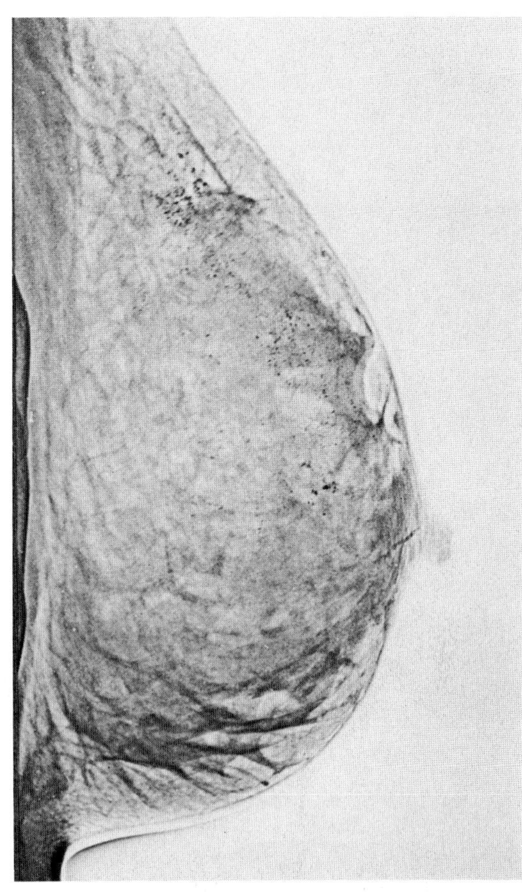

B

Figure 2-16. Evaluating positive-mode image quality. A. Properly exposed xeromammogram. B. Underexposed image of the same breast. White halo peripheral to skin is wider than skin, and dark blue (black in figure) pseudo-skin ring is present. There is inadequate penetration of thicker tissues, particularly near chest wall.

entire breast except the skin and subcutaneous tissue. Mid-breast dose is the dose received at a point in the exact center of the breast. Since it represents the dose to a less representative volume, it is not as reliable an index of risk as is mean glandular dose.

Beam Hardening

The development of low-dose screen-film mammography, as well as concern regarding radiation risk, led to the introduction of reduced-dose xeromammography in 1976. Entrance exposures were reduced from those arising from previous xeromammography methods by means of increasing the aluminum filtration of the x-ray beam, thereby causing a preferential reduction in lower-energy radiation. The "softer" radiation previously used had contributed more to absorbed dose than to image detail. To compensate for the added filtration, the kVp was raised from 35–45 kVp to 45–55 kVp. (If milliamperes rather than kVp had been increased, lengthened exposure times could have created motion problems.) Unlike screen-film mammography, xeromammography can be performed at higher kVp ranges, because the edge enhancement effect partially offsets the decreased image contrast. In fact, in large or dense breasts, the "hardened" beam results in improved penetration.[18] The decreased image contrast resulting from the increased kVp is partially restored by lowering the back-bias voltage setting of the Xerox processor.

In xeromammography, the reduction in skin dosage is primarily a function of increasing the thickness of added aluminum filtration of the x-ray beam. Aluminum filtration thicker than 2.5 mm should not be used, however, as it produces a "flat," low-contrast image of suboptimal diagnostic quality, with negligible additional dose reduction.[13,28,39] Dose reduction results from "hardening" of the x-ray beam (higher kV) so that the falloff in absorbed dose with increasing tissue depth (depth-dose curve) becomes less steep than with a "softer" (lower kV) beam. The reduction in absorbed dose is proportionately less than the reduction in skin

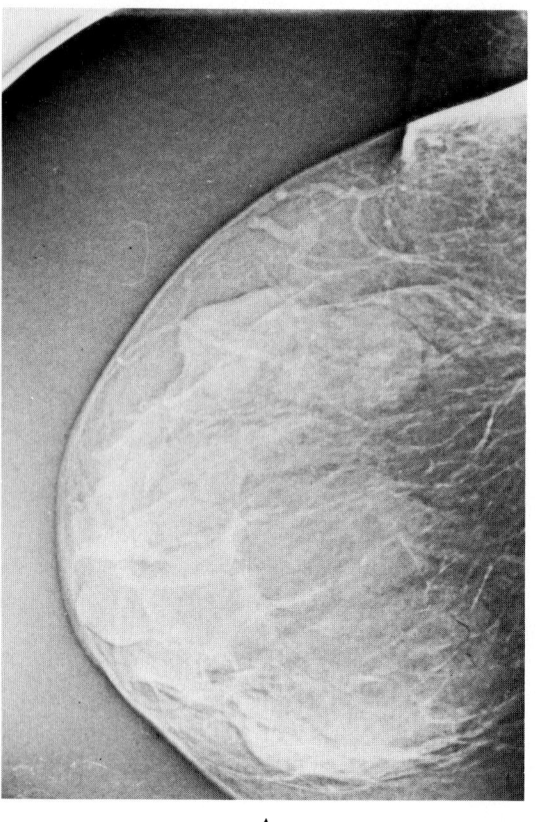

A

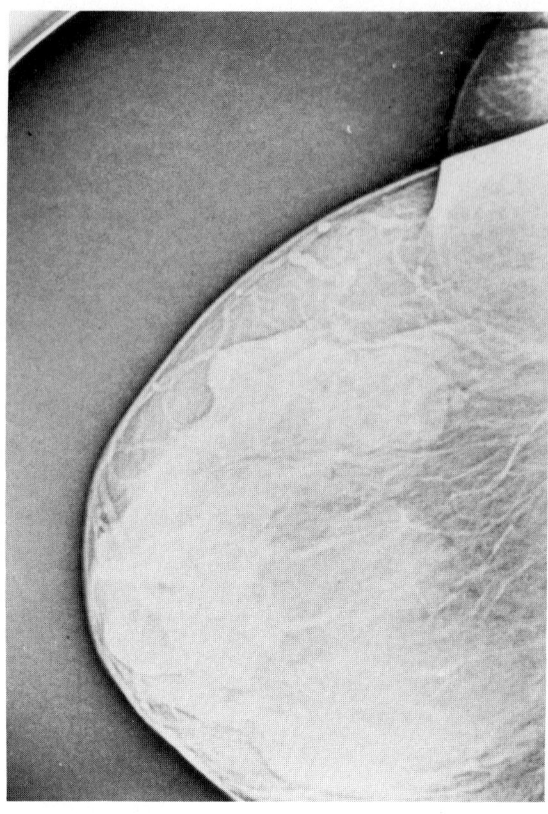

B

Figure 2-17. Evaluating negative-mode image quality. A. Properly exposed image. B. Underexposed image is too white and shows excessive contrast.

dose[13] (Fig. 2-20). Doses from xeromammography imaging systems are shown in Table 2-2.

Negative Mode

Employment of negative-mode development[8,18,28,41] may allow a 20–25 percent dose reduction from that of the conventional positive mode. To change from a positive- to a negative-mode technique, the mAS is reduced by one-third with a 1–2 kVp increase. The negative back bias should be set approximately 1300 V higher than the corresponding positive-mode back bias.

175 System

Further dose reduction has been made possible through the Xerox 175 system (Figs. 2-21 and 2-22), which was announced in late 1985 and which should be commercially available in mid 1987. The system is based on a photoreceptor plate that enables an increase in x-ray absorption due to increased thickness of the selenium alloy photoreceptor as well as more efficient conversion of absorbed x-rays to electrical charge signals due to changes in the manufacturing process.

Although the new photoreceptor plate requires decreased dosage, it would have resulted in nonuniform image density due to the higher voltage operation, decreased resolution, and increased image graininess. To counteract these problems, a new liquid toner system was also developed (Figs. 2-23 and 2-24) that possesses the following advantages compared with the previous powder-cloud toner:

1. higher resolution and less image noise due to generally smaller-size toner particles, fewer charges per particle, and decreased turbulence of the liquid toner fountain compared with the powder cloud chamber
2. lower dose, increased contrast, and ability to operate at lower charging potentials due to high optical density/charge density.

Overall, the combination of the new photoreceptor and liquid toner in the 175 system results in a 50 percent reduction in absorbed dose compared with the 126 system. Resolution, edge-enhancement, and broad area contrast are equivalent or better. Image noise is similar or decreased[11] (Fig. 2-25).

A recent study by Speiser, et al.[24] indicates that the

mean glandular dose for a 2-view study of a 5-cm-thick breast is 0.26 rad. The mean glandular dose for a 2-view study of a 4-cm-thick breast (more vigorous compression used in screen-film mammography) with Min R screen-Ortho M Film combination would be 0.23 rad with a grid and 0.10 rad for a non-grid study. Thus, the mean glandular dose for the Xerox 175 liquid toner system would be similar to that from the Kodak Min R-Ortho M System used with a grid and 2.5 times that of the same system used without a grid,[24] and would be 2.5 times that of a new double-screen/double-emulsion film system (Kodak Min-R fast screens/Kodak T-Mat M Film) used with a grid (0.09 rad).[8]

DETECTION SENSITIVITY

Although experiments with breast phantoms and tissue specimens suggest that xeromammography can detect smaller calcifications and spiculations than can screen-film mammography,[16,23,26,27,36,38] this advantage may not be retained in patient studies that involve factors such as high kVp, high filtration (more than 1.0 mm aluminum), negative-mode development, and increased distance of the object from the image receptor due to use of a sponge and/or moderate instead of vigorous compression. Results from a recent in vitro study suggest that when these factors are taken into account, detection of microcalcifications by radiography and screen-film mammography are practically equivalent.[21]

Early clinical experience indicated that microcalcifications and spiculations in dense breasts were more easily demonstrated by xeromammography than by screen-film mammography, due to higher kVp and edge enhancement.[5,18] Subsequently, the use of grids in screen-film mammography improved its performance in such breasts.[22] However, no comparative study of

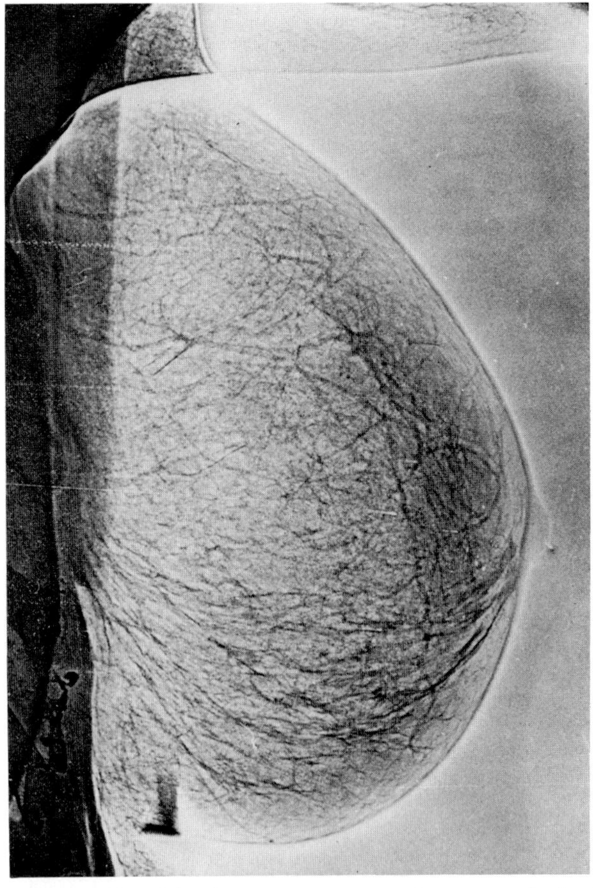

Figure 2-18. The image was properly exposed, but plate defects caused powder deficient spots (PDSs) seen here as horizontal white lines across the upper half of the breast. Improper positioning resulted in skin fold which partially obscures the upper posterior breast near the rib cage.

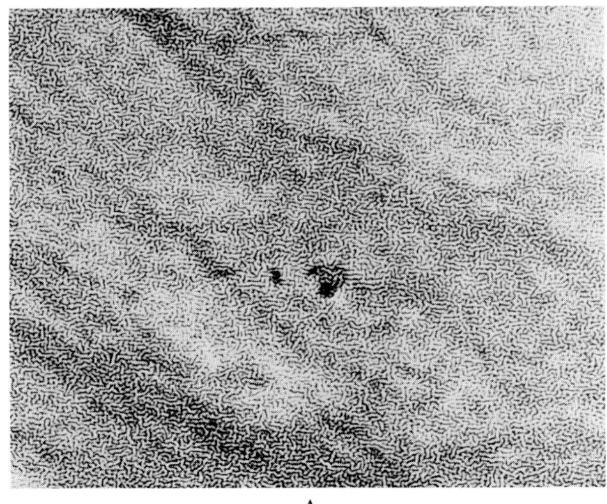

A

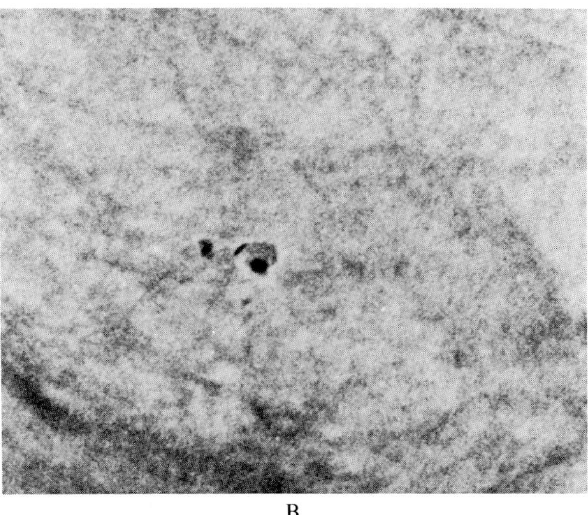

B

Figure 2-19. A. Reticulation defect in selenium plate obscures image detail. B. Xeroradiograph of same breast taken with good plate provides better image of calcifications and breast markings.

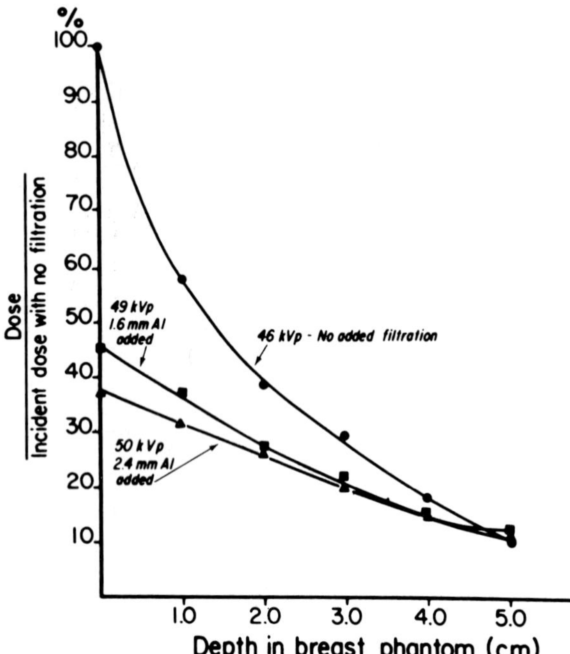

Figure 2-20. Relationship of incident skin dose and depth dose to kVp and filtration in a tungsten target glass window tube. Increase in kVp and filtration will reduce skin dose and mean glandular dose while same dose of radiation will reach image receptor. From Milbrath JR: Reduced-dose xeromammography. In Logan WW, (ed): Breast Carcinoma. The Radiologist's Expanded Role. New York, John Wiley, 1977, p 144. With permission.

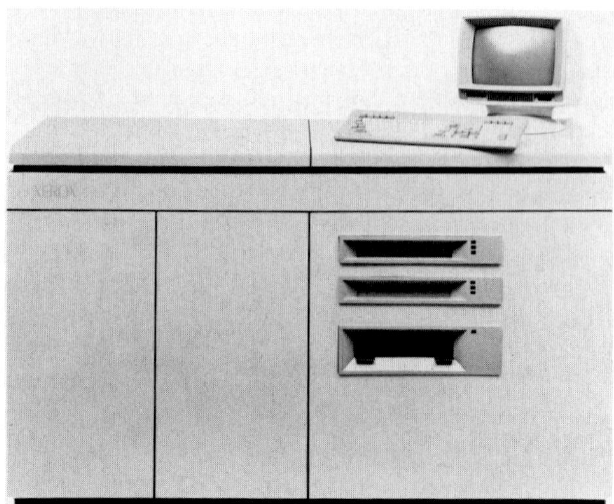

Figure 2-21. Xerox 175 system. The conditioner and processor are combined. (Courtesy, Xerox Corporation.)

xeromammography and grid-assisted screen-film mammography in dense breasts has yet been reported.

Secondary signs of cancer such as skin thickening and skin and nipple retraction may be more readily appreciated on xeromammography than on screen-film mammography due to the wide recording latitude of xeromammography. By the same token, poorly defined, low-density breast masses are less easily seen on xeromammography than on the higher-contrast screen-film studies.

Unlike screen-film mammography, xeromammography is able to image the entire breast from nipple to chest wall on a single mediolateral radiograph. It is not, however, clear whether more posterior breast tissue is visualized on a chest wall lateral xeromammogram than on a properly positoned oblique-lateral screen-film mammogram.[12] A study by Bassett, et al.[2,17] indicated that some posteriorly located cancers detected in chest wall lateral xeromammograms could be projected off the edge of a mediolateral screen-film image. In the same study, some posterior breast cancers that were readily identified on mediolateral screen-film studies were not seen on chest wall lateral xeromammograms, due to obscuration by the overlying rib cage and/or dense juxtathoracic tissues. Although the oblique lateral screen-film projection results in visualization of tumors located more posteriorly than those visualized by the standard mediolateral screen film projection,[1] no studies comparing the oblique lateral screen-film projection with the chest wall lateral xeromammogram have been reported.

Table 2-2
Dose Reduction in Xeromammography

Year Introduced	Technique	Skin Dose (R per exposure)	Mean Glandular Dose (rads per 2-view exam)
1971	Xeromammography	3	1.6
1976	Reduced-dose xeromammography		
	positive mode	0.75	0.64
	negative mode	0.60	0.51
1987	175 system	0.30	0.26

Data from Haus;[7] Muntz, Wilkinson, George;[14] National Council on Radiation Protection and Measurements;[15] Speiser, Zanrosso, Jeromin, et al;[24] Stanton, Villafana, Day, et al;[25] Van De Riet, Wolfe;[28] Xerox Corporation.[39,41]

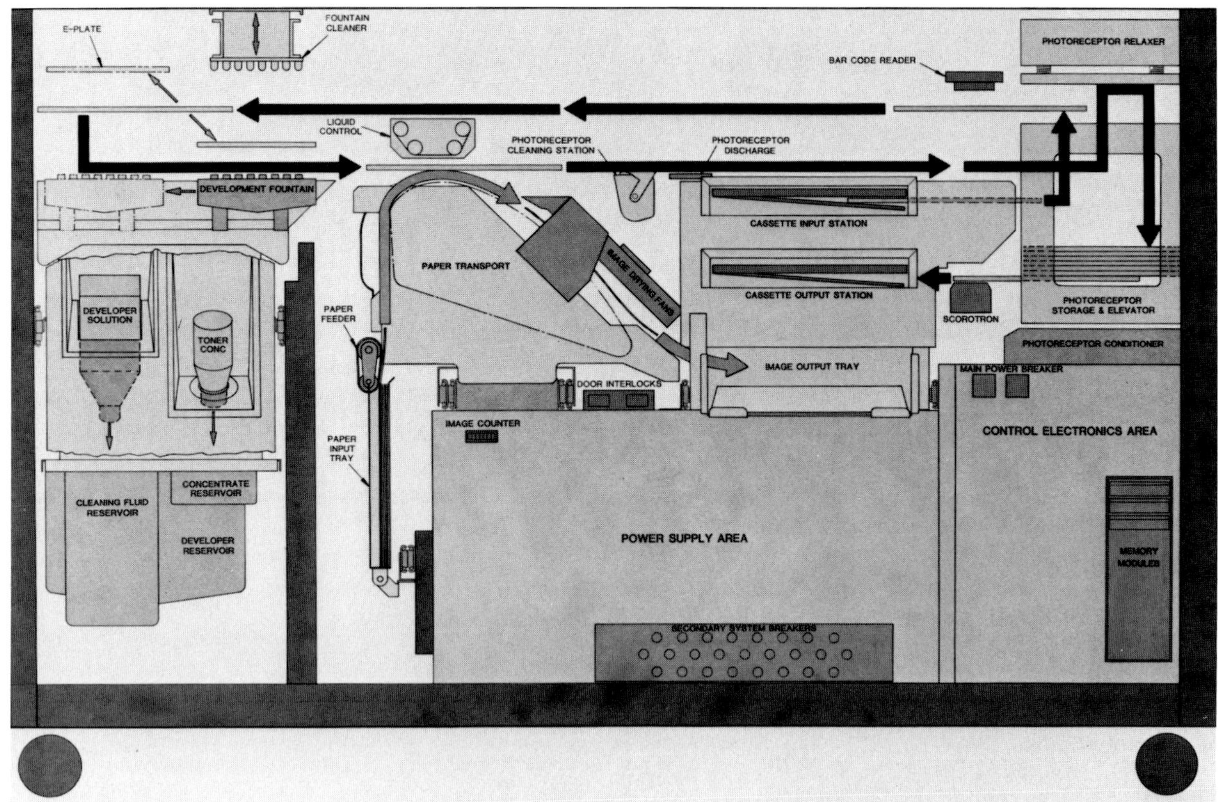

Figure 2-22. Schematic drawing of Xerox 175 System. (Courtesy, Xerox Corporation.)

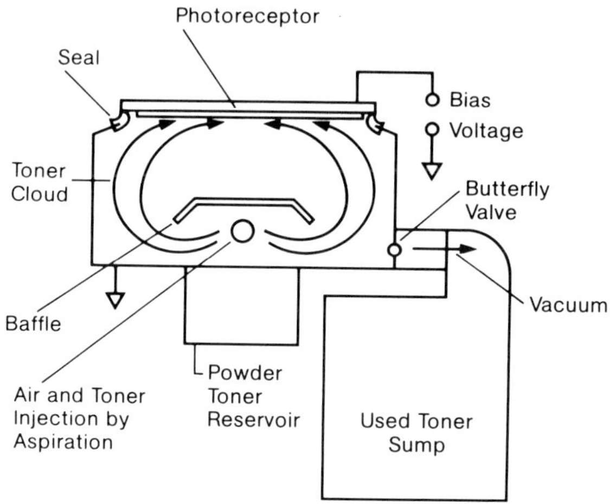

Figure 2-23. Powder cloud development system. Though not desirable from a development standpoint, turbulence is necessary in order to generate a uniform powder cloud over the large area of the photoreceptor. (Courtesy, Xerox Corporation.)

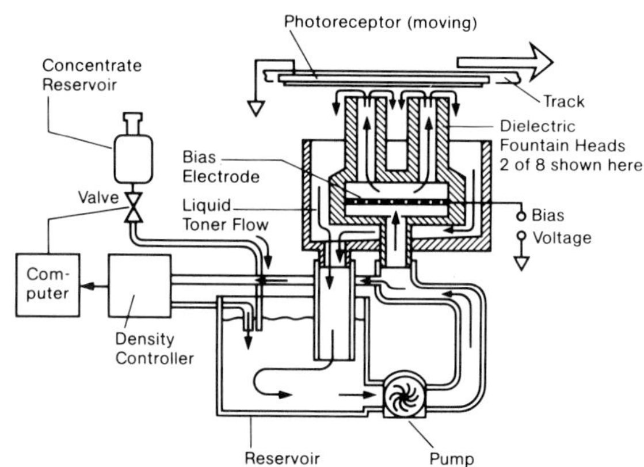

Figure 2-24. Liquid toner fountain development system. Reduced turbulence is an advantage of this system. (Courtesy, Xerox Corporation.)

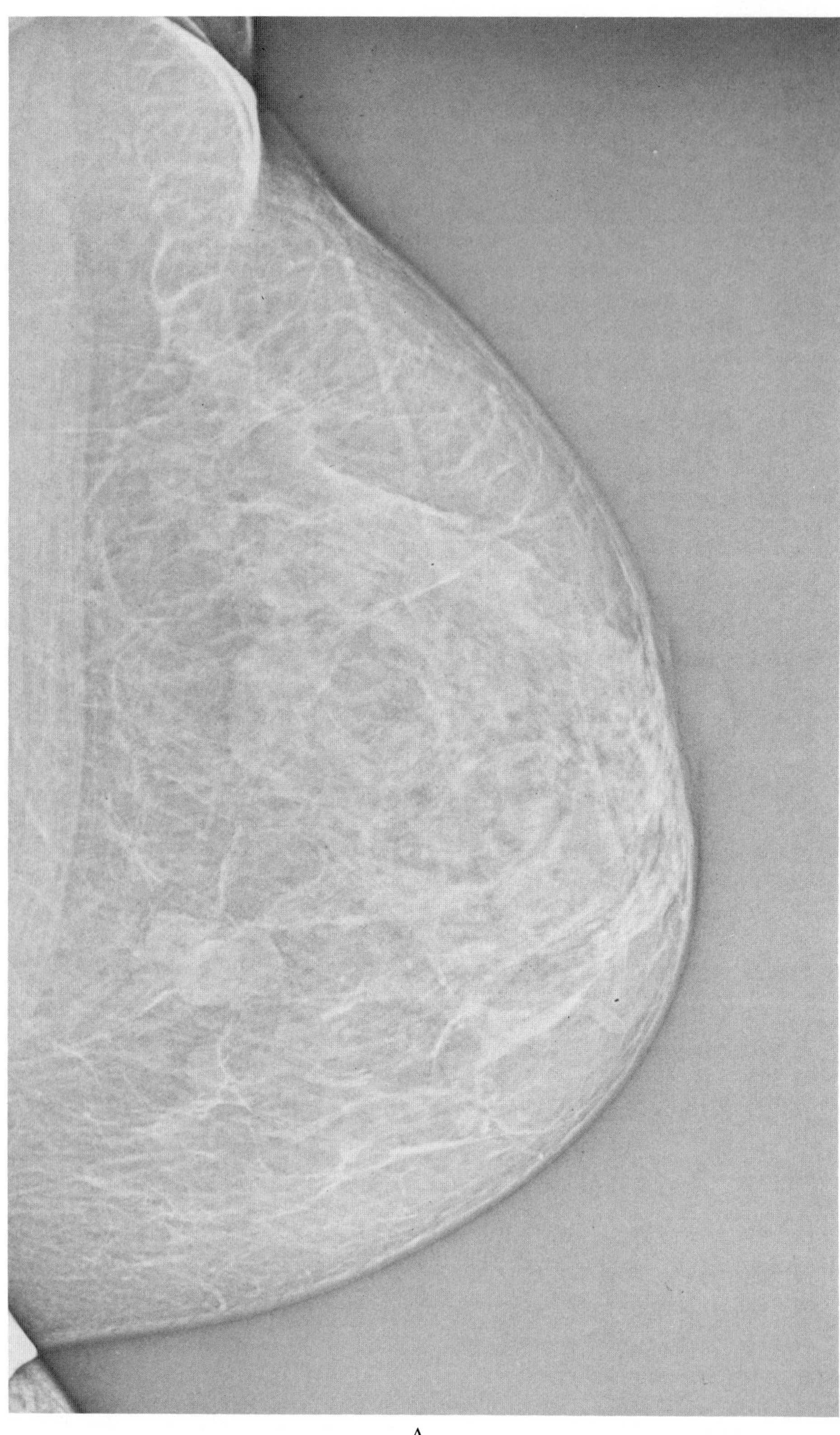

A

Figure 2-25. Images of the same breast taken with (A) 126 and (B) 175 Systems. Masses are better seen on 175 system due to increased broad-area contrast. Smaller details such as trabeculae are also better visualized as a result of better resolution and edge enhancement. (Courtesy, John N. Wolfe, M.D., Hutzel Hospital, Detroit, MI.)

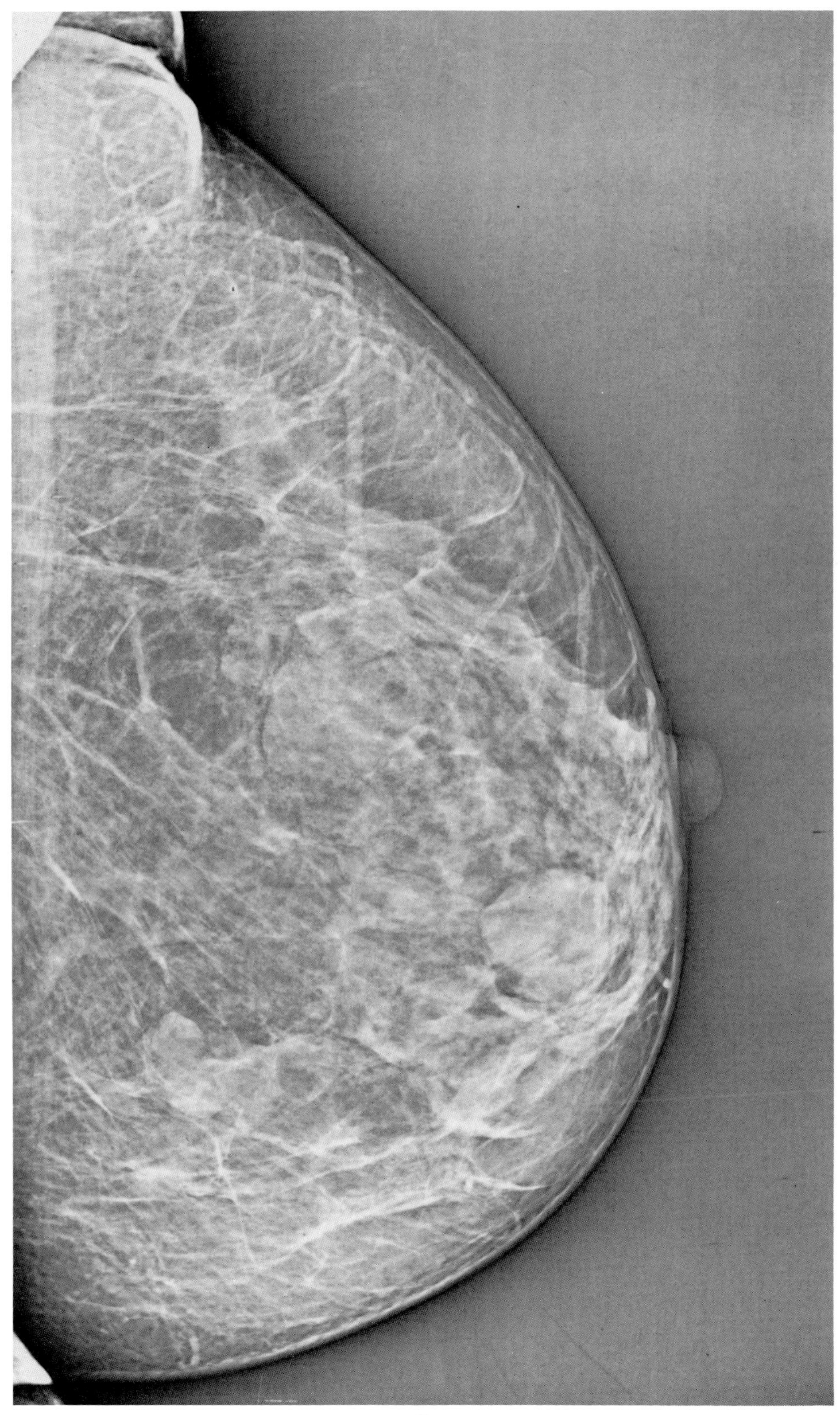

B

REFERENCES

1. Bassett LW, Gold RH: Breast radiography using the oblique projection. Radiology 149:585–587, 1983
2. Bassett LW, Pagani JJ, Gold RH: Pitfalls in mammography. Demonstrating deep lesions. Radiology 136:641–645, 1980
3. Curry TS, Dowdey JE, Murry RC: Christiansen's Introduction to the Physics of Diagnostic Radiology. (3rd ed.) Xeroradiography. Philadelphia, Lea and Febiger, 1984, pp 300–319
4. DeWerd LA: Quality assurance in mammography—Diagnosis of artifact sources in the xeroradiographic systems. NIH Publication No. 79-1684. Bethesda, MD: U.S. Dept. of Health, Education and Welfare, Public Health Service, National Institutes of Health, National Cancer Institute, 1979
5. Dodd GD: Radiation detection and diagnosis of breast cancer. Cancer 47:1766–1769, 1981
6. Fatouros PP, Rao GUV: Xeroradiography and electron radiography. In Coulam CM, Erickson JJ, Rollo FD, et al. (eds): The Physical Basis of Medical Imaging. New York, Appleton-Century-Crofts, 1981, pp 265–278
7. Haus AG: Physical principles and radiation dose in mammography. In Feig SA, McLelland R (eds): Breast Carcinoma: Current Diagnosis and Treatment. New York, Masson USA—American College of Radiology, 1983, pp 99–114
8. Haus AG: Trends in screen/film mammography: Grids, small focal spots, high-speed screen-film combination, controlled film processing, reduced radiation dose. Eastman Kodak Company Publications NoN-196. Rochester NY: Eastman Kodak Company, Health Sciences Division, 1986
9. Haus AG, Doi K, Metz CE, et al: Image quality in mammography. Radiology 125:77–85, 1977
10. Haus AG, Metz CE, Chiles JT: The effect of x-ray spectra from molybdenum and tungsten target tubes on image quality in mammography. Radiology 118:705–709, 1976
11. Jeromin LS, Speiser RC: Process studies on higher sensitivity xeromammography. Medical Imaging and Instrumentation '85. SPIE Proceedings, vol. 555, Bellingham WA, Society of Photo-Optical Instrumentation Engineers, 1985, pp 127–136
12. Logan WW, Norlund AW: Screen-film mammography technique. Compression and other factors. In Logan WW, Muntz EP (eds): Reduced Dose Mammography. New York, Masson USA, 1979, pp 415–428
13. Milbrath JR: Reduced-dose xeromammography. In Logan WW, (ed): Breast Carcinoma. The Radiologist's Expanded Role. New York, John Wiley, 1977, pp 143–151
14. Muntz EP, Wilkinson E, George FW: Mammography at reduced doses: Present performance and future possibilities. AJR 134:741–747, 1980
15. National Council on Radiation Protection and Measurements. Scientific Committee 72 on Radiation Protection in Mammography: Mammography—A user's guide. NCRP Report no. 85. Bethesda, MD, National Council on Radiation Protection and Measurements, 1986
16. Nguyen MT, Sickles EA: Radiographic detectability of breast microcalcifications: In vitro studies using a wide variety of mammography techniques. In Gray JE (ed): Application of Optical Instrumentation in Medicine VII. SPIE Proceedings, vol. 173, Bellingham, WA, Society of Photo-Optical Instrumentation Engineers, 1979, pp 120–128
17. Pagani JJ, Bassett LW, Gold RH, et al: Efficacy of combined film/screen xeromammography: Preliminary report. AJR 135:141–146, 1980
18. Paulus DD: Xeroradiography. An in-depth review. CRC Crit Rev Diagn Imaging 12:309–384, 1980
19. Rao GUV, Fatouros PP: Dose reduction in xeromammography. In Logan WW, Muntz EP (eds): Reduced Dose Mammography. New York, Masson USA, 1979, pp 347–356
20. Ratliff F: Contour and contrast. Sci Am 226:91–101, 1972
21. Sickles EA: Mammographic detectability of breast microcalcifications. AJR 139:913–918, 1982
22. Sickles EA, Weber WN: High-contrast mammography with a moving grid: Assessment of clinical utility. AJR 146:1137–1140, 1986
23. Smathers RL, Bush E, Drace J, et al: Mammographic microcalcifications: Detection with xerography, screen-film, and digitized film display. Radiology 159:673–677, 1986
24. Speiser RC, Zanrosso EM, Jeromin LS, et al: Dose comparisons for mammographic systems. Medical Physics 13:667–673, 1986
25. Stanton L, Villafana T, Day JL, et al: Dosage evaluation in mammography. Radiology 150:577–584, 1984
26. Stanton L, Villafana T, Day JL, et al: A study of mammographic exposure and detail visibility using three systems: Xerox 125, Min-R, and Xonics XERG. Radiology 132:455–462, 1979
27. Tonge KA, Davis R: The problem of discrimination in mammography. Arguments for using a biological test object. Br J Radiol 49:678–685, 1976
28. Van De Riet WG, Wolfe JN: Dose reduction in xeromammography of the breast. AJR 128:821–823, 1977
29. Wilson O: Mammographic technique. In Parsons CA (ed): Diagnosis of Breast Disease. Imaging, Clinical Features and Pathology. Baltimore, University Park Press, 1983, pp 54–75
30. Wolfe JN: Xeroradiography of the Breast (1st ed). Springfield, IL, Charles C. Thomas, 1972
31. Wolfe JN: Xeroradiography of the Breast (2nd ed). Springfield, IL, Charles C. Thomas, 1983
32. Wolfe JN, Quello C: Xeroradiography Technologist Manual. Pasadena, CA, Xerox Corporation, 1971
33. Xerox Corporation: An Illustrated Guide to Image Analysis. Pasadena, CA, Xerox Corporation, 1973
34. Xerox Corporation: The Principles of the Xeroradiographic Process. Pasadena, CA, Xerox Corporation, 1975
35. Xerox Corporation: Technical Application Bulletin 1: What is Edge Enhancement and How Does It Affect the Mammographic Image? Pasadena, CA, Xerox Corporation, 1974
36. Xerox Corporation: Technical Application Bulletin 2: How Does the Resolution Capability of Xeroradiography Compare With That of Films Used in Mammography? Pasadena, CA, Xerox Corporation, 1975
37. Xerox Corporation: Technical Application Bulletin 3: What are the Most Common Xeroradiographic Terms and What do They Mean? Pasadena, CA, Xerox Corporation, 1975
38. Xerox Corporation: Technical Application Bulletin 4:

How Does Calcification Visibility in Xeroradiography Compare With That in Film Mammography? Pasadena, CA, Xerox Corporation, 1975

39. Xerox Corporation: Technical Application Bulletin 5: Reducing Radiation Exposure in Xeroradiography. Pasadena, CA, Xerox Corporation, 1976
40. Xerox Corporation: Technical Application Bulletin 6: How Does the Recording Latitude of Xeroradiography Compare with That of Films Used in Mammography? Pasadena, CA, Xerox Corporation, 1977
41. Xerox Corporation: Technical Application Bulletin 7: Negative Development in Xeroradiography of the Breast. Pasadena, CA, Xerox Corporation, 1977
42. Xerox Corporation: Technical Application Bulletin 8: Exposure and Development Criteria in Xeroradiography of the Breast. Pasadena, CA, Xerox Corporation, 1977

Edward A. Sickles, M.D.

3

Magnification Mammography

Conventional screen-film mammography and xeromammography are the most successful imaging techniques for the detection and diagnosis of breast cancer. To make a confident diagnosis of cancer, mammographers usually rely on the demonstration either of a breast mass having poorly defined spiculated or knobby margins[12,23] or of a cluster of tiny calcifications that are linear, curvilinear, or branching in shape.[11,24] Benign breast lesions also have typical mammographic features: benign masses have sharply defined margins and smooth contours,[12,23] while benign calcifications, if tiny and clustered, are round or oval in shape.[11,24]

Unfortunately, many breast lesions do not exhibit these characteristically benign or malignant features, primarily because of the inherent unsharpness of conventional mammography images. Indeed, to distinguish benign from malignant breast masses often requires unusually finely detailed images to portray the nature of their margins with optimal clarity; equally finely detailed images frequently are needed to demonstrate the specific shapes of breast microcalcifications. Lack of detail, a situation commonly encountered, renders unreliable the diagnostic criteria described above, leading to equivocal radiographic interpretations. Standard practice calls for biopsy of such equivocal lesions in order to rule out malignancy; indeed, this is necessary to detect as many small cancers as possible. An unfortunate consequence of this approach, however, is that several benign lesions have to be removed for each cancer discovered. In some circumstances, especially when malignancy is thought to be unlikely, biopsy is deferred in favor of a series of follow-up mammographic examinations. It is even more unfortunate, if this latter course of action is chosen, when the underlying lesion proves to be cancerous and appropriate treatment is thereby delayed.

One potential solution to this double-edged problem of equivocal interpretations is to substantially improve the sharpness and detail of the radiographic image, thus permitting one to utilize more fully the standard mammographic interpretive criteria that otherwise might be ignored. If this approach proves successful, some equivocal interpretations will be converted into more definitive diagnoses, either benign or malignant.

The technique of direct radiographic magnification has been shown to be very helpful in this regard. Not only are magnification images known to display improved sharpness and detail,[3,13] but magnification techniques have already been applied successfully to mammography, angiography, and skeletal radiography, resulting in increased diagnostic accuracy for these examinations.[2,4–6,9,14,16–22]

BREAST CANCER DETECTION
ISBN 0-8089-1842-7

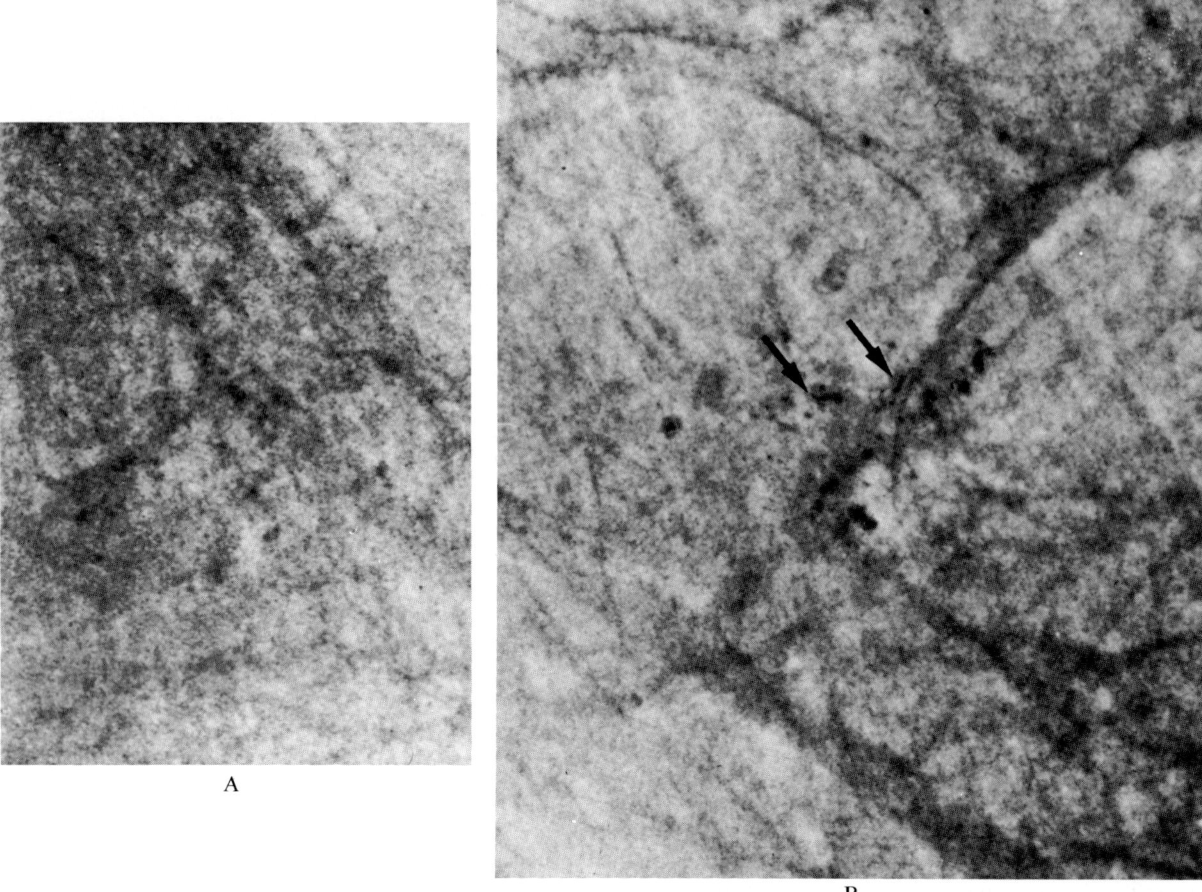

Figure 3-1. Conventional (A) and magnification (B) xeromammograms of 46-year-old woman with benign mass in opposite breast. Only magnification mammogram demonstrates cluster of microcalcifications, with some thin linear shapes (arrows), indicating malignancy (biopsy-proven intraductal carcinoma, not palpable even in retrospect). From Sickles EA: Microfocal spot magnification mammography using xeroradiographic and screen-film recording systems. Radiology 131:605, 1979. With permission.

TECHNICAL CONSIDERATIONS

Conventional mammograms are taken with the x-ray film in contact with the breast, producing an essentially life-size image. By increasing the distance between breast and film, an enlarged (magnified) x-ray image results. Magnification radiography, however, will not be successful unless done with a specialized x-ray tube that has an extremely small x-ray source (focal spot) to minimize the blurring that accompanies geometric image enlargement.[7,14] Laboratory data suggest that the largest acceptable focal-spot size for magnification mammography is 0.3 mm in greatest diameter,[13] a condition met by some, but not all, dedicated mammography units currently being promoted as having magnification capability.[16] Magnification mammography also requires firm breast compression to prevent even the slightest motion of the breast during the relatively long (1–4 seconds) exposures that are needed.

Laboratory evaluation of microfocal-spot mammography equipment has also determined the optimal degree of magnification to be approximately 1.5 times life size.[15,19] It has been shown both qualitatively and quantitatively that the improved sharpness of magnification mammograms results from both increased resolution and reduced effective noise.[15,19] Although there also is the potential for improved contrast with magnification mammography, the limited air gap used is usually not sufficient to significantly reduce scattered radiation.[18]

CLINICAL EXPERIENCE

The most extensive published experience with magnification mammography is a prospective clinical trial to determine the ability of 1.5×-magnification imaging to increase the accuracy of the conventional mam-

A

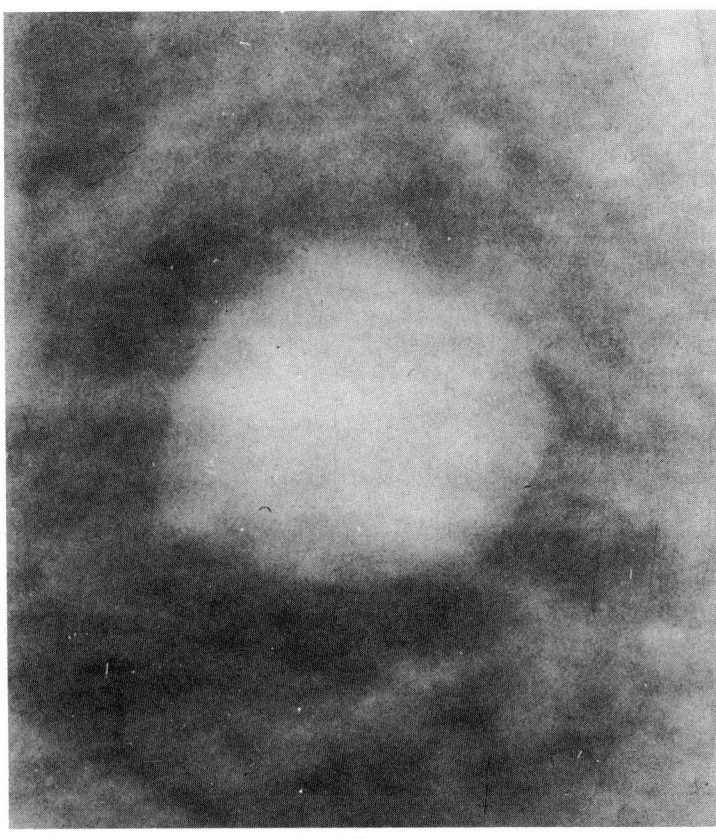

B

Figure 3-2. Conventional (A) and magnification (B) screen-film mammograms showing 1.7 × 2.3-cm mass. Only magnification image demonstrates sharply defined, smooth-contoured margins of mass with sufficient clarity to permit confident diagnosis of benignity (biopsy-proven fibroadenoma). From Sickles EA: Microfocal spot magnification mammography using xeroradiographic and screen-film recording systems. Radiology 131:601, 1979. With permission.

mography examination.[17,18] Patients were selected for study either because conventional mammograms were given an equivocal interpretation (suspicious for but not diagnostic of malignancy) or because it was known that biopsy was planned in the near future and hence pathologic proof could be expected. A single additional magnification mammogram was taken using the same recording system (screen-film or xerographic) that had been used for conventional mammography. The conventional-plus-magnification examination was then reinterpreted by the same observers, who recorded any changes in overall diagnostic impression.

The study involved 750 patients, approximately equal numbers examined with xerographic and screen-film imaging systems. No differences in results were found between these two imaging systems in any of the subsequent data breakdowns. For almost every patient studied, the single additional 1.5×-magnification mammogram produced a sharper, more detailed image of the breast than its conventional (1×) counterparts. Magnification mammography detected 9 breast cancers that had been missed completely on the entire standard examination (Fig. 3-1). These cancers were found by serendipity, since in each case the magnification mammogram was done to investigate a lesion elsewhere in the breast. The principal impact of magnification mammography, however, was found in the evaluation of lesions interpreted as equivocal on conventional examination. Margins of breast masses and the shapes of clustered breast microcalcifications were often portrayed with so much greater clarity that a definitively benign or malignant diagnosis could be made (Figs. 3-2–3-4). Overall, approximately 70 percent of the cases initially read as equivocal were reinterpreted definitively with the addition of a single magnification mammogram (Table 3-1). Radiographic–histopathologic correlation was done on the 251 patients who underwent biopsy within 1 month of study. These data, shown in Table 3-2, indicate the striking increase in diagnostic accuracy of magnification mammography among patients whose conventional mammograms were interpreted as equivocal. Of the 48 cases read as frankly malignant because of the additional magnification mammogram, only 1 interpretation proved to be in error; and all of the 57 cases read as benign after magnification mammography were indeed benign at biopsy.

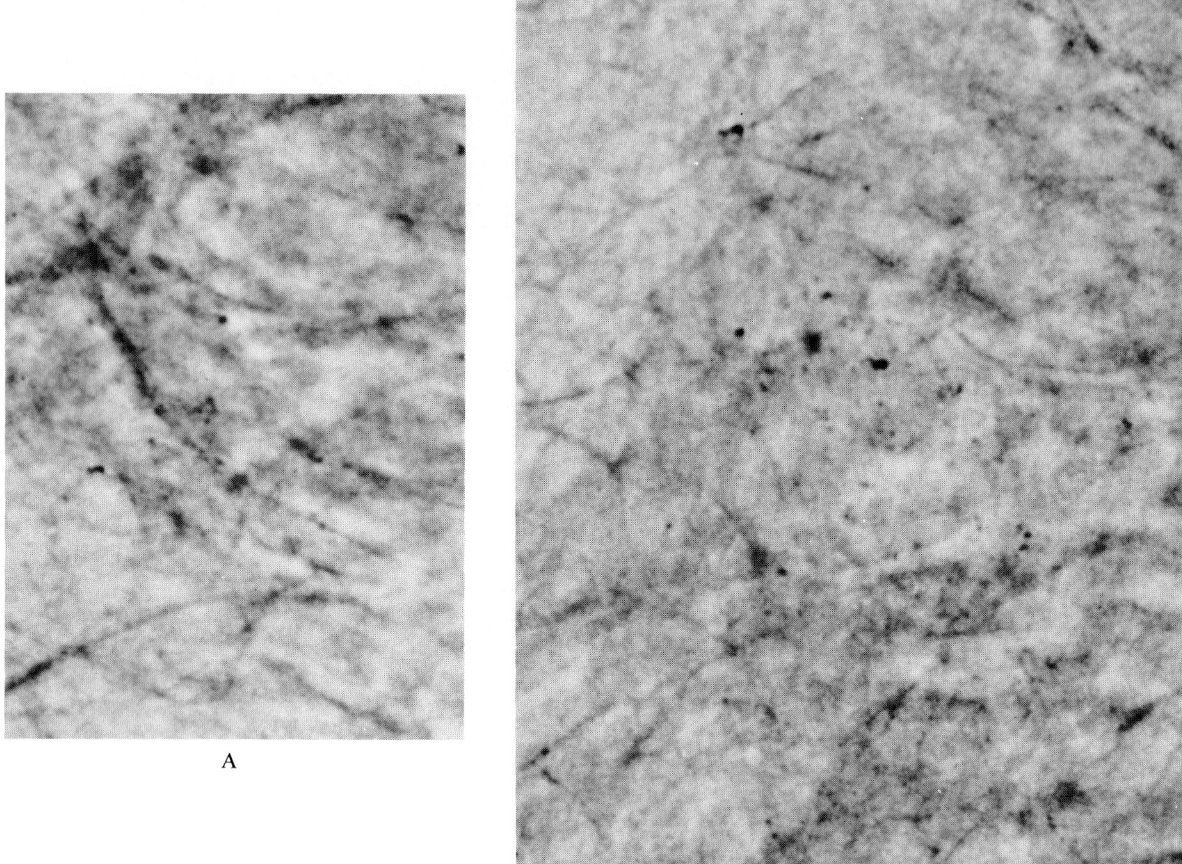

A

B

Figure 3-3. A. Conventional xeromammogram. Isolated cluster of microcalcifications of indeterminate nature is identified. Mammographic diagnosis: equivocal for malignancy. B. Magnification xeromammogram. Many more microcalcifications are evident. Since all particles appear round or oval in shape, mammographic diagnosis was changed to benign. Biopsy revealed mammary dysplasia with foci of sclerosing adenosis. From Sickles EA: Further experience with microfocal spot magnification mammography in the assessment of clustered breast microcalcifications. Radiology 137:13, 1980. With permission.

The increased diagnostic accuracy of magnification imaging translates readily into improved patient management. Magnification mammography causes some cancers to be removed more promptly than would be done otherwise, either because it detects malignant lesions that are not even suspected on conventional mammograms, or because it definitively demonstrates malignancy in lesions that are judged to be equivocal by conventional mammography. (Despite the suggestion to biopsy all equivocal lesions, occasionally the surgeon or the patient elects to defer biopsy in favor of clinical observation.) A much more substantial effect of magnification mammography, however, is a considerable reduction in the number of biopsies for benign lesions, i.e., cases in which the magnification mammogram substantially reduces or completely eliminates the suspicion of malignancy that had been indicated by conventional examination. As a result, these patients safely can be followed with repeat magnification mammographic examinations instead of undergoing biopsy. Although there is no pathological proof in these cases, I am now following more than 1000 such women, some for as long as 9 years, and none have developed cancer in or adjacent to the area where conventional mammograms initially suggested some suspicion of malignancy.

PRACTICAL APPLICATIONS

The most clearly established role of magnification mammography is as an adjunct to conventional mammography when the initial study is interpreted as equiv-

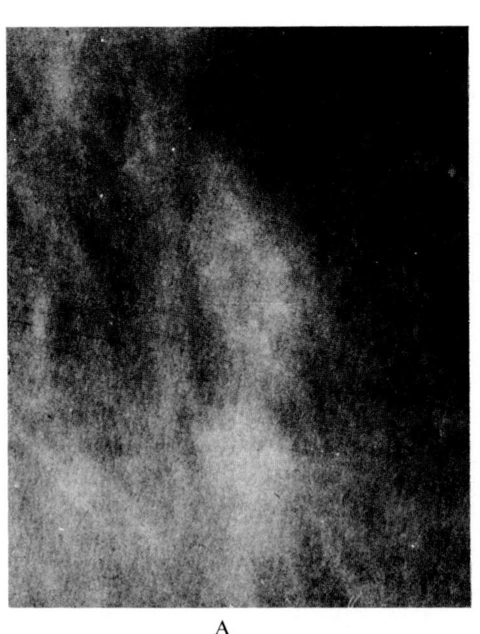

A

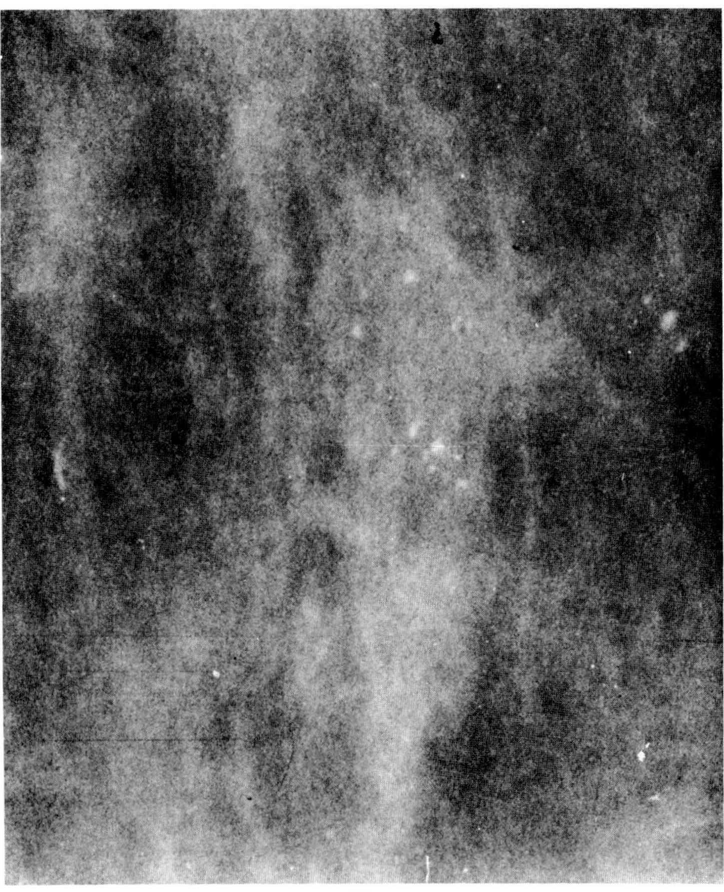

B

Figure 3-4. Conventional (A) and magnification (B) screen-film mammograms showing cluster of microcalcifications within and adjacent to poorly defined area of increased density. Only magnification image demonstrates calcifications with sufficient clarity to make mammographic diagnosis of malignancy (biopsy-proven infiltrating ductal carcinoma). From Sickles EA: Microfocal spot magnification mammography using xeroradiographic and screen-film recording systems. Radiology 131:604, 1979. With permission.

ocal for malignancy. My own ongoing experience with magnification mammography, now comprising well over 5000 cases, continues to confirm its ability to facilitate definitive diagnosis among cases otherwise considered equivocal. Similar anecdotal experience has been reported by others.[2,9,14,21]

I have also defined several other uses for magnification mammography: (1) It may clearly demonstrate on two projections a nonpalpable yet suspicious lesion shown on only one projection by conventional mammography, thereby permitting prompt radiographic localization for biopsy. All too often the only alternative to this approach is to wait for the lesion to grow further, until it either becomes palpable or is visible on more than one mammographic view. (2) Even when conventional mammography indicates the presence of malignancy, magnification mammography may demonstrate the existence of otherwise unsuspected multicentric foci of tumor, thereby more accurately delineating the tumor size and extent. This information is very useful in determining whether excisional biopsy and comprehensive radiation therapy could represent an acceptable alternative to mastectomy.[20] (3) When conventional mammograms show barely perceptible abnormalities not sufficiently worrisome to consider "equivocal," magnification mammography may permit visualization of more suspicious features, prompting earlier biopsy of lesions that prove to be small cancers. This occurs most frequently when only 2 or 3 adjacent nondescript calcific particles are seen on conventional images but magnification mammograms demonstrate a cluster of 5 or more suspicious microcalcifications.

FURTHER CONSIDERATIONS

Despite the experience that magnification mammography outperforms conventional techniques in several specific circumstances, magnification examinations are not currently recommended in place of conventional

Table 3-1
Mammographic Interpretations for All 750 Patients studied

Conventional Mammography	Conventional + Magnification Mammography
227 Benign	201 Benign
	19 Equivocal
	7 Malignant
496 Equivocal	297 Benign
	151 Equivocal
	48 Malignant
27 Malignant	27 Malignant

mammography. The primary reason is that one would expect a much lower number of improved diagnoses in a consecutive series of unselected patients than the dramatic increase in accuracy observed in the controlled study described above, which was heavily weighted with difficult-to-evaluate patients. Another valid concern is that magnification mammography results in a radiation dose to the breast 1.5–4 times higher than that of standard contact mammography.[18] Each magnification exposure produces a breast dose of 0.25–0.50 rad, a dose that is entirely acceptable for the one-time evaluation of a radiographically suspicious lesion, for which the likelihood of malignancy is relatively high. On the other hand, a complete examination with magnification technique would require at least four exposures, and twice as many for large-breasted women in order to include all the breast tissue on available recording systems. Especially if repeated examinations are planned for an asymptomatic patient population, in which a very low yield of breast cancer is expected, lower-dose conventional (1×) mammography seems a more prudent alternative. Although magnification mammography is also quite feasible using screen-film systems faster than those now used for conventional examinations, resulting in substantially reduced radiation doses, such low-dose magnification techniques have not yet been adequately evaluated to determine whether improved diagnostic accuracy is observed at a radiation dose equal to or lower than that of conventional mammography.[1,2,8,18]

In most major medical centers and private radiology offices, breast imaging now is being done with conventional dedicated mammography units. As this equipment wears out or otherwise becomes obsolete, replacement with a microfocal-spot unit represents an attractive alternative, since microfocal-spot systems not only offer the capability for magnification imaging, but also do excellent contact (1×) mammography. Indeed, the resolution of microfocal-spot contact screen-film mammograms is slightly better than that of contact screen-film mammograms taken with conventional dedicated equipment, while the radiation dose, image contrast, and background noise are essentially identical.[18] As discussed previously, magnification mammography can be done successfully only with an x-ray tube having a focal spot no larger than 0.3 mm in greatest diameter. In this regard it is important to know that there often is a substantial difference between true (measured) focal spot size and the (nominal) size claimed by the manufacturer. In practice, the measured focal spot size usually is almost twice that of the nominal size, suggesting that magnification imaging will work reliably only for x-ray tubes nominally 0.1 mm in size or smaller. Fortunately, there are several commercially available x-ray units that currently meet this specification. However, because nominal size is such an unreliable indicator of imaging performance, prospective buyers should insist on purchase specifications that guarantee measured focal spot size.[10]

CONCLUSIONS

Successful magnification mammography requires proper x-ray equipment and careful attention to radiographic technique. Magnification imaging is a useful adjunct to conventional mammography, producing radiographs that have increased sharpness and detail. It is

Table 3-2
Radiographic-Pathologic Correlations for the 251 Biopsy-proven Cases

Mammographic Diagnosis		Pathological Diagnosis	
Conventional	Conventional + Magnification		
56 Benign	38 Benign	36 Benign	2 Malignant
	12 Equivocal	9 Benign	3 Malignant
	6 Malignant	6 Malignant	
168 Equivocal	57 Benign	57 Benign	
	63 Equivocal	44 Benign	19 Malignant
	48 Malignant	1 Benign	47 Malignant
27 Malignant	27 Malignant	27 Malignant	

most helpful when conventional mammography results in equivocal diagnostic interpretation, frequently eliminating the need to biopsy breast lesions that subsequently prove to be benign after clinical and mammographic observation.

REFERENCES

1. Arnold BA, Eisenberg H, Bjärngard BE: Magnification mammography: A low-dose technique. Radiology 131: 743–749, 1979
2. Bassett LW, Arnold BA, Borger D, et al: Reduced dose magnification mammography. Radiology 141:665–670, 1981
3. Bookstein JJ, Voegeli E: A critical analysis of magnification radiography: Laboratory investigation. Radiology 98:23–30, 1971
4. Genant HK, Doi K, Mall JC: Optical versus radiographic magnification for fine-detail skeletal radiography. Invest Radiol 10:160–172, 1975
5. Genant HK, Doi K, Mall JC, et al: Direct radiographic magnification for skeletal radiography: An assessment of image quality and clinical application. Radiology 123:47–55, 1977
6. Greenspan RH, Simon AL, Ricketts HJ, et al: In vivo magnification angiography. Invest Radiol 2:419–431, 1967
7. Haus AG, Paulus DD, Dodd GD, et al: Magnification mammography: Evaluation of screen-film and xeroradiographic techniques. Radiology 133:223–226, 1979
8. Kubo K: Recent development of magnification technique in mammography and its diagnostic significance. Twelfth International Cancer Congress, Buenos Aires, Oct 5–11, 1978
9. Logan WW: Overview of the radiologist's role in breast cancer detection. In Logan WW (ed): Breast Carcinoma: The Radiologist's Expanded Role. New York, Wiley, 1977, pp 343–365
10. Logan WW: Screen-film mammography: Technique. In Feig SA, McLelland R (eds): Breast Carcinoma. Current Diagnosis and Treatment. New York, Masson, 1983, pp 141–160
11. Martin JE: Benign vs. malignant calcifications. In Margulis AR, Gooding CA (eds): Diagnostic Radiology 1977. San Francisco, University of California, 1977, pp 831–836
12. Martin JE: Correlations of mammography and histology of the breast, benign and malignant. In Margulis AR, Gooding CA (eds): Diagnostic Radiology 1977. San Francisco, University of California, 1977, pp 807–821
13. Milne ENC: The role and performance of minute focal spots in roentgenology with special reference to magnification. CRC Crit Rev Radiol Sci 2:269–310, 1971
14. Muntz EP, Logan WW: Focal spot size and scatter suppression in magnification mammography. AJR 133: 453–459, 1979
15. Nguyen MT, Sickles EA: Radiographic detectability of breast microcalcifications: *in vitro* studies using a wide variety of mammography techniques. In Gray JE (ed): Application of Optical Instrumentation in Medicine VII, SPIE Proceedings, vol. 173. Bellingham, WA, Society of Photo-Optical Instrumentation Engineers, 1979, pp 129–134
16. Sickles EA: Dedicated mammography equipment. In Syllabus for the Categorical Course on Mammography. Chevy Chase, MD, American College of Radiology, 1984, pp 1–7
17. Sickles EA: Further experience with microfocal spot magnification mammography in the assessment of clustered breast microcalcifications. Radiology 137:9–14, 1980
18. Sickles EA: Microfocal spot magnification mammography using xeroradiographic and screen-film recording systems. Radiology 131:599–607, 1979
19. Sickles EA, Doi K, Genant HK: Magnification film mammography: Image quality and clinical studies. Radiology 125:69–76, 1977
20. Sickles, EA, Weber WN: Magnification mammography to evaluate extent of breast cancer in women desiring alternative treatments to mastectomy. Radiology 157(P):174, 1985
21. Tabár L: Microfocal spot magnification mammography. In Brünner S, Langfeldt B, Andersen PE (eds): Early Detection of Breast Cancer. New York, Springer-Verlag, 1984, pp 62–68
22. Takahashi S, Sakuma S, Kaneko M, et al: Angiography at four-fold magnification with special reference to the examination of tumours. Acta Radiol (Diagn) 4:206–216, 1966
23. Wolfe JN: Xeroradiography: Uncalcified Breast Masses. Springfield, IL, CC Thomas, 1977, pp 3–41
24. Wolfe JN: Xeroradiography: Breast Calcifications. Springfield, IL, CC Thomas, 1977, pp 3–43

Barbara Threatt, M.D.

4

Ductography

Ductography or galactography (radiography following mammary duct injection with radiopaque contrast material) is useful in the evaluation of spontaneous nipple discharge from a nonlactating breast. Bloody, serous, and serosanguinous are the most common and significant of these spontaneous discharges. Although carcinoma is the cause of the discharge in only a comparatively small percentage of patients, a thorough evaluation followed by surgical identification and removal of the causative lesion, with subsequent histologic analysis, is imperative to exclude that possibility.[13] (Haagensen[5(pp276–291)] has described a rare benign bilateral bloody discharge occurring in late pregnancy and lactation, probably related to hyperplasia of ductal tissue, and requiring only clinical follow-up to regression.) Although these discharges are associated with a mass in about 50 percent of cases, identifying and excising the appropriate area can sometimes be difficult. Careful palpation may cause expression of the discharge, thus identifying its source even in the absence of a palpable mass. Blind excision can only be deplored, since excessive tissue is often removed in seeking a small, usually benign lesion. Ductography is useful to accurately identify the involved ductal system.

HISTORICAL BACKGROUND

Ductography was first described by Ries[11] in 1930. Hicken[6] and Leborgne[8] subsequently elaborated on the procedure and the anatomic findings. Following the report of Romano and McFetridge[12] on complications secondary to the contrast agents employed, the procedure was virtually abandoned until the 1960s when, with the advent of improved contrast agents, Funderburk and Syphax[4] reintroduced it. Since then, other authors[2,4,5(p102),7,12,13–15] have reported their techniques and findings. Today, ductography is considered a safe and simple method of identifying the discharging ductal system in three dimensions, allowing for the precise localization of the suspicious area prior to biopsy.

CLINICO-PATHOLOGIC FEATURES OF DISCHARGES

Discharges can be divided into those that are spontaneous and those that are manually expressible. In a population with breast symptoms, approximately 25 percent of patients will have either or both types. Although a spontaneous discharge in a nonlactating asymptomatic breast is infrequent, it occurs in as many as 10 percent of women with breast symptoms.[3,5(p102),8,9] Approximately 40–60 percent of patients with spontaneous discharge will have an associated palpable mass that reproduces the discharge on pressure.[5(p102),8] The percentage of women with an expressible breast discharge in an asymptomatic population is difficult to estimate but probably runs about 10 to 15 percent (figures based on data from the University of Michigan Breast Cancer Detection Demonstration Project). Such discharges are typically of benign origin, usually associated with

BREAST CANCER DETECTION
ISBN 0-8089-1842-7

Table 4-1
Diagnostic Evaluation of Patients with Discharge

Color Discharge	HX	PE	Mammography	Duct Injection	Biopsy	Management
White	X	X	Not specifically indicated under age 40	Not indicated	Not indicated	BSE; annual PE; annual mammogram if over age 40
Creamy	X	X	Not specifically indicated under age 40	Not indicated	Not indicated	BSE; annual PE; annual mammogram if over age 40
Grumous	X	X	Not specifically indicated under age 40	Not indicated	Not indicated	BSE; annual PE; annual mammogram if over age 40
Greenish-black	X	X	X	X	Not indicated unless mass or specific abnormality on PE	BSE; annual PE; annual mammogram if over age 40
Serous	X	X	X	X	If specific mass or abnormality on mammogram or PE mass	BSE; annual PE (may be more frequent, depending on histologic findings); annual mammogram if over age 40
Bloody	X	X	X*	X*	X*	BSE; annual PE (may be more frequent, depending on histologic findings); annual mammogram if over age 40
Clear	X	X	X	X	If X-ray abnormality and/or PE mass	BSE; annual PE (may be more frequent, depending on histologic findings); annual mammogram if over age 40
Pus	X	X	X	Not indicated unless chronic condition	Not indicated unless chronic condition; may be acute mastitis	Antibiotics; soaks; follow-up PE

HX = history; PE = physical examination; BSE = breast self-examination
* not in pregnant or lactational, bilateral bloody-discharge patients

fibrocystic disease or inappropriate response to estrogen–progesterone stimulation.

Spontaneous Discharges

Nipple discharge in the nonlactating breast may be white, creamy, grumous, greenish-black, clear, serous, serosanguinous, or frankly bloody. The most significant discharges are those that are serous, serosanguinous, or bloody. In the past, surgery for such discharges has varied from local excision to mastectomy. Radical surgery was performed in many cases because the lesion producing the discharge could not be identified by physical examination or at surgical exploration.

While intraductal papilloma, single or multiple, is the single most common cause of bloody, serous, or serosanguinous discharges at all ages,[5(pp250–291)] the incidence of cancer as the cause increases with age.[13] Cancer is responsible in only 12–15 percent of cases overall. Although papillomas and papillomatosis are benign, Buhl-Jorgensen et al.[1] reported an increased incidence of carcinoma in patients with these lesions, solitary papillomas being associated with the higher incidence. They considered the intraductal papilloma to be a premalignant lesion. McPherson and MacKenzie,[10] however, were unable to find an increased incidence of carcinoma in patients with an intraductal papilloma followed over a 10-year period. Haagensen reported an association between multiple papillomas and carcinoma.[5(pp276–291)]

The indicated workup for a patient with a spontaneous discharge depends upon the medical history, type

Table 4-2
Material for Mammary Duct Injection

Alcohol wipes
Sterile gauze pads
Betadine
Sterile gloves
Sterile aperture drape
5-cc syringe
18-gauge needle
60% Renografin (3 cc)
30-gauge blunt lymphangiogram needle*
Gooseneck lamp
Cellophane tape

* Blunt #30-gauge needles can be ordered from the Becton-Dickinson Company. Lymphangiogram needles can be blunted by machine; however, this method is time-consuming and frequently results in occlusion or "hooks." Sharp lymphangiogram needles should not be used since they can produce bleeding and/or pierce the duct wall.

of discharge, physical findings, and age (Table 4-1). In patients with serous, serosanguinous, or bloody discharges, however, two considerations are paramount: (1) identification and removal of the source of the discharge; and (2) histological evaluation of the causative lesion. The evaluation of each patient should be individualized and tailored to the patient's particular problem.

Manually Expressible Discharges

Patients with white or creamy discharges typically present with encrusted nipples and/or multiple discharging ducts. The discharge is usually obtained only by manual expression from the nipple, is not associated with a mass, and results either from an abnormal response of the breasts to hormonal stimulation or from fibrocystic disease. A serum prolactin level should be obtained in cases of profuse milky discharge to exclude a prolactin-secreting pituitary tumor. Milky discharges tend to occur most commonly in women who have had one or more pregnancies. Further evaluation is unnecessary unless other abnormalities are documented by history, physical examination, or mammography.

The grumous (thick, grayish) discharge, as described by Haagensen,[5(p102)] is typically found in women during the premenopausal period. It usually occurs upon manual expression and regresses after the menopause.

A greenish-black discharge, at times misdiagnosed as bloody, and typically seen exuding from multiple ducts of both breasts, is usually associated with secretory disease (duct ectasia) in menopausal and early postmenopausal women. Its color, which varies from pale green to darkest black, is best determined by

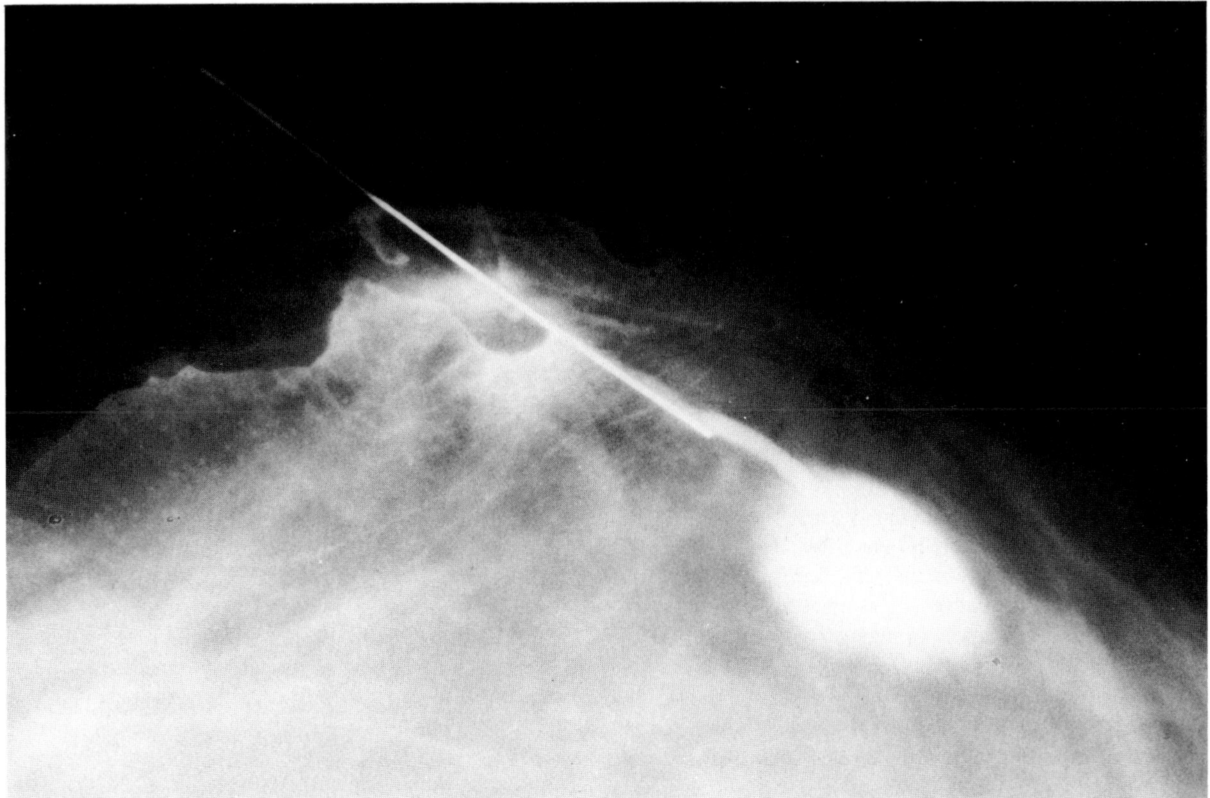

Figure 4-1. Extravasation of contrast material during ductography, signified by white shadow with fuzzy borders.

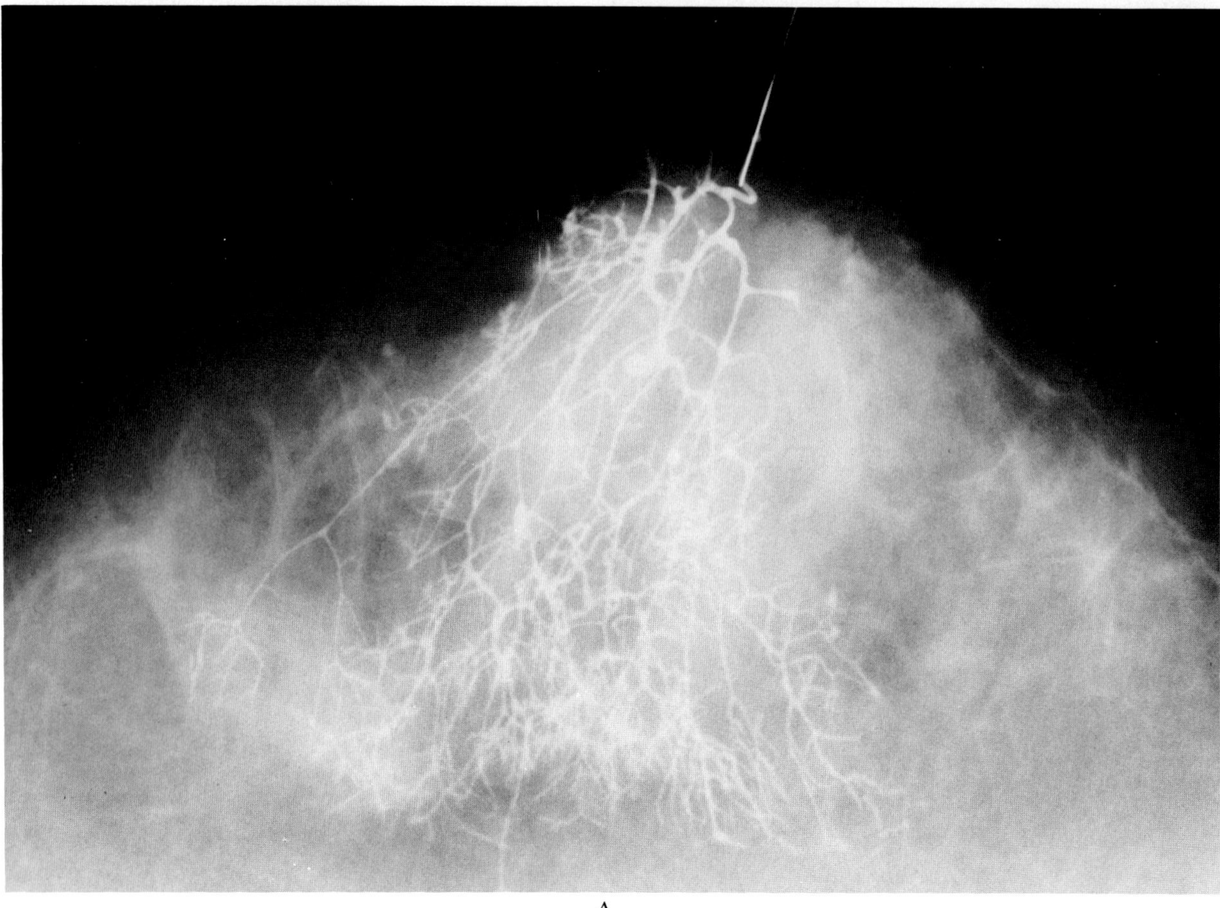

A

Figure 4-2. Postinjection mammograms showing variation in width of normal ducts. A. Ducts of fine caliber, normal in size and distribution. B. Ducts of larger caliber, but still normal. Caliber of ducts gradually diminishes as they branch and extend posteriorly.

placing a small drop on sterile gauze. Gradually progressive nipple retraction ultimately becomes bilateral and may be severe. Occasionally a spontaneous greenish-black discharge from a single duct may result from a papilloma.[16]

A clear, watery discharge is rare, even for one that is manually expressible. Although it has been reported by Haagensen in association with carcinoma,[5(p74)] a watery discharge is rarely the initial symptom of carcinoma.

A thick, yellowish, sometimes blood-tinged, occasionally foul-smelling discharge is pus. It is infrequent and is usually associated with acute mastitis, especially during lactation. A sudden onset of pain and warmth in the breast and a discharge of pus are the classic symptoms and signs. All such women should be evaluated and treated with antibiotics. Mammograms, especially for women over age 40, are indicated to look for signs of carcinoma. Ductography is not indicated in the acute phase, but should be performed if the discharge does not clear after resolution of the mastitis.

TECHNIQUE OF DUCTOGRAPHY

First, a thorough medical history is obtained, and a physical examination is performed. Then mammograms are obtained. Even if a mass or other abnormality is identified in the mammograms, galactography is indicated to exclude a nonvisualized, separate abnormality. To perform galactography, the patient is placed supine on an examining table. The materials needed for ductography are listed in Table 4-2. The nipple is cleansed with alcohol, and the discharging duct is identified. The breast is cleansed with Betadine and covered with a sterile plastic aperture drape. The discharging duct is cannulated with a blunt needle. This process is usually accomplished easily, since a discharging duct has an enlarged ostium. Probing is sometimes necessary when the orifice is partially obscured by encrustation or when it is oriented obliquely to the nipple surface. It is helpful to express a minimal amount of discharge before attempting cannulation. Once the needle tip is in the ostium, it usually enters the duct easily and without pressure. In fact, a delicate, light

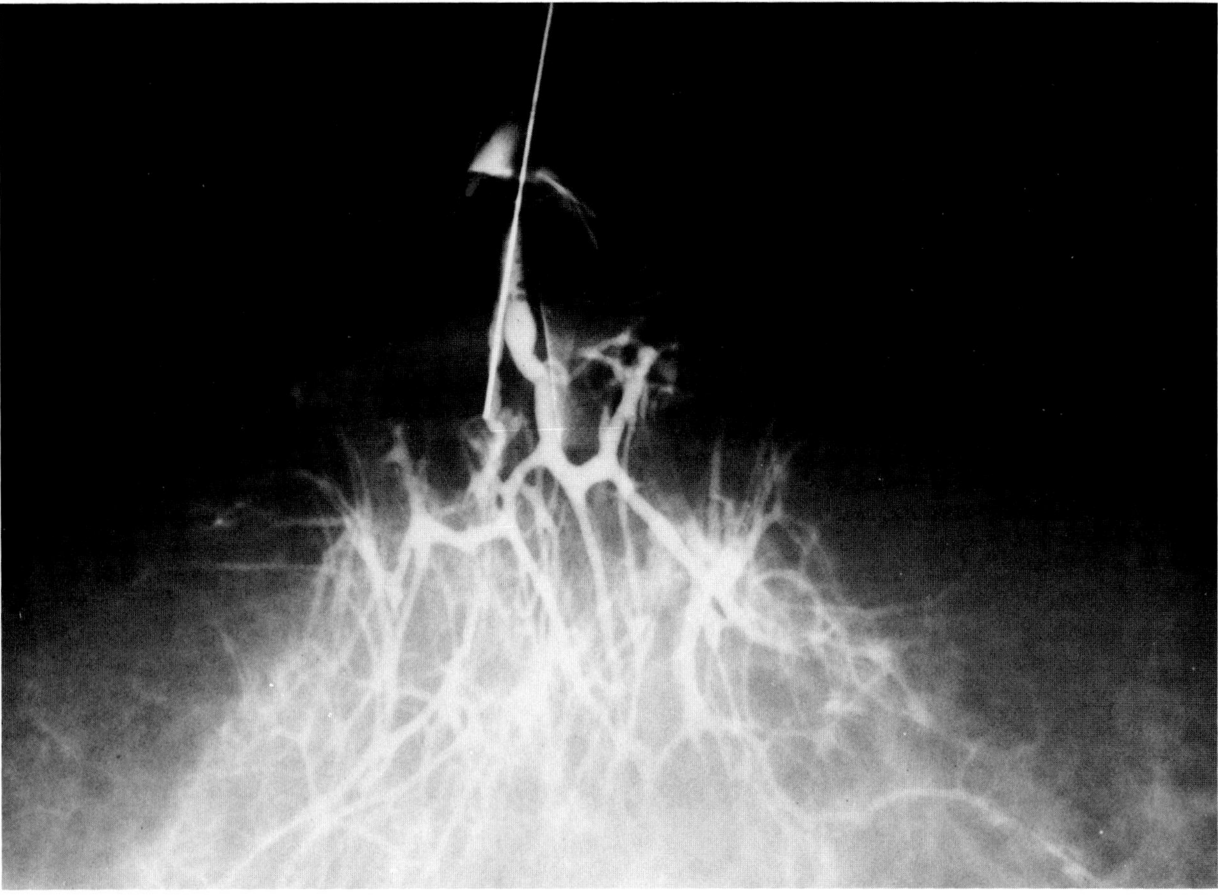

B

touch is essential to avoid penetration of the duct wall. The needle is inserted to its hub and taped securely in place.

After secure needle placement, the patient is positioned as for mammography. The breast is placed in profile, and 0.1–0.3 ml of a 60 percent solution of Renografin is injected initially. While the response of the patient is variable and dependent upon the duct size (injection of small duct systems produces more discomfort), there should be no sharp pain. Although a slightly uncomfortable, sometimes warm sensation is predictable, sharp pain indicates extravasation of contrast material (Fig. 4-1). If the needle has been properly positioned, as implied by a painless preliminary injection, another 0.5 ml or so is injected, the exact volume depending upon the capacity of the ductal system. A total volume of 3.0 ml may be required for complete filling, which is usually signaled when the patient experiences a fullness or tightness in the breast.

Cephalocaudal and mediolateral mammograms are performed with minimal compression of the breast. If incomplete filling is apparent, or should areas of narrowing be identified, additional contrast is injected. If the subareolar ampullary portion of the duct has not been filled, further contrast agent should be injected during needle withdrawal and any excess contrast material on the skin wiped away prior to obtaining an additional radiograph. Generally, we obtain four radiographs in various stages of duct filling. A single set of two films is insufficient, since areas of incomplete duct filling or even air bubbles are often present initially and require further evaluation.

RADIOGRAPHIC APPEARANCE

The preinjection and postinjection mammograms are reviewed. Typical postinjection mammograms are shown in Figures 4-2A and B. The subareolar portion of the ducts is 2–3 mm in diameter, with the ampulla slightly wider. The more posterior branches become progressively smaller in caliber, the appearance reminiscent of a bronchogram or cholangiogram. The walls should be smooth, without beading, angulation, or narrowing. Changes in size and direction should be smooth and progressive. There is a normal variation in diameter, and ducts of large caliber may be normal (Fig. 4-2).

Extreme dilatation, sometimes to 7 or 8 mm in

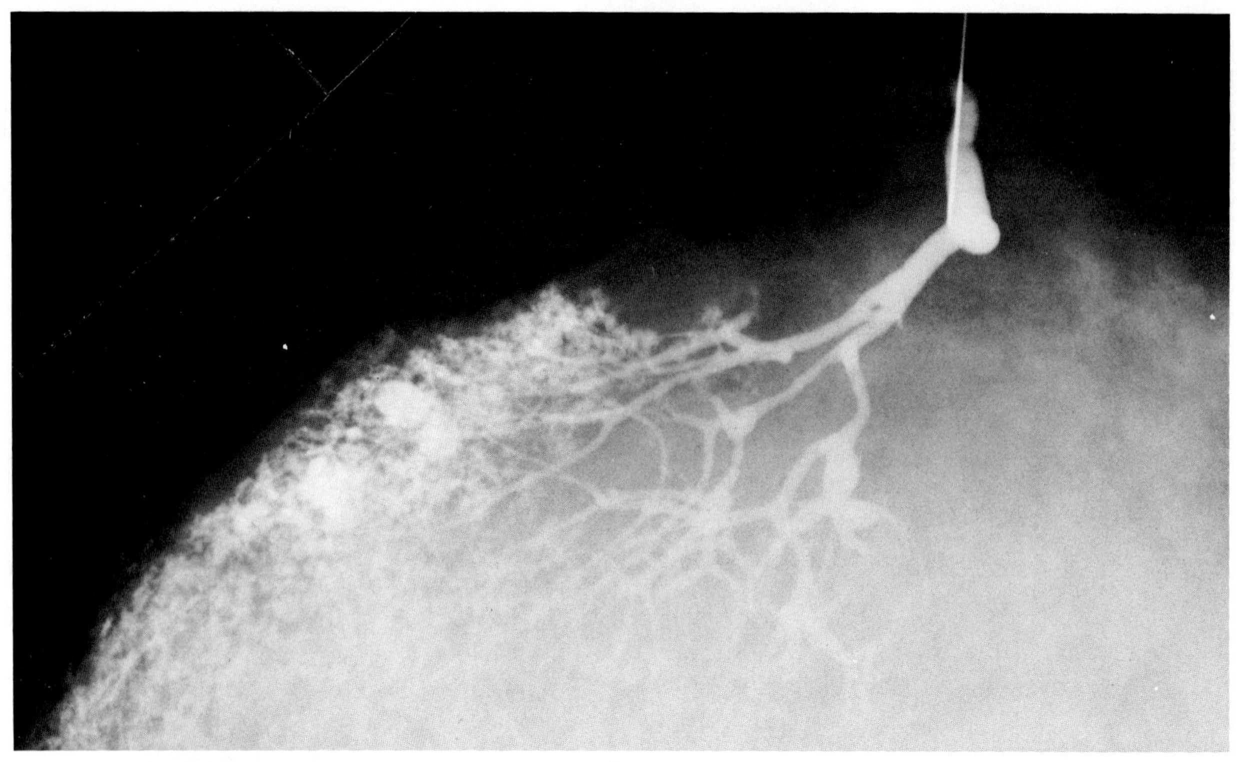
A

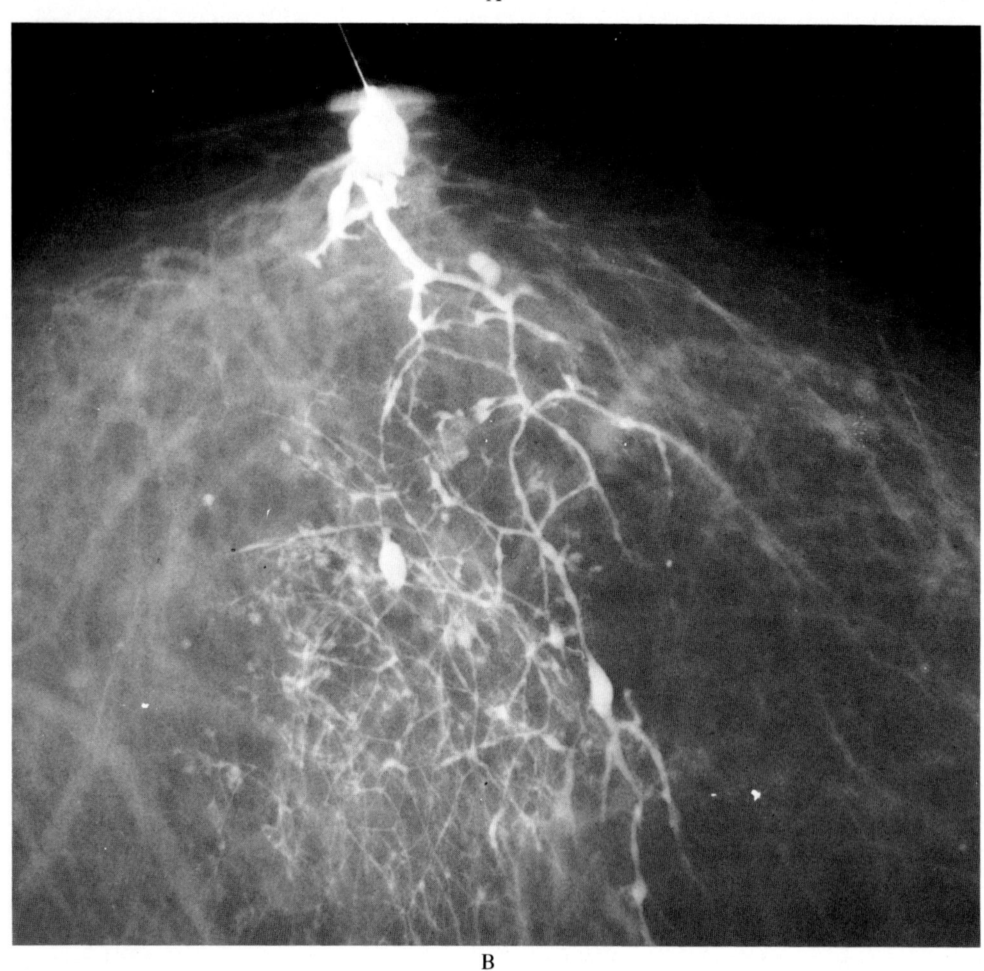
B

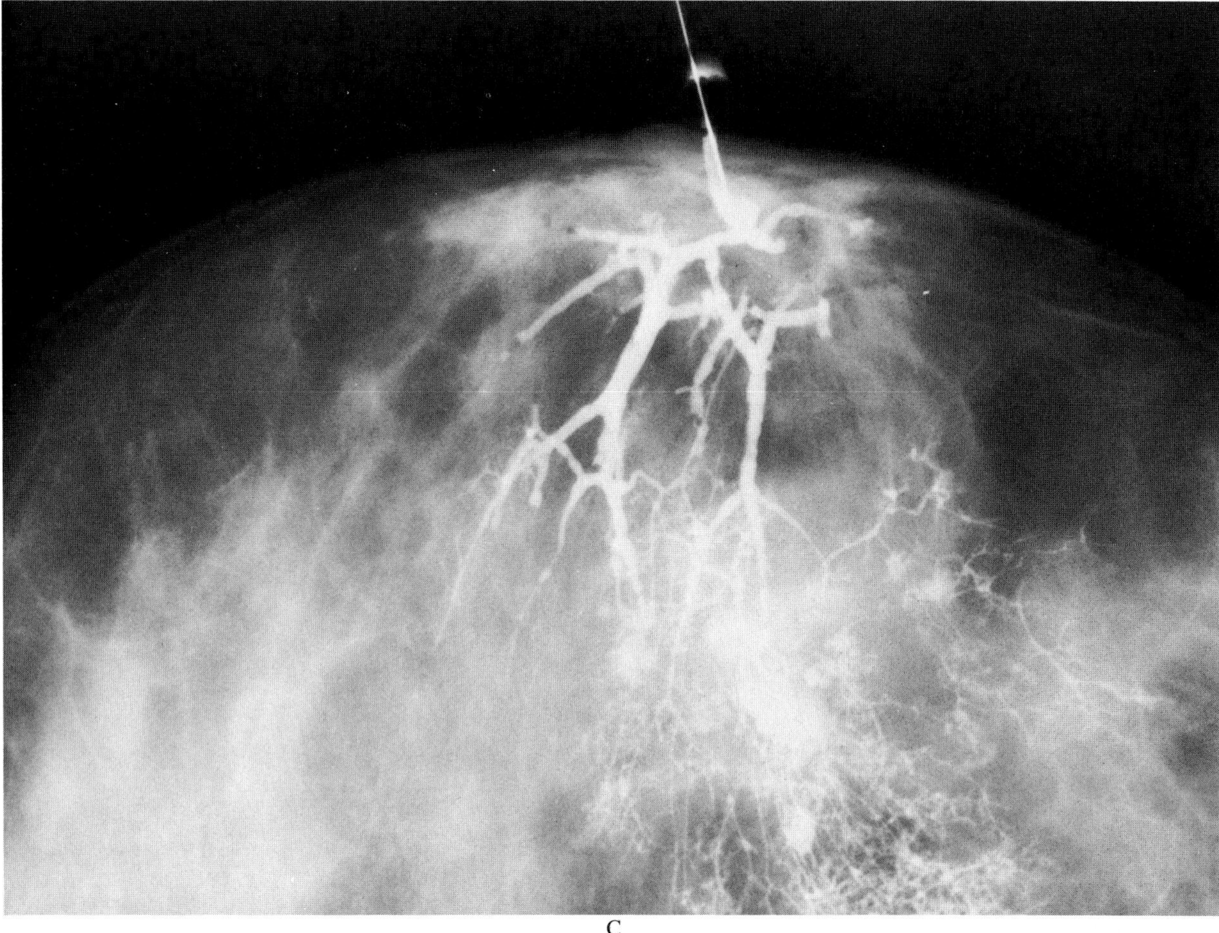

C

Figure 4-3. Secretory disease (ductal ectasia). A. Dilated ducts are most prominent in subareolar region. More flocculent foci of opacification represent lobules. B. Dilated subareolar and central ductal systems, with strikingly narrowed and beaded posterior ductal system. C. Subareolar and central ductal systems are dilated, while foci of narrowing, beading, and obstruction affect posterior system.

diameter, especially in the subareolar and ampullary portions, is characteristic of secretory disease (ductal ectasia). The walls of the dilated ducts are usually smooth, but may occasionally be beaded, with areas of narrowing separated by dilated segments. Figure 4-3A demonstrates a dilated duct system, and Figure 4-3B yet another dilated system with beading in association with secretory disease. Normal opacified branches as well as obstructed branches can be seen. The latter must be carefully evaluated since they could signify malignancy. Figure 4-3C also demonstrates the features of benign secretory disease.

Intraductal masses are easily demonstrated by ductography and typically take two forms: The first is a well-circumscribed radiolucent defect within the duct, varying in size from 1 to 8 mm in diameter and typically closely related to the duct wall (Fig. 4-4A). The second is represented by multiple small to large radiolucent defects (Figs. 4-4B and C). The solitary defect is most often an intraductal papilloma, usually occurring in the ampullary portion of a duct or in an immediately underlying branch. The intranipple portion of the duct system must be carefully filled, since papillomas occasionally occur there. Intraductal hyperplasia may be reflected in multiple small filling defects (Fig. 4-4D), as may clots of blood.

Cysts may opacify during injection (Fig. 4-5), as befits their origin from dilated ducts. The cysts tend to be small, multiple, and in the deep or central portion of the breast.

Occult carcinomas are occasionally identified by ductography (Figs. 4-4D and 4-6). They may appear as irregular masses, usually under 1 cm in diameter. Most commonly, however, they result in a combination of multiple intraluminal defects, ductal strictures and distortions, and blunted foci of obstruction. The ductographic features of breast cancer are similar to the vascular changes seen in angiograms of cancerous organs: regions of distortion, narrowing, and obstruction.

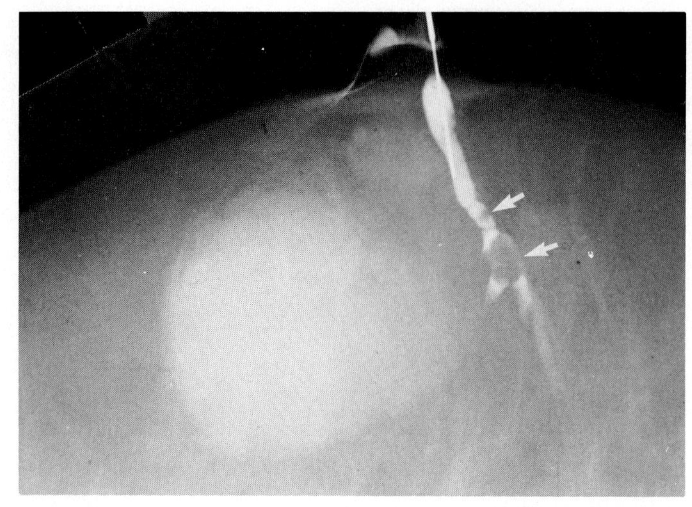

A

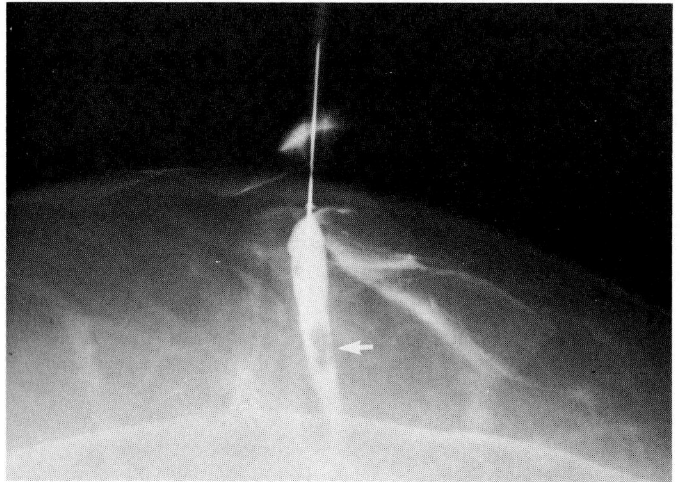

B

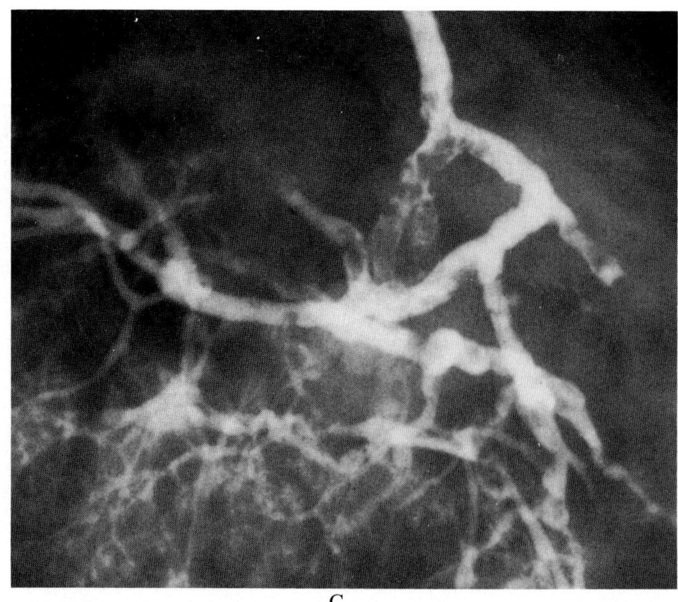

C

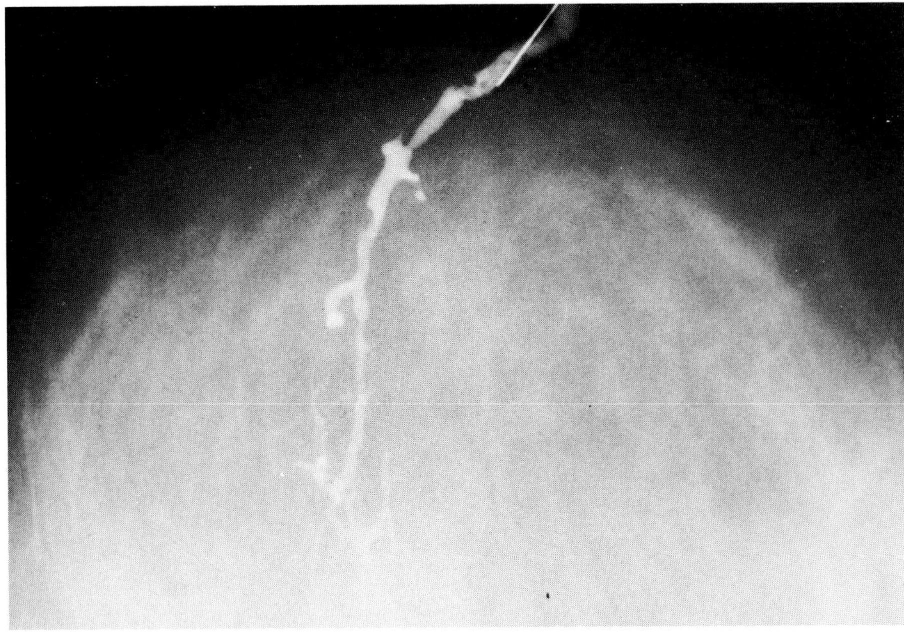

D

Figure 4-4. Intraductal lesions. A. Well-circumscribed filling defects (arrows) are typical of benign lesions. Biopsy yielded intraductal papillomas. B. Large nodular filling defect closely related to duct wall is typical of intraductal papilloma (arrow). Tiny air bubble present in more anterior part of duct was not a constant feature from one exposure to the next. C. Extensive filling defects throughout opacified ducts represent papillomatosis. D. Dilated subareolar duct containing several well-circumscribed radiolucent nodules is typical of intraductal hyperplasia and papillomas. Posteriorly, however, ducts are narrow and irregular, suspicious of their involvement and encasement by malignancy. Biopsy disclosed intraductal hyperplasia in addition to extensive multifocal intraductal carcinoma.

Invasive carcinoma often fails to be outlined by duct injection because the associated fibrous connective tissue envelops the ducts, closing off their lumens. However, some of the opacified ducts in the vicinity of the carcinoma are usually irregular in outline and are discontinuous.

It may be impossible to determine from duct injection whether an abnormality is benign or malignant. Even when ductograms have localized a suspicious area, precise biopsy may be difficult, particularly when the abnormality is not in a major duct. Re-evaluation in 6–12 months with physical examination, mammography, and ductography is essential should any question exist regarding the adequacy of the biopsy.

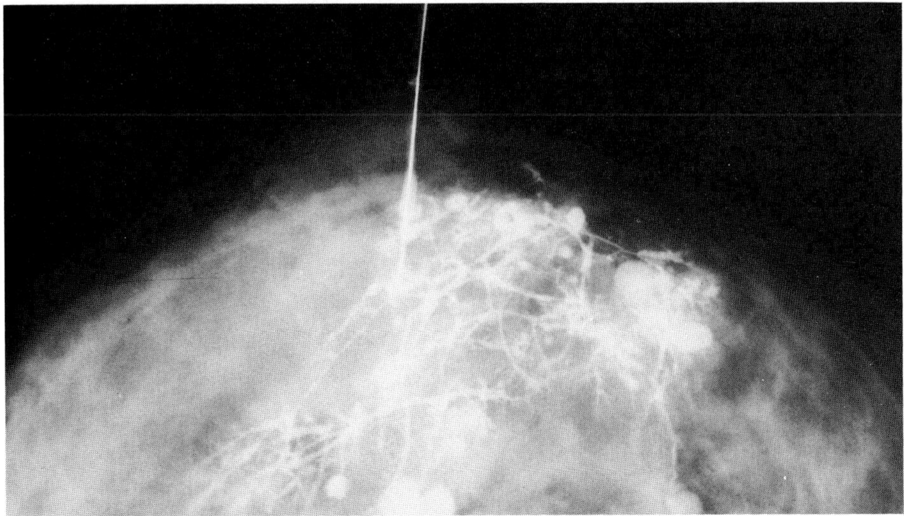

Figure 4-5. Opacification of multiple cysts communicating with ductal system.

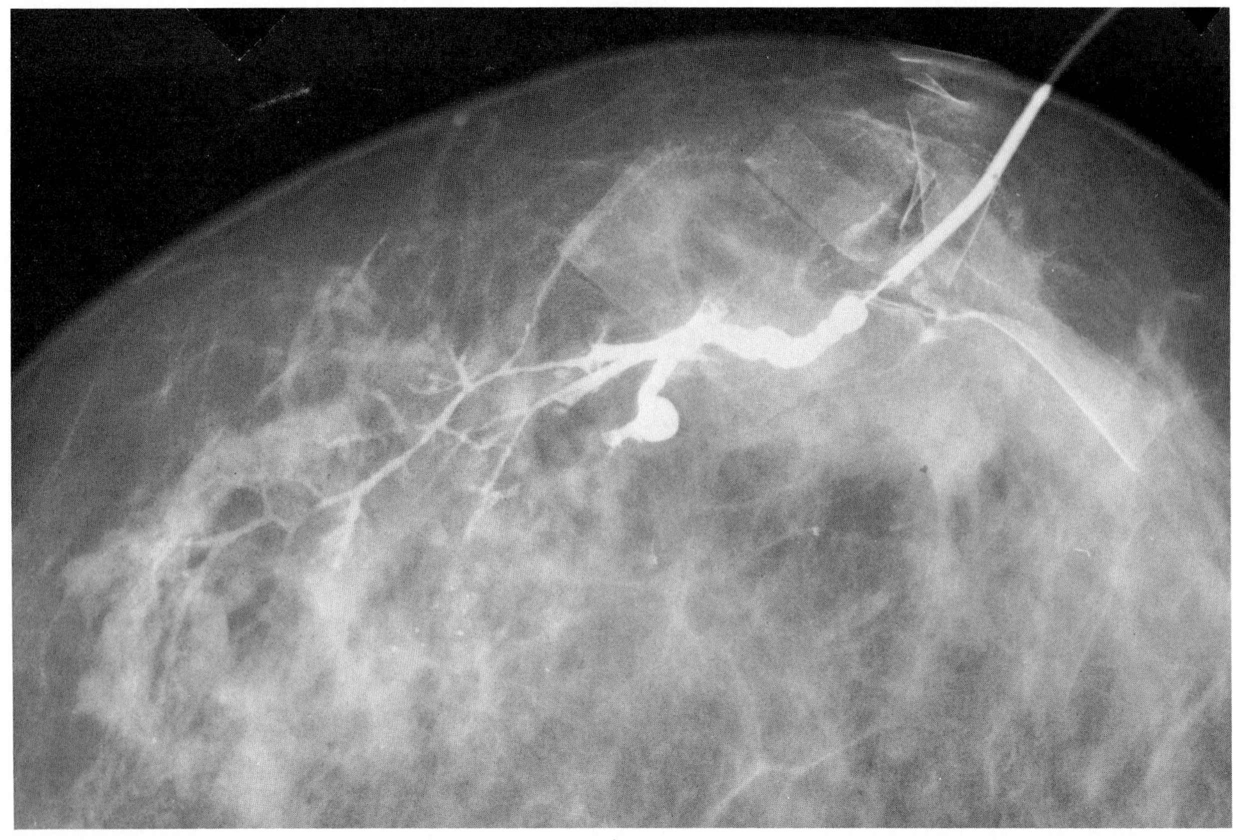

A

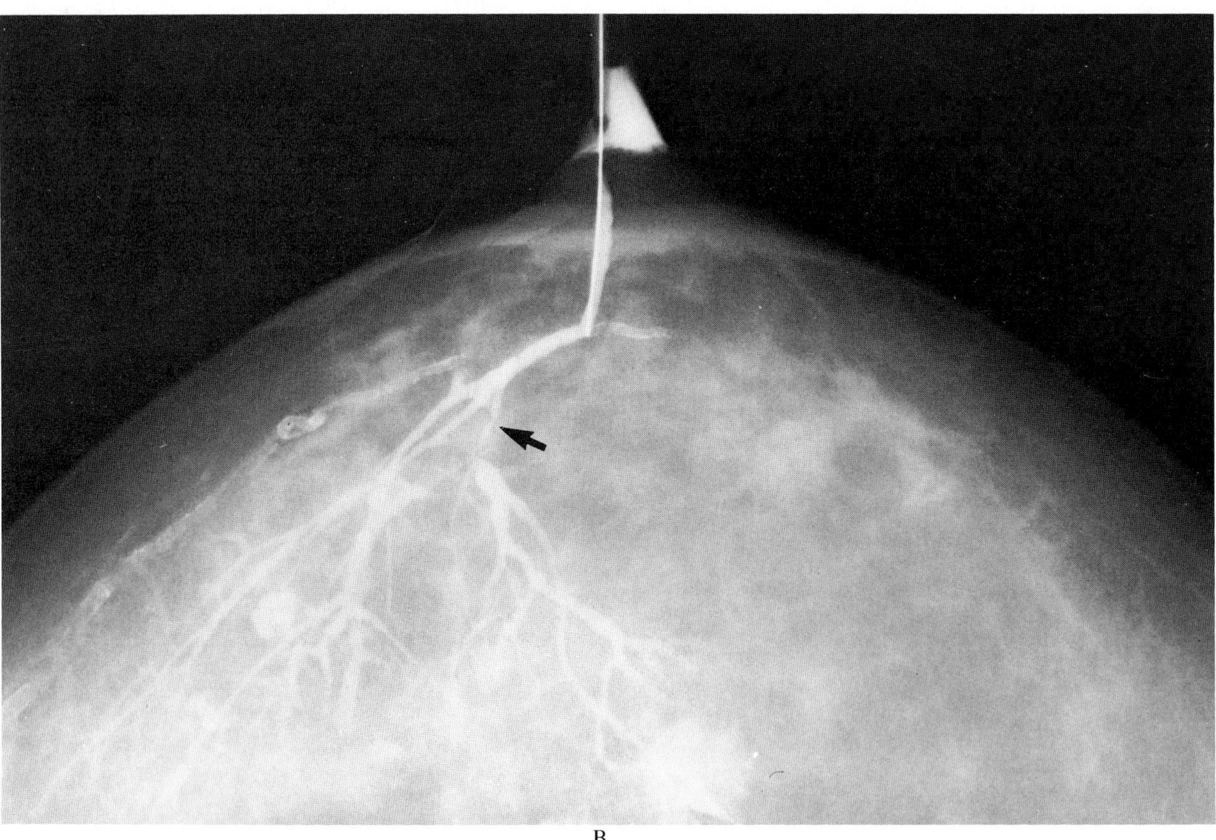

B

Figure 4-6. Occult carcinomas. A. Central ductal system is dilated anteriorly, then abruptly becomes narrow and irregular in contour, and finally becomes obstructed. Narrowed branches reflect intraductal carcinoma. B. Duct near its origin is of normal caliber, but one of its branches is irregularly narrowed (arrow), with distal poststenotic dilatation, findings suspicious of carcinoma. Biopsy revealed intraductal carcinoma.

CONCLUSIONS

We have performed over 400 ductograms between 1970 and 1981. There have been no known reactions, immediate or late, to the contrast material, and no known late sequelae, even in those women in whom extravasation occurred. Ductography is a safe, simple technique for visualization of the duct system in women with significant discharges. It may provide a diagnosis (mass or suspicion of carcinoma), and it localizes the origin of the discharge prior to biopsy. Spontaneous serous, serosanguinous, or bloody discharges (other than bilateral during pregnancy or lactation) necessitate biopsy, utilizing ductography as a guide.

REFERENCES

1. Buhl-Jorgensen SE, Fischermann K, Johansen H, et al: Cancer risk in intraductal papilloma and papillomatosis. Surg Gynecol Obstet 127:1307–1312, 1968
2. DiPietro S, Coopmans D, Gianfranco G, et al: Nipple discharge as a sign of preneoplastic lesion and occult carcinoma of the breast: Clinical and galactographic study in 103 consecutive patients. Tumori 65:317–327, 1979
3. Donnelly B: Nipple discharge: Its clinical and pathologic significance. Ann Surg 131:342–355, 1950
4. Funderburk WW, Syphax B: Evaluation of nipple discharge in benign and malignant disease. Cancer 24:1290–1296, 1969
5. Haagensen CD: Diseases of the Breast. Philadelphia, Saunders, 1971
6. Hicken NF: The roentgenographic diagnosis of breast tumors by means of contrast media. Surg Gynecol Obstet 65:593–603, 1937
7. Kindermann G, Patenok E, Weishaar J, et al: Early detection of ductal breast cancer: The diagnostic procedure for pathological discharge from the nipple. Tumori 65:555–562, 1979
8. Leborgne RA: The Breast in Roentgen Diagnosis. Montevideo, Uruguay, Impresora Uruguaya, 1953
9. Leis HP Jr, Pilnik S, Dursi J, et al: Nipple discharge. Int Surg 58:162–165, 1973
10. McPherson VA, MacKenzie WC: Lesions of the breast associated with nipple discharge: Prognosis after local excision of benign lesions. Can J Surg 5:6–11, 1962
11. Ries E: Diagnostic lipiodol injection into the milk ducts followed by abscess formation. Am J Obstet Gynecol 20:414–416, 1930
12. Romano SA, McFetridge EM: Limitations and dangers of mammography by contrast medium. JAMA 110:1905–1910, 1938
13. Seltzer M, Perloff LJ, Kelley RI, et al: The significance of age in patients with nipple discharge. Surg Gynecol Obstet 131:519–522, 1970
14. Tabár L, Márton Z, Kádas I, et al: Galactography in the examination of secretory breasts. Am J Surg 127:282–286, 1974
15. Threatt BA, Appelman HD: Mammary duct injection. Radiology 108:71–76, 1973
16. Weshler Z, Horn Y, Siew F, et al: Experience with contrast mammography in the diagnosis of various breast diseases. Israel J Med Sci 11:448–457, 1975

Section 4
Benefit and Risk

Myron M. Moskowitz, M.D.

DEFINITION OF TERMS

Aggressive screening by mammography Takes cognizance not only of the classical mammographic signs of malignancy but of indirect signs as well (asymmetrical density, localized architectural distortion, etc.) that could reflect minimal, presymptomatic cancer.

BCDDP The multicenter Breast Cancer Detection Demonstration Project, funded by the American Cancer Society and the National Cancer Institute in the mid-1970s. Volunteer asymptomatic women were screened for breast cancer with mammography, thermography, and physical examination.

Biopsy yield ratios The number of positive results (proven cancers) per number of biopsies performed. Can be expressed as a percentage.

Breast self-examination (BSE) Women are taught to systematically palpate their own breasts. Performed monthly, this practice will, it is to be hoped, reveal breast cancer at the earliest time it is palpable.

Cincinnati BCDDP One of the 27 centers participating in the BCDDP project.

Clinically occult cancer Cancer evident on mammography but not on physical examination. Physical examination has limitations in breasts that are large, that manifest fibrocystic disease, or that contain tumors deep in the breast. Therefore, clinically occult tumors are not necessarily small, and for larger occult tumors the prognosis may not be as good as for minimal cancers.

HIP Breast cancer screening study undertaken by the Health Insurance Plan (HIP) of Greater New York in the 1960s. Randomly selected and matched cohorts of screened (yearly mammography and physical examination) and nonscreened groups were compared.

Incidence screening Regular annual screening examinations following the initial or prevalence screen.

Interval cancer Cancer detected in the course of a usual clinical case finding after a *completely negative screening examination* and before the next regularly scheduled annual examination.

Lead-time bias The concept that detecting a lesion earlier than usual may result only in an *apparent* increased survival rather than really adding years to the total lifetime. This concept would be especially true if many tiny cancers detected by screening would *never* reach clinical threshold if left undetected and untreated.

Length-bias sampling Since breast cancers grow at different rates, the efficacy of screening examinations depends on the biology of the cancer (rate of growth), the effectiveness of the screening modality (how small a cancer can be detected by the modality, i.e., threshold sensitivity), and the time interval between screens.

Linear hypothesis of the carcinogenic effects of ionizing radiation The carcinogenic effects of radiation observed at very high dose levels can be expected to apply in linear extrapolation to very low levels of radiation, but on a much smaller scale. This is a conservative estimate of the dose-response relationship at low levels of radiation.

Minimal breast cancers Noninvasive cancers, whether wholly intraductal or in situ lobular, or, if invasive, 5 mm or less in size without demonstrable spread beyond the breast. When treated, these cancers are considered to have an excellent chance for cure.

Mortality analysis Based on a comparison between the number of patients in a control population of well persons who die because of a disease, e.g., breast cancer, and the number who die with this same disease in a study population of well women.

BREAST CANCER DETECTION
ISBN 0-8089-1842-7

Prevalence screen The initial screening examination of a population.

Screening examinations Survey examinations conducted to detect abnormalities in asymptomatic people, either in the general population or in specific groups. The subject population may be selected because of its proclivity to a condition, e.g., women in a high-risk category for breast cancer.

Staging (clinical) of breast cancer A method to indicate the extent of disease prior to therapy by assessment of tumor growth, spread to primary lymph nodes, and metastasis. Staging assists in communicating clinical information, deciding on treatment, and judging prognosis. (See Table 1-1.)

Survival data Based on the percentage of patients with a particular disease, e.g., breast cancer, who are alive at any defined point in time after discovery and/or treatment.

BENEFITS OF MAMMOGRAPHY

One of the most perplexing problems facing mammographers is to critically define and quantify the benefit from their work. While early diagnosis or detection of breast cancer may be a laudable goal, does it truly benefit the patient? This section will attempt to clarify some of the problems associated with estimating benefits. Using available data, we will try to point out reasonable answers to questions posed by these problems.

First, let us assume that a patient had a palpable mass, with no other significant clinical signs, and that mammography was not done. The mass was unsuccessfully aspirated, and subsequent biopsy showed cancer.

Now, let us assume another scenario for the same patient. Mammography was done, the mammographic diagnosis was cancer, and biopsy verified the diagnosis. Can this be defined as a benefit resulting from mammography? Biopsy was still necessary, the stage at detection was not altered, the ultimate outcome for the patient was not changed, and the total cost was increased.

If a negative or benign mammographic diagnosis had been rendered and biopsy had been deferred, it is possible that the ultimate outcome would have been altered for the worse. In point of fact, the data of Burns et al.,[15] Devitt,[19] and Lesnick[44] show that deferred biopsy is a potential risk of mammography. A review of 13 reported series[2,5,16,17,25,26,31,41,43,53,59,72,81] indicates that the true-positive (sensitivity) rate of mammography for the diagnosis of cancer ranged from a low of 65 percent to a high of 97 percent. The true-positive rate in 11 of the 13 series was in the 70–88 percent range, and the average true-positive rate was 83 percent. In most of the reports, a negative mammogram did not sufficiently exclude neoplasm to preclude biopsy of a palpable abnormality.

In our experience with an asymptomatic, self-selected population in the Cincinnati Breast Cancer Detection Demonstration Project, a negative mammogram reduced the likelihood of cancer being present by a factor of 10. Of 600 radiographically benign masses over 1 cm in size, palpable and nonpalpable, only 2 percent were malignant. Of these malignancies, however, 6 were highly curable minimal cancers. While it might be argued that these statistics favor mammographic observation over biopsy, one could equally argue that biopsy and/or aspiration are the preferred diagnostic procedures.

What, then, is the benefit of mammography? Mammography can do what no other available test can do: consistently detect a significant number of cancers of the breast at an earlier stage of development than heretofore possible.[1–3,8,10,12,14,18,21,30,36,37,41–43,46,49,51–53,56–58,61–63,66,71,75,76,83,84]

It has been generally assumed by most of the medical community that this early detection and diagnosis of breast cancer would alter the natural history of the disease and add years to patients' lives. Until recently, however, due to certain reasonable, theoretical considerations (to be discussed below), we have not been able, without reservation, to state this as the case. We now, without equivocation, can state that, for breast cancer, earlier detection does improve patient outcome and, even more important, that screening for breast cancer is an effective tool for control of breast cancer in a population of women over age 40.

This statement can be made without equivocation because of two landmark, controlled trials,[68,79] and the outcome of two other case control studies.[18,84] Let us examine this a little further.

One cannot assume that earlier detection, and an apparent increased survival, is meaningful, because of the Scylla and Charybdis of lead-time bias and length-bias sampling. These biases will be discussed in more detail subsequently. Suffice it to say that: (1) lead-time bias assumes that earlier detection than the usual state-of-affairs (lead-time) adds only time from observation to the usual detection level, and that no time is added to true survival (Figs. 1-1 and 1-2); and (2) length-bias sampling assumes that periodic screening tends to find slower-growing cancers, and that the more rapidly growing cancers become evident between screens or as advanced disease on follow-up screening (Fig. 1-3).

Both of these biases preclude using survival as an endpoint of benefit. In order to satisfactorily eliminate these biases from consideration, one needs to perform a controlled trial of early detection and use mortality outcome as a measure of effectiveness.

Because the dependent variable, mortality (the number of breast cancer deaths in a defined population of women, most of whom do not have breast cancer) represents an otherwise constant "force," any alteration linked to changing an independent variable, i.e., screening, indicates a meaningful effect. Use of a control group, and including for analysis all women offered

Table 1-1
Clinical Staging of Breast Cancer

Primary Tumor (T)	
TX	Tumor cannot be assessed
T0	No evidence of primary tumor
TIS	Paget's disease of the nipple with no demonstrable tumor
	(Note: Paget's disease with a demonstrable tumor is classified according to the size of the tumor.)
T1*	Tumor 2 cm or less in greatest diameter
T1a	No fixation to underlying pectoral fascia or muscle
T1b	Fixation to underlying pectoral fascia and/or muscle
	i tumor ≤ 0.5 cm i tumor > 0.5 ≤ 1.0 cm iii tumor > 1.0 ≤ 2.0 cm
T2*	Tumor more than 2 cm but not more than 5 cm in its greatest dimension
T2a	No fixation to underlying pectoral fascia or muscle
T2b	Fixation to underlying pectoral fascia and/or muscle
T3*	Tumor more than 5 cm in its greatest dimension
T3a	No fixation to underlying pectoral fascia or muscle
T3b	Fixation to underlying pectoral fascia and/or muscle
T4	Tumor of any size with direct extension to chest wall or skin
	(Note: Chest wall includes ribs, intercostal muscles, and serratus anterior muscle, but not pectoral muscle.)
T4a	Fixation to chest wall
T4b	Edema (including peau d' orange), ulceration of the skin of the breast, or satellite skin nodules confined to the same breast
T4c	Both of the above

Lymph Nodes (N)	
NX	Regional lymph nodes cannot be assessed clinically
N0	Homolateral axillary lymph nodes not considered to contain growth
N1	Movable homolateral axillary nodes considered to contain growth
N2	Homolateral axillary nodes considered to contain growth and fixed to one another or to other structures
N3	Homolateral supraclavicular or infraclavicular nodes considered to contain growth, or edema fo the arm.†

Distant Metastases (M)	
MX	Minimum requirements to assess the presence of distant metastasis cannot be met
M0	No (known) distant metastasis
M1	Distant metastasis present

Clinical Diagnostic stage

Stage TIS	in situ
Stage X	Cannot stage

	Tumor growth	Spread to lymph nodes	Metastasis
Stage I	T1ai	N0	M0
	T1ii	N0	M0
	T1aiii	N0	M0
	T1bi	N0	M0
	T1bii	N0	M0
	Tbiii	N0	M0
Stage II	T0	N1a or 1b	M0
	T1a or T1b	N1a or 1b	M0
	T2a or T2b	N0	M0
	T2a or T2b	N1a or 1b	M0
Stage IIIa	T0	N2	M0
	T1a or T1b	N2	M0
	T2a or T2b	N2	M0
	T3a or T3b	N0	M0
	T3a or T3b	N1	M0
	T3a or T3b	N2	M0
Stage IIIb	Ant T	N3	Any M
	Any T4	Any N	Any M
Stage VI	Any T	Any N	Any M1

From Manual for Staging of Cancer. second edition. American Joint Committee on Cancer, Philadelphia, Lippincott, 1983, pp 127–133. With permission.

Note: Cases of inflammatory carcinoma should be reported separately.

* Dimpling of the skin, nipple retraction, or any skin changes except those in T4b may occur in T1, T2, or T3 without affecting the classification.

† Edema of the arm may be caused by lymphatic obstruction and lymph nodes may not then be palpable.

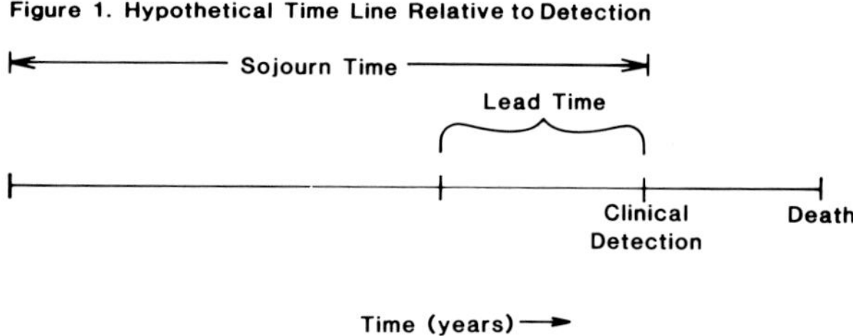

Figure 1-1. Hypothetical time line relative to detection.

screening in the study group, controls for the effects of: (1) length-bias sampling; (2) lead-time bias; (3) self-selection bias; (4) diagnostic bias; and (5) secular trends. There are now reported two such prospective, controlled trials.

The first study, the HIP project, was a matched cohort study, and the second study, the Falun, Sweden study, was a population-based trial. Two case control studies from Nijmegen[83,84] and Utrecht[18] in the Netherlands have also been done. All studies demonstrate a 30–40 percent reduction in the mortality associated with breast cancer.

However, while screening was offered to women over age 40 in the HIP, Falun, and Nijmegen trials, early- and intermediate-term mortality reduction has been shown only for women age 50 and older at entry. In HIP, the only study available for longer term follow-up (10 years or more), there is a delayed mortality reduction in younger women. It begins at the seventh year after entry and is equal in incremental difference from the controls to the difference from the controls seen in older women. Although this difference in mortality is not statistically significant, statistical significance in this age group would not be expected because insufficient numbers of young women were enrolled in the HIP study. It is estimated that for women age 40–49, about 300,000–700,000 women would have been needed in both the control and study groups in order to see a statistically significant difference at a reasonable confidence level. In this study only 60,000 women were present in the entire cohort at all ages, about two-thirds of whom were age 40–49.

Another interesting side-finding that is developing from the Falun data[79] is that the rate of advanced cancers in the study group also decreased over time, and that this decrease appears to begin about one year prior to the decrease in deaths. Thus, it may be possible to judge the effectiveness of screening by substituting the number of advanced cancers as a surrogate for mortality when comparing the study and control populations.

Therefore, taken as a whole, these data mean that early detection undoubtedly adds time to life and, in some cases, the patients may be cured. For populations of women over age 50, screening, as done in the aforementioned studies, can impinge on sufficient numbers of cases in the total population examined to exert a salutary effect on the whole population.

While it is possible to attribute the lack of demonstrable, short-term benefit in young women to the biology of the disease, it seems unlikely that this is the whole explanation. In the Cincinnati BCDDP, for women age 35–49 at entry, the 10-year survival of all cases that occurred during the time that screening was offered (*including* those detected as interval cases within 1–11 months after the last screen) was 95 percent. If one excludes noninvasive cancers, the 10-year survival was 88 percent. Therefore, biology alone does not seem to be the sole answer to the question as to why evidence of short-term benefit in younger women was lacking. Let us look for other possible explanations.

You will recall that length-bias and lead-time bias have been invoked in the past to explain why screening, theoretically, *would not* work. Failure to account for these biases in design and conduct of the experiment *will assure* that screening will not work.

Lead-time Bias

Remember that lead time (Fig. 1-1) represents the added time one gains by detecting cancers when they are generally smaller than the usual size detected under

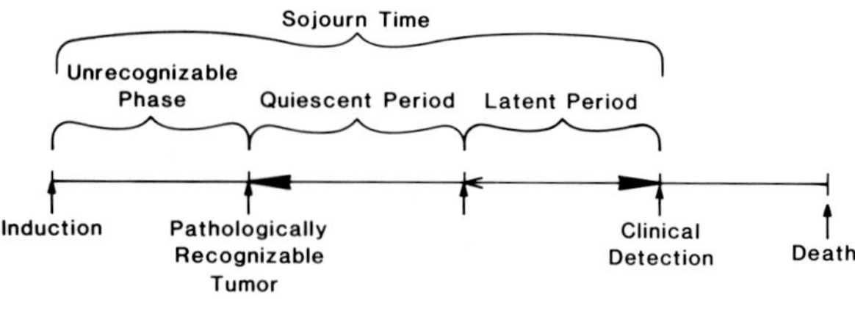

Figure 1-2. Hypothetical time line of breast cancer.

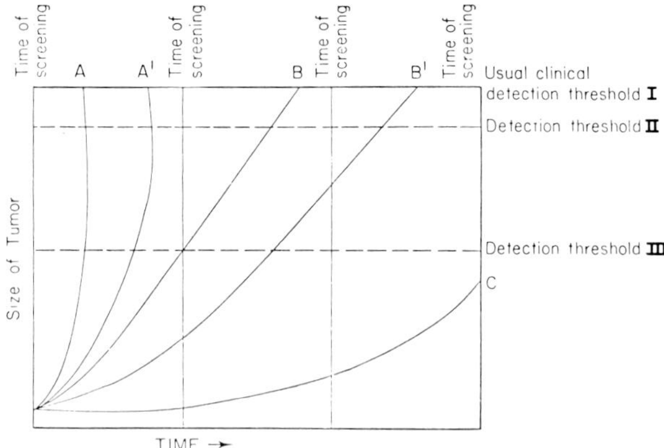

Figure 1-3. Relationship between tumor growth rate, threshold sensitivity, time between screens, and interval cancers. From Milbrath JR, Moskowitz M, Bauermeister DE: Breast cancer screening. CRC Crit Rev Diagn Imaging 16:207, 1981. With permission.

normal clinical conditions. It is the *goal* of screening to achieve this gain in time and, by lowering the threshold at detection, dip into future incidence, i.e., detect cases that would have presented as larger tumors at some time in the future. It is possible, however, that instead of dipping into a pool of potential future incident cancers, we are dipping into a pool of stagnant, inactive lesions, never-to-become clinical cancers.

For example (Fig. 1-2), let us assume that the point of induction of the normal cell begins the presymptomatic period of tumor growth. However, until morphologic changes appear which are recognizable as cancer by light microscopy, one cannot know when this happens. The time from the point of induction to that of clinical detection can be considered the sojourn time. Within the period of sojourn time, there is a phase during which tumor cells proliferate, regress, or, perhaps, remain stable. At some point in this period, however, a change in the equation occurs, and the equilibrium shifts "to the right." Of those lesions that reach this second phase, a few may stabilize or regress, but most will proceed inexorably to clinical detection. They proceed at varying rates depending on the host and the biology of the tumor.[35] This period, within the sojourn time, might well be called the "latent" period, and the first period could be called the "resting" or "quiescent" period.

In this scenario, under ideal circumstances the lead time and latent period will superimpose and become one and the same. A shift too far to the left in screening sensitivity will identify an excess number of cases that would otherwise never reach clinical detection. A minimal shift to the left will detect cases that, although clinically occult, will have passed beyond the point of curability.

In our series, most of the cancer cases detected by screening seem to have been detected in *this latent period* of the sojourn time. For example, in young women during the time of screening, about 35–40 percent of the cases were contributed by "minimal" breast cancers. If these cancers were in the quiescent phase and incapable of progressing, then the cancer detection rate *after* the cessation of screening should be only 60–65 percent of the screening rate. However, within 17–18 months of cessation, the incidence rate in these women was slightly higher than the screened rate.

Therefore, while screening by mammography and clinical examination is far from perfect, it would appear that aggressive screening in women age 40–49 with mammography and clinical examination detects cancers which, if left unattended, would go on to present as "killing" cancers. This is also borne out by recent autopsy data.[60] Therefore, it appears that for these women the lead time gained by current screening methods is probably not longer than the latency period.

Length-bias Sampling

Fox has suggested that there are two types of breast cancers: fast growers and slow growers.[33] Periodic screening will tend to detect the slower growing tumors at an early stage, while rapidly growing tumors may present betweens screens or may be detected at an advanced stage, even in the face of regular annual screening.[50] The implication is that the ultimate outcome for a given patient may be more dependent on tumor biology than on early detection. This is obviously correct to some degree.

However, the effect of length-biased sampling reflects the interplay of: (1) the biology of the tumor (rate of growth); (2) the effectiveness of the screen; and (3) the interval between examinations. If the time interval selected is equal to or longer than the lead time over usual clinical detection, gained by screening, much of the benefit of screening will be vitiated.

The effect of length-biased sampling can be estimated by (1) interval cancer rate, and (2) the *overall* threshold sensitivity of the screening examination. If many cancers in a given population have rapid growth rates, one should expect to see an increased number of interval cancers. Interval cancers can be defined as those that are detected in the course of usual clinical case finding after a *completely negative screen* and before the next regularly scheduled annual examination. (A cancer that has been detected as a result of a short-term follow-up of an abnormality detected on a screening visit is not considered an interval cancer.)

While rapid tumor growth rate or inordinately long intervals between screens may be reasons for interval cancers to appear, another reason may be the failure to maximize the threshold-lowering effect of the screening examination. In Figure 1-3, tumor size is plotted against time, and several hypothetical tumor rates are presented. Threshold I represents the size of tumor found at the usual clinical threshold; threshold II represents a screen whose sensitivity for size is not much below usual clinical threshold; and threshold III represents a screen whose size threshold is markedly smaller than that of either of the first two. For simplicity, all tumors are represented as starting at point 0. Periodic screens are indicated by vertical lines. For a tumor having a growth rate of either A or A′, neither of the two depicted screens is effective in detecting the tumor before it reaches the clinical threshold. A tumor growth rate of C would be found by both screens. A tumor growing at the rate of B or B′ would develop as an interval cancer for a screen with threshold II, while a screen with threshold III would have found the tumor when it was a small lesion. A screen of threshold II would thus only detect one of these hypothetical tumors and would leave all the rest as interval cancers. A screen with threshold III would detect more of the lesions, would detect them at a much earlier stage, and would leave only a few as interval lesions. It is obvious from this example that if many of the tumors have growth rates A or A′, all the screens would have a high-interval cancer rate.

It is also obvious that if the interval between screens were increased, even in the case of screens with threshold III, interval cancers would increase. It is

Table 1-2
Mean Detection Lead Time Gained by Screening a Randomly Selected Population

Age	Projected by Model of Fox, Moskowitz, et al.[34] years	Observed in Controlled Study (Tábar)[79] years
Under 50	2.1 ± 0.5	2.52
45–54	2.0 ± 0.5	. . .
50–54	. . .	1.52
55–64	3.2 ± 0.6	. . .
55–69	. . .	3.27
60–69	. . .	4.52
65–74	4.7 ± 1.3	. . .
70+	. . .	4.08

therefore imperative to screen at intervals significantly shorter than the lead time gained over usual clinical detection. A reasonable rule of thumb would be to screen at intervals equal to one-half of the expected lead time.

It should be parenthetically noted that the effect of length-bias sampling is best seen in the initial or prevalence year. Here, slower growing tumors, present for a long time, are relatively abundant.

Expected Effects of Failing to Account for These Biases When Designing and Conducting A Screen

1. The rate of interval cancers would be excessive.
2. An excessive number of advanced cancers would develop.
3. The survival of cases detected at the second screen (i.e., first incidence year) would be poorer than the survival of cases detected at the first screen and poorer than the survival of those interval cases occurring between screens.

Observed Impact of Length-bias and Lead-time Effects

In order to evaluate these effects, we need to know a little more about the controlled studies already cited.

The HIP study was performed in the 1960s, and mammography and clinical examination were offered annually. However, due to the technology extant at that time, mammography alone did not detect many of the cases in women under age 50. In HIP women over age 50, about 42 percent of cases were found by mammography alone,[3] while less than 20 percent of cases in younger women were found by mammography alone. In the BCDDP, started a decade later,[3] mammography alone was responsible for detecting about 40 percent of cases in both age groups.

The Swedish and Dutch studies did not offer clinical examination. Only a single mediolateral oblique mammogram was performed. For younger women it was done ever 2 years, and for older women every 3 years. How do these planned screen intervals compare with lead time that is gained by screening?

Using early data generated by several Breast Cancer Detection Demonstration Projects, Fox and I developed a model projecting lead-time estimates gained by screening a randomly selected population (Table 1-2). We estimated that for women age 35–49 at entry, the mean lead time gained over usual clinical detection would be about 2.1 ± .5 years, and for women over age 50 at entry about 3.2 ± .6 years.[55]

It can be estimated from the BCDDP data[3] that the range of lead-time estimates varies with the age at screening (Table 1-3). While admittedly these data are derived from a self-selected population, the population base is huge, i.e., 280,000. The number of cancers is similarly large, in excess of 5000. For women age 35–39 at entry, the maximum lead time gained can be estimated to be about one year. As the patient population ages, lead times approaching 3 years are gained.

Schwartz[64] has reported a model estimating the effect of lead-time and length-biased sampling. This model estimates a 2-year lead time for the HIP study and a 3-year lead time for current screens. Using the same data, Hutchinson and Shapiro estimated a lead time of 10 months, Zelen 2.36 years, and Kirch and Klein 14 months.[64] Considering the size and stage of tumors detected in the HIP study and the interval cancer rate, I believe that a shorter lead time for that study is more likely, perhaps as short as 1 year.

Thus far, the lead times noted above have been estimates based on mathematical calculations. A more direct way to estimate lead time is to determine the incidence of breast cancer during screening and in the post-screening years. Since screening should dip into future incidence, there should be a drop in annual incidence for some period until the newly appearing cancers reach the size for detection threshold extant in the general community. When that point is reached, annual incidence will equal screen incidence. The time

Table 1-3
Age-specific Lead Time*

	All BCDDPs
35–39	1
40–44	1.5
45–49	1.8
50–54	2.4
55–59	2.25
60–64	2.6
65–69	2.6
70–74	2.6

* in years

required to reach the usual incidence will represent the mean lead time gained over usual clinical detection.

We have done this direct measurement in Cincinnati, and the age-specific lead times are: age 35–49, about 2 years, and for age 50 and older about 3.5–4 years.

The variation in lead time is important in relation to interval cancers. One would expect that if the lead time gained over usual clinical detection is shorter in one age group and the screen interval is not correspondingly shortened to account for this, more cases of cancer would occur between screens than would if the lead time is longer. Thus, if one screened at the end of lead time or beyond, there would be an excess number of interval cases.

In the BCDDP, where women of all ages were screened at annual intervals, there is a decreasing rate of interval cancers with increasing age (Table 1-2), coinciding with a prolongation of lead time. In the youngest women, screened at the end of their expected lead time, a higher rate of interval cancers did indeed occur. When the screen interval was half of the lead time, the interval cancer rates were the lowest.

The Swedish trial and the Dutch study used a screen interval of a little over 2 years for younger women and about 3 years for older women. The age-specific interval rates are not yet published from the Falun trial, but note that in the *younger* women in the Dutch trial (Table 1-4) the reported interval cancer rate is 56 percent. In the older women, the interval cancer rate is only 28 percent. In both age groups these interval rates are several times greater than the corresponding interval rate occurring between annual screens in Cincinnati, and are greater than the interval cancer rates already shown by age in the whole BCDDP.

There is another pernicious effect of extending the lead time beyond appropriate intervals. If this is done a meaningful portion of cancers that are of intermediate-to-longer growth rates will be detected at screening, however, they will be found at a point in their life cycle beyond which cure is possible. The combination of these two effects should result in an overall excess in stage II cancers. In the Nijmegen study, *excluding in situ cancers*, 49 percent of cases occurring in young women were stage II disease. In older women, 36 percent were stage II.

In the HIP breast cancer screening program in the 1960s, only 60 percent of the cancers were detected through the screening process.[65,67,73,74] A significant number of minimal cancers were not found.[80] In the Cincinnati BCDDP, 10 years after the HIP study, when 40 percent of the cancers were minimal, 93 percent of the cancers were found by the combined mammography/physical examination screen, including those found during the prevalence year. In a screen[38,39] consisting of physical breast examination alone, only 55 percent of cancers were found.

During the years 1973–1975, the importance of finding minimal breast cancers was not widely appreciated. Indeed, the mammographic criteria for identifying minimal cancers were not widely known.[36,37] Up to that time, the emphasis was on detecting "clinically occult" lesions.

Table 1-4
Screen Sensitivity by Age in Nijmegen*

	# of TP	TP Rate	FP Rate	% of Stage 2+
Birth cohort 1925–1939	42/96	44%	56%	49%
Birth cohort 1910–1924	100/138	72%	28%	36%

* Note that in younger women, 56% of cases occurred between screens (interval cancers), while in older women this rate was halved.
TP = true positive; FP = false positive.

In the combined BCDDPs (1973–1975), 25 percent of all prevalent cancers occurred as interval cancers within 3 months of a negative screening examination.[6–8] In that same time in Cincinnati, where aggressive screening was performed, about 5 percent of cancers occurred within 12 months of a negative screen. In Tabar's current screening project in Sweden,[78] only about 3 percent of cancers were found within 12 months of a negative prevalence screen.

Clearly, altering the threshold sensitivity can alter interval cancer rates. Improvements in mammographic technology and interpretation are the major factors in detecting earlier cancers.

Recall that according to the theory of length-bias sampling, screening tends to detect the slower growing cancers, and the most rapidly growing tumors occur between screens. It is these interval cancers that should have the poorest prognosis. If, however, one artificially increases the effect of length-bias sampling by increasing the lead time between screens, some relatively slower growing tumors will present as interval cancers and an apparent improvement in the survival of the interval cases will occur. Conversely, some number of cases detected at the artificially delayed second screening will be more advanced than anticipated, and this should decrease the overall survival for the incidence group. This, of course, is the opposite of the anticipated effect of screening.

The survival rate of prevalence cases should be best because a significant portion of prevalence cases will be slower growing tumors. Indeed, in the Nijmegen screen, where, we suggest, that for young women the interval between screening exceeds the appropriate interval by a factor of two, the worst survival rate occurs not in the interval cases, but in the cases detected at the incidence or second screening, again reinforcing our hypothesis about appropriate screen intervals.

Even in the older women in the Swedish trial, the effect of a long screening interval is suggested. For example, in HIP, where screening was done every year with mammography and clinical examination, a mortality decrease first became apparent at 3 years and was quite clear by 5. In the Swedish study, where intervals were 3 years and no clinical examination was performed, mortality reduction is really not clear until 7 years post-entry. Since it would be difficult to repeat either of these two studies, screening every 2 years for women over age 50 would probably be a safer strategy.

Summary

Thus far, we have clearly seen that experimental evidence proves that screening women over age 40 for breast cancer reduces mortality by about 30–40 percent. While the maximal early effect has been shown to occur in women over age 50, a delayed benefit has been seen in the 40–49 age group in one such controlled trial.

If an early mortality reduction in the 40–49 age group is to be achieved, it will probably be necessary to: screen the women yearly; to use two-view breast mammography; to offer clinical examination as well as mammography; and to utilize high-quality, low-dose mammography performed by highly skilled technologists, and interpreted by radiologists dedicated to the concept of breast imaging. For women over age 50, screening with only a mediolateral oblique view every 3 years has been shown to be effective. Screening at least every 2 years in this age group would probably offer a wider margin of safety and would be more cost effective than annual screening.

In younger women the margin for error is relatively slim; if the medical community is not willing to accept the difficult challenge posed by these women, it would be better to defer screening until age 50.

RISKS OF MAMMOGRAPHY

Detailed descriptions of the methods for estimating the risks associated with mammography, as well as the controversy surrounding these estimates, have been published elsewhere.[9,13,27–29,45,69,70,77,82] Rather than concentrate on a detailed critique or evaluation of that ongoing scientific ferment, we will present a summary of the salient theoretical points:

1. Ionizing radiation at high-dose levels is a carcinogen.
2. The breast is sensitive to radiation.
3. Risk estimates for breast cancer induction at high x-ray dose rates and total doses have been made, and in several different series there is a striking linkage of data suggesting that the risk estimates for high-dose radiation are real. In the high-dose ranges, the effects seem to be linear.
4. Little is known about the oncogenic effect of radiation in the diagnostic low-energy, low-dose range used in mammography. In this low-dose range, it is not known whether the effects are linear.[27,70] Recently reported work by Miller et al.[48] strongly suggests that the effect of radiation at low-dose rates is quadratic, or quadratic-linear. This implies a threshold effect, and the dose at this threshold is 50–75 rads. Considering that modern mammography, when well controlled and monitored, delivers about 0.06–0.15 rads per exam, 167 annual exams could be given before this threshold was reached.
5. For breast cancer induction there is unquestionably an age relationship as well as a dose relationship. It would seem from the data generated by the atomic bomb blast in Japan,[9,27,29,45,70,82] the data of Baral et al.,[4] in Sweden, as well as re-evaluation of the work of Myrden and Hiltz,[47] that the risk of oncogenesis for women over age 40 at the time of initial radiation is perhaps half the risk of women age 10–19. Indeed re-evaluation of the Nova Scotia fluoroscopy series demonstrates no increased risk of breast cancer beyond that naturally expected for women over age 40 at the time of initial radiation.[47] The results of the Rochester postpartum mastitis series[69] suggest that the breasts of recently pregnant older, premenopausal women have their oncogenic sensitivity increased to the same level as do young menarchal women age 10–19.
6. The effects of each unit of absorbed dose are cumulative and operative throughout the remaining life span of the individual. Therefore, not only are the breasts of younger women more sensitive than those of older women, but the numbers of years over which each unit of energy exerts its influence is greater for younger than for older women.

These observations suggest that there is a point in time when each additional rad of radiation has a decreasing oncogenic effect, although it is cumulative from each preceding rad. On the other hand, the risk of developing non-radiation-related sporadic cancer steeply increases with each year after age 35.

BENEFIT/RISK RATIOS

It should be emphasized that: (1) the data for estimating risk do not result from controlled experiments and, because of the high rate of sporadic breast cancer, cannot be determined with great certainty; and (2) there is a large body of clinical, albeit anecdotal, data that supports the need for early detection. In other words, data supporting the benefit of early detection, while not sufficient to satisfy absolute scientific purity, are at least equal to the quality of the data that support risk. To ignore one side of the equation in favor of the other is, at best, imprudent.

Many models have been developed and some are cited below for historical interest. Note that even using the worst-case linear assumptions, radiation effect is negligible at today's dose levels.

For women age 40 and over, radiation risk is negligible. For younger women, if symptomatic, the individual radiation risk is so low as not to warrant clinical consideration.

Widespread screening for low-risk, asymptomatic women younger than age 40 is not recommended, simply because there are too few cancers extant[60] to justify the cost or minimal radiation exposure to large populations of young women.

Table 1-5 presents the most likely benefit/risk ratios for the independent added value of mammography in an asymptomatic, randomly selected population exposed for 5 years at 1 rad per year, based on a model developed by Fox.[34]

Dose rates per mammographic exposure have decreased markedly over the past 15 years, particularly during the past 7 years. In the early 1960s, exposures of 10 rads per image were common. Today it is possible to do a *two-view screen-film mammogram combined with a single lateral view xeromammogram for a total midline absorbed dose of 0.43 rad in a 6-cm-thick breast.* When these lower-dose figures are applied to calculations of risk, the benefit/risk ratios noted in Table 1-4 increase by 200 percent. Using only screen-film mammography, presuming that the equal sensitivity for stage at detection were maintained, the benefit/risk ratio would be increased by 550 percent.

As a result of extensive mathematical modeling, Eddy[22–24] has estimated the impact of the radiation hazard at 1 rad per year for women both over age 50 and under age 50. This estimate assumes that women receive mammograms and physical examinations annually from age 50 in one group and from age 35 in the other group, and that these screening examinations continue for the rest of their lives. For women over age 50, if one assumes no hazard from the radiation, Eddy estimates that the increase in life expectancy offered by screening would be an average of 60.5 days. Even assuming the usual worst-case risk of 6 excess cancers per rad per million women per year, after 10 years of screening, the increase in life expectancy per woman would be 60.2 days. If the radiation hazard were doubled, the increase in life expectancy per woman would be 59.8 days. (Since the added radiation risk to women over age 40 is probably no more than half of the original worst-case risk, and more likely near zero, the increase in life expectancy is essentially the same as if we assume no hazard at all.)

For women over age 35, using the same risk estimates as above and assuming the benefits are equal to the benefits demonstrated for women over age 50 in the HIP study, Eddy estimates that, with no hazard, an average of 96.9 days would be added to each woman's life. Assuming the usual worst-case risk of 6 excess cancers per rad per million women per year, 88.4 days would be added, and if the risk were doubled, 77.1 days would be added. If the benefit of aggressive screening for younger women is what it appears to be in our Cincinnati BCDDP series, the time added to each woman's life would be greater than the Eddy estimates from the HIP study results.

Table 1-5
Benefit/risk Ratios of Mammography for Asymptomatic Women

Age	Benefit/risk Ratio
35–49	8.0 ± 3.1
45–54	11.2 ± 4.0
over 50	31.0 ± 8.8

COST-BENEFIT ANALYSIS

Although it is currently in vogue to invoke the importance of cost-benefit analyses in medical care, such analyses raise important ethical and humanitarian questions. Before we as a society acquiesce to this approach, we must know exactly what we are buying.

Bierman[11] has stated, "Ultimately, when the scent is of flesh rather than figures, even the economist concedes that it will be important to insulate the individual practitioner [from cost-benefit/cost-effectiveness analysis] on a day-to-day basis because of potential conflict with the commitment to do what is best for each patient. Here is the crux. The economist's reference to the 'nation's health' is at best ambiguous and more likely meaningless. The physician's commitment to the patient's health is neither of these: it is clear, undeniable, and profoundly meaningful."

In his model, Eddy[23] estimates that the cost per person-year gained by screening with physical examination is about $1000. With estimated mammographic costs added, the cost per person-year gained rises to $7000. Substituting our own mammographic costs into Eddy's model, the cost per person-year gained by screening is only $1900. We have previously estimated[54] in our own model that the cost per person-year gained for screening with physical examination alone is in excess of $4500. If mammography were added to our screening process, the cost would drop to about $3300 per person-year gained because of a greater yield of smaller cancers detected.

The Cincinnati approach to screening requires that a definitive diagnosis be established for any persistent abnormality. For subtle mammographic findings, this approach requires biopsy. The cause of many physical findings can often be determined with aspiration, with or without cytology. We have nevertheless calculated the cost of all such procedures on the basis of the most expensive procedure, i.e., biopsy. While biopsy-yield ratios of 20–30 percent are standard, we accept a ratio of 10 percent as not unreasonable if 30 percent or more of the invasive cancers are 5 mm or smaller in size or are in situ lobular or intraductal carcinomas. It has been claimed that our aggressive approach is too expensive. We feel, however, that the cost of the added biopsies is trivial compared with the other costs of screening.[54]

On the basis of the HIP data, Eddy[23] estimates that annual clinical screening will increase the average woman's life expectancy by 38 days. Annual clinical examination plus annual mammography would increase her life expectancy by 60 days. For this incremental gain in longevity, there is about a 12-fold increase in cost—i.e., from $100 to $1200. Eddy also estimated the costs resulting from improvements in mammography. He theorized that mammograms could detect 80 percent of malignant lesions before they are detected by physical examination an average of 1 year earlier, and 20 percent 2 years earlier. Under this new set of circumstances, a strategy of annual physical examination and mammography every other year would increase life expectancy from 38 days to about 80 days at a cost of approximately $637. Annual physical examination and annual mammography increase the benefit to almost 100 days at a cost of about $1200. Our own data[34] suggest that 60 percent of malignant lesions are detected before they are found by physical examination, and on the average, they are detected 2 years earlier by mammography than physical examination in women age 40–49. These data would also imply that a strategy of annual screening would increase the life expectancy over 100 days for less than $1200. For women age 50 and older, screening every other year is cheaper and probably equally effective due to the 3-year lead time gained.

Other pragmatic problems arise in estimating cost effectiveness of a given procedure. Doberneck,[20] for example, analyzed the cost of finding cancer in 1064 women seen at the University of New Mexico from 1972 to 1978 for breast pain, fibrocystic disease, or breast neoplasm. For 516 biopsies done, the cost per cancer was found to be $6411, compared with $11,175 reported by Feig and $24,482 reported by Lewis. Doberneck concluded that the present state of the surgical art is more cost-effective than is screening for breast cancer.

We believe the foregoing is an incorrect comparison. If it is assumed that the role of screening is to detect cancer when it is still small in size and most amenable to cure, examination of symptomatic women is case finding and cannot be compared with screening. In our view, the correct comparison would have been the cost per highly curable cancer found by screening versus the cost per highly curable cancer found in the symptomatic setting. If the distribution of cancers in Doberneck's series is in line with other analyses of nonscreened populations,[32,40,58] the number of curable breast cancers detected probably does not comprise more than 3–9 percent of the total cancers. In a personal communication, Doberneck has verified that only 2 cancers in his series were minimal; the cost per minimal cancer found therefore was $224,397, *ten times* the cost of even aggressive screening![54]

SUMMARY

Quantifying the benefits of mammography is tricky and must take into account many factors (e.g., lead-time bias, length-bias sampling, patient self-selection, efficacy of screening tools) in order to be meaningful. If there are risks in mammographic screening with modern technologies, they are theoretical and small. Calculated benefit/risk ratios of mammographic screening for breast cancer vary with the age of the screenee, but are strongly in favor of screening. Although the costs of screening have to be considered, cost-benefit analyses give rise to important ethical and philosophical questions.

REFERENCES

1. Andersson I: Mammographic Screening for Breast Carcinoma. A Cross-sectional Randomized Study of 45–69 Year-old Women. Malmo, Sweden, Litos Retrtryck, 1980
2. Andersson I, Andrén L, Hilldell J, et al: Breast cancer screening and mammography: A population-based randomized trial with mammography as the only screening mode. Radiology 132:273-276, 1979
3. Baker L: Breast Cancer Detection Demonstration Project: 5 year summary report. CA 32:4-35, 1982
4. Baral E, Larsson LE, Mattson B: Breast cancer following irradiation of the breast. Cancer 40-2905-2910, 1977
5. Barrett AH, Myers PC, Sadowsky ML: Microwave thermography in the detection of breast cancer. AJR 134:365–368, 1980
6. Beahrs OH, Shapiro S, Smart C, et al: Report of the Working Group to Review the National Cancer Institute-American Cancer Society Breast Cancer Detection Demonstration Projects. J Natl Cancer Inst 62:639-698, 1979
7. Beahrs OH, Shapiro S, Smart C, et al: Supplemental and concluding report of the Working Group to Review the National Cancer Institute-American Cancer Society Breast Cancer Detection Demonstration Projects. J Natl Cancer Inst 62:699-709, 1979
8. Beahrs OH, Smart CR: Diagnosis of minimal breast cancers in the BCDDP: The 66 questionable cases. Cancer 43:848-850, 1979
9. BEIR Report, Advisory Committee on the Biological Effects of Ionizing Radiation: The effects on populations of exposure to low levels of ionizing radiation. National Academy of Sciences, National Research Council, 1972
10. Berlin NI: Breast cancer screening: The case for screening women younger than 50 years of age. JAMA 245:1060, 1981
11. Bierman SF: Letter to the editor. NEJM 304:432, 1981
12. Blan KI, Buchanan JB, Mills DL, et al: Analysis of breast cancer screening in women younger than 50 years of age. JAMA 245:1037-1042, 1981
13. Boice JD, Monson RR: Breast cancer in women after repeated fluoroscopic examinations of the chest. J Natl Cancer Inst 59:823-832, 1977
14. Buchanan JB: Mammography in the practice of medicine. Int J Dermatol 19:400-404, 1980
15. Burns PE, Grace MGA, Lees AW, et al: False negative

mammograms causing delay in breast cancer diagnosis. J Can Assoc Radiol 30:74-76, 1979

16. Chamberlain J, Rogers P, Price JL, et al: Validity of clinical examination and mammography as screening tests for breast cancer. Lancet 2:1026-1030, 22 Nov., 1975
17. Clark RL, Copeland MM, Egan RL, et al: Reproducibility of the technique of mammography (Egan) for cancer of the breast. Am J Surg 109:127-133, 1965
18. Collette HJA, Day NE, Rombach JJ, et al: Evaluation of screening for breast cancer in a non-randomized study (The DOM Project) by means of a case-controlled study. Lancet 1:1224-1226, 2 June, 1984
19. Devitt JE: Mammography: A surgeon's experience. Can Med Assoc J 120:1370-1372, 1979
20. Doberneck RC: Breast biopsy: A study of cost effectiveness. Ann Surg 192:152-156, 1980
21. Dodd GD: Radiation detection and diagnosis of breast cancer. Cancer 47:1766-1769, 1981
22. Eddy D: Guidelines for the cancer-related checkup: Recommendations and rationale. CA 30:194-240, 1980
23. Eddy DM: A Mathematical Model on the Efficacy of Breast Cancer Screening. In Feig SA, McLelland R (eds): Breast Carcinoma. Current Diagnosis and Treatment. New York, Masson USA, 1983, pp 339-349
24. Eddy DM: Screening for Cancer: Theory, Analysis, and Design. Englewood Cliffs, NJ, Prentice Hall, 1980
25. Egan RL: Experience with mammography in a tumor institution: Evaluation of 1000 cases. Radiology 75:894-900, 1960
26. Egan RL, Goldstein GT, McSweeney MM: Conventional mammography, physical examination, thermography and xeroradiography in the detection of breast cancer. Cancer 39:1984-1992, 1977
27. Fabrikant JI: The BEIR III Report: Origin of the controversy. AJR 136:209-214, 1981
28. Feig SA: Biologic determinations of radiation induced human breast cancer. CRC Crit Rev Diagn Imaging 13:229-248, 1980
29. Feig SA: Ionizing radiation and human breast cancer. CRC Crit Rev Diagn Imaging 11:145-166, 1978
30. Feig SA, Shaber GS, Schwartz GF, et al: Thermography, mammography and clinical examination in breast cancer screening: Review of 16,000 studies. Radiology 122:123-127, 1977
31. Forrest APM: Cancer of the breast: Early diagnosis. Br Med J 2:265-267, 1970
32. Foster RS, Lang SP, Constanza MC, et al: Breast self examination practices and breast cancer stage. NEJM 299:265-270, 1978
33. Fox MS: On the diagnosis and treatment of breast cancer. JAMA 241:489-494, 1979
34. Fox SH, Moskowitz M, Saenger EL, et al: Benefit/risk analysis of aggressive mammographic screening. Radiology 128:350-365, 1978
35. Gallager HS, Martin JE: Early phases in the development of breast cancer. Cancer 24:1170-1178, 1969
36. Gallager HS, Martin JE: An orientation to the concept of minimal breast cancer. Cancer 28:1505-1507, 1971
37. Gallager HS, Martin JE, Moore DL, et al: The detection and diagnosis of early occult and minimal breast cancer. Curr Probl Cancer 3:1-32, 1979
38. Gilbertsen VA: The earlier detection of breast cancer. Semin Oncol 1:87-89, 1974
39. Gilbertsen VA, Nelms JM: Breast cancer: Improving long term survival. Minn Med 63:160A-160C, 1980
40. Greenwald P, Nasca PC, Laurence CE, et al: Estimated effect of breast self-examination and routine physical examination on breast cancer mortality. NEJM 299:270-273, 1978
41. Hicks MJ, Davis JR, Layton JM, et al: Sensitivity of mammography and physical examination of the breast for detecting breast cancer. JAMA 242:2080-2083, 1979
42. Kalisher L, Schaffer DL: Xeromammography in early detection of breast cancer. JAMA 234:60-63, 1975
43. Karsell PR: Mammography at Mayo Clinic: A year's experience. Mayo Clin Proc 49:954-957, 1974
44. Lesnick GJ: Detection of breast cancer in young women. JAMA 237:967-969, 1977
45. McGregor DH, Land CE, Choi K, et al: Breast cancer incidence among atomic bomb survivors, Hiroshima and Nagasaki, 1950-1969. J Natl Cancer Inst 59:799-811, 1977
46. Milbrath JR, Moskowitz M, Bauermeister DE: Breast cancer screening. CRC Crit Rev Diagn Imaging 16:181-218, 1981
47. Miller AB: Personal communication, 1980
48. Miller AB, Howe GR, Sherman GJ, et al: The Canadian study of cancer following multiple fluoroscopies. I. Mortality from breast cancer in women 1950-1980. Presented at Imaging Technologies in Breast Cancer Control. World Health Organization committee meeting, Moscow, USSR, October, 1985
49. Moskowitz M: Breast cancer detection and treatment revisited. JAMA 242:1037-1038, 1979
50. Moskowitz M: Heroic positives and false negatives panel. In Logan WW, Muntz EP (eds): Reduced Dose Mammography. New York, Masson USA, 1979, pp 453-462
51. Moskowitz M: How can we decrease breast cancer mortality? CA 30:272-276, 1980
52. Moskowitz M: The importance of finding minimal breast cancer. In Logan WW, Muntz EP (eds): Reduced Dose Mammography. New York, Masson USA, 1979, pp 97-110
53. Moskowitz M: Screening for breast cancer: How effective are our tests? 33:26-39, 1983
54. Moskowitz M, Fox SH: Cost analysis of aggressive breast cancer screening. Radiology 130:253-256, 1979
55. Moskowitz M, Gartside PS: Evidence on breast cancer mortality reduction by aggressive screening in women under age 50. AJR 138:911-916, 1982
56. Moskowitz M, Garstide PS, Gardella L, et al: The breast cancer screening controversy: A perspective. In Logan WW (ed): Breast Carcinoma: The Radiologist's Expanded Role. New York, Wiley, 1977, pp 35-52
57. Moskowitz M, Pemmaraju S, Russel P, et al: Observations on the natural history of carcinoma of the breast: Its precursors and mammography counterparts. Part. I: National history. Breast 3:14-19, 1977
58. Moskowitz M, Russel P, Fidler J, et al: Breast cancer screening: Preliminary report of 207 biopsies performed in 4,128 volunteer screenees. Cancer 36:2245-2250, 1975
59. Nathan BE, Burn JI, Doyle FH: An evaluation of mammography in a breast clinic. Clin Radiol 23:87–92, 1972
60. Pollei SR, Mettler FA, Bartow S, et al: Radiographic appearance and detectability of occult breast cancer. (Submitted for publication)
61. Rodes N, Farrell C, Blackwell CW: Missouri's role in breast cancer detection. Mo Med 74:689-694, 1977

62. Rombach JJ: Breast Cancer Screening: Results and Implications for Diagnostic Decision Making. Alphen Aan Den Rijn/Brussels, Stafleu's Scientific Publishing Co., 1980
63. Roselli del Turco M, Giannardi G, Villari N: The diagnostic efficacy of mammography and palpation in early detection of breast cancer. Tumori 66:85-92, 1980
64. Schwartz M: Estimates of lead time and length bias in a breast cancer screening program. Cancer 46:844-851, 1980
65. Shapiro S: Evidence on screening for breast cancer from a randomized trial. Cancer 39:2772-2782, 1977
66. Shapiro S: Screening for early detection of cancer and heart disease. Bull NY Acad Med 51:80-95, 1975
67. Shapiro S, Strax P, Venet L, et al: Changes in 5-year breast cancer mortality in a breast cancer screening program. In Seventh National Cancer Conference Proceedings. Philadelphia, Lippincott, 1973
68. Shapiro S, Venet W, Strax P, et al: Ten to fourteen year effects of breast cancer screening on mortality. J Natl Cancer Inst 69:349-355, 1982
69. Shore RE, Hempelmann LH, Kowaluk E, et al: Breast neoplasms in women treated with x-rays for acute postpartum mastitis. J Natl Cancer Inst 59:813-822, 1977
70. Sinclair W: Effects of low level radiation and comparative risk. Radiology 138:1-10, 1981
71. Stevenson TD, Batley F, Blakemore WS, et al: Recognition and management of breast cancer. Ohio State Med J 73:677-690, 1977
72. Stewart GR, Ryan J, Raffles B, et al: Early detection of breast cancer. Med J Aust 2:419-423, 1977
73. Strax P: Control of breast cancer through mass screening. JAMA 235:1600-1602, 1976
74. Strax P: Evaluation of screening programs for the early diagnosis of breast cancer. Surg Clin North Am 58:667-679, 1978
75. Strax P: Screening for breast cancer. Clin Obstet Gynecol 20:781-801, 1977
76. Strax P, Venet L, Shapiro S: Value of mammography in reduction of mortality from breast cancer in mass screening. AJR 117:686-689, 1973
77. Swartz HM, Reichling BA: The risks of mammograms. JAMA 237:965-966, 1977
78. Tábar L: Personal communication
79. Tábar L, Fagerberg CJG, Gad A, et al: Reduction in mortality from breast cancer after mass screening with mammography. Randomized trial from the Breast Cancer Screening Working Group of the Swedish National Board of Health and Welfare Lancet (April 13) 1:829-832, 1985
80. Thomas LB, Ackerman LV, McDivitt RW, et al: Report of NCI Ad Hoc Pathology Working Group to Review the Gross and Microscopic Findings of Breast Cancer Cases in the HIP study (Health Insurance Plan of Greater New York). J Natl Cancer Inst 59:495-541, 1977
81. Thoreau M, Fitzharris BM, Redding WH, et al: Clinical examination, xeromammography, and fine needle aspiration cytology in diagnosis of breast tumors. Br Med J 2:1139-1141, 1978
82. Upton AC, Beebe GW, Brown JM, et al: Report of NCI Ad Hoc Working Group on the Risks Associated with Mammography in Mass Screening for the Detection of Breast Cancer. J Natl Cancer Inst 59:479-493, 1977
83. Verbeek ALM. Population screening for breast cancer in Nijmegen: An evaluation of the period 1975-1982. Publ Dept of Social Medicine, Katholieke Universiteit Nijmegen, 1985
84. Verbeek ALM, Hendriks JHCL, Peeters PHM, et al: Mammographic breast pattern and the risk of breast cancer. Lancet (March 17) 1:591-593, 1984

PART II

Thermography, Ultrasound, Lightscanning, and Magnetic Resonance Imaging

John R. Milbrath, M.D.

1

Thermography

The fact that disease processes are frequently accompanied by a rise in body temperature has been known since antiquity. The first thermometer was constructed in 1595 by Galileo, who called his crude instrument a thermoscope. The thermoscope was versatile, being useful also as a barometer, but it had the disadvantage of requiring recalibration at each use. In the 18th century, thermometry was first used in a clinical setting by the Dutch physician-investigator, Boerhaave, who had obtained several thermometers from Fahrenheit. DeHaen, a student of Boerhaave, discovered the diurnal fluctuations of body temperature. In 1851 Wunderlich began to regularly measure the temperature of his patients and thereby gave thermometry a permanent place in clinical examination.

Thermography was first utilized for breast disease in 1956, when Lawson made the observation that breast cancers were associated with an elevation of the temperature of the overlying skin.[10] A technical breakthrough occurred when electronic scanners used by the military in bombing and surveillance missions were modified for use in evaluating skin temperature. Throughout its 30-year history, the use of thermography for breast cancer detection has been controversial.

FUNDAMENTALS OF THERMOGRAPHY

All objects emit infrared radiations, electromagnetic waves with wavelengths from 0.75μ to 1 mm. Infrared radiation was discovered in 1800 by the astronomer Sir William Herschel. The radiation emitted by an object is proportional to the area and emissivity of the object and to the fourth power of its absolute temperature. Although the human body emits infrared energy with wavelengths of 3μ to 75μ, the peak emission is at 9.3μ. Since infrared radiation is invisible, special instruments utilizing photoelectric or photochemical phenomena are necessary to detect it.

One can also measure longer wavelength radiation emanating from the body. Preliminary data have shown that microwave radiometers may be able to sense small temperature changes emanating from some depth below the surface of the skin. The major disadvantage of this technique is that only a small amount of radiation is emitted by the body at the longer wavelengths. Consequently, detection devices must be extremely sensitive and very large. According to a recent review of microwave and millimeter wavelength thermography, the potential disadvantages of this technique were considered to far outweigh its advantages.[17] Technical problems are largely unresolved, and widespread clinical acceptance is unlikely in the near future.

The mechanism of tumor thermogenesis and heat transfer is still poorly understood. Until recently, conduction of heat was considered to play the primary role in the recording of superficially located abnormalities, resulting in a so-called overlying "hot spot" on the thermogram. Conversely, venous convection was thought to be the primary mode of heat transfer for deeper-seated abnormalities.[4] The deeper cancers were believed to increase the temperature of adjacent blood,

BREAST CANCER DETECTION
ISBN 0-8089-1842-7

which then coursed from deep veins to superficial veins on its way to a plexus of rich venous anastomoses beneath the areola. Love, however, has disputed these theories and has shown that the metabolic rate of most cancers is too low to account for the measured temperature increase.[11] According to Love, blood perfusion, and not the local heat from the tumor, is the main factor controlling the variation in local skin temperature, which becomes a direct indicator of subsurface blood flow. According to this theory, the increased blood perfusion is part of a generalized response to the tumor.

Current Methods of Infrared Breast Thermography

Breast thermography is usually performed by one of three methods: telethermography, contact thermography, or computerized thermography. Since cooling the breasts accentuates abnormal heat patterns, all thermographic examinations should take place in a draft-free room in which the humidity is controlled and the temperature is a constant 20°C. The patient should disrobe to the waist for about 10 minutes prior to the examination.

Telethermography

In telethermography, infrared radiation emitted from the body is measured by an electronic infrared detector.

In one method, called "graphic stress thermography," an infrared sensor is placed over specific data-collection points both before and after immersion of the patient's hands in ice water for 15 seconds. This variation purports to take advantage of the lack of normal physiologic constriction by tumor vessels.

In the other, more common, method of telethermography, infrared radiation is focused by an optical mirror on a thermistor that converts infrared energy to an electrical signal displayed on a cathode ray tube (CRT). The CRT image may then be photographed for a permanent record. A mechanical scanning system permits the energy to be collected in small increments in rapid succession. The thermistor (usually mercury-cadmium-telluride or indium antimonide) must be continuously cooled by liquid nitrogen.

In the scanning method of telethermography, anteroposterior and oblique projections are routinely made of both breasts (Fig. 1-1). While some thermographers prefer black-and-white images with black representing warmer foci and white cooler foci, others prefer to view images in which these shades are reversed. A number of thermographers prefer to view the images in color. Although some thermographers prefer real-time images, the final interpretation is usually performed off-line using static photographs. While the examination is usually performed with the patient upright, a supine position may be necessary to completely visualize larger breasts.

In the United States, telethermographic images

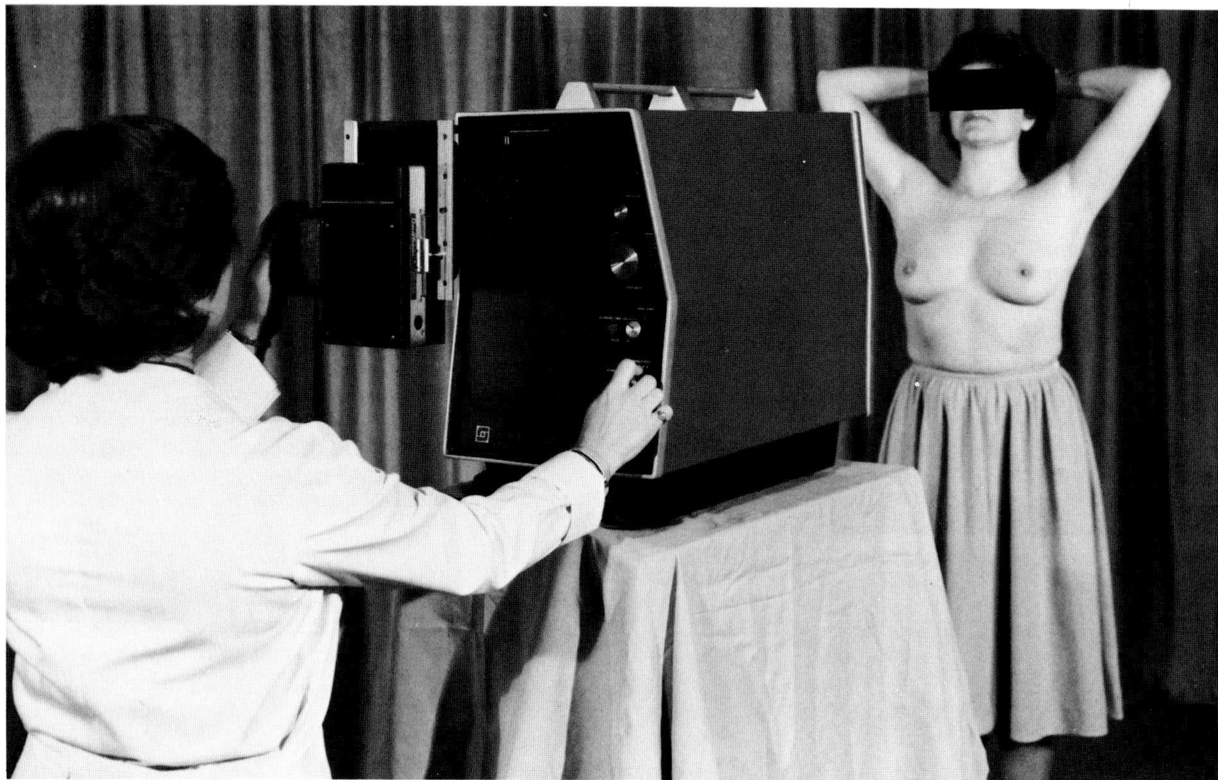

Figure 1-1. Telethermography. Infrared radiation emitted from breasts is photoelectrically converted to a visible image that is photographed for permanent record.

have usually been analyzed in a qualitative fashion. Corresponding areas in each breast are compared, and a judgment is made on the basis of the symmetry of the heat patterns (Fig. 1-2). If very asymmetric, the thermogram is considered abnormal (Fig. 1-3), while lesser degrees of asymmetry may be considered equivocal or even normal. Because this method of interpretation is excessively subjective, there has been great variation in intraobserver and interobserver interpretation. In 1976, the American Thermographic Society published a consensus interpretive classification of several recognized experts (Table 1-1).[9] Although the system has not been adopted by all thermographers, the report was a step forward in the standardization of diagnostic criteria. Isard's "edge sign" is one criterion of malignancy that is independent of vascularity or infrared emission.[8] It is the telethermographic image of flattening of the contour of the breast due to skin retraction. Unfortunately, this sign is usually associated with locally advanced cancer. Isard has also reported the as-yet-unexplained observation that some cancers may be associated with foci of *hypo*thermia rather than with focal or diffuse hyperthermia.[7] In Europe, telethermographic interpretation has been more quantitative, with actual temperature measurements being used as diagnostic critiera. Many European centers and, more recently, some centers in the United States have adapted a classification system devised by Amalric et al.[1] This system uses five categories that are reported to correlate with the presence or absence of cancer.

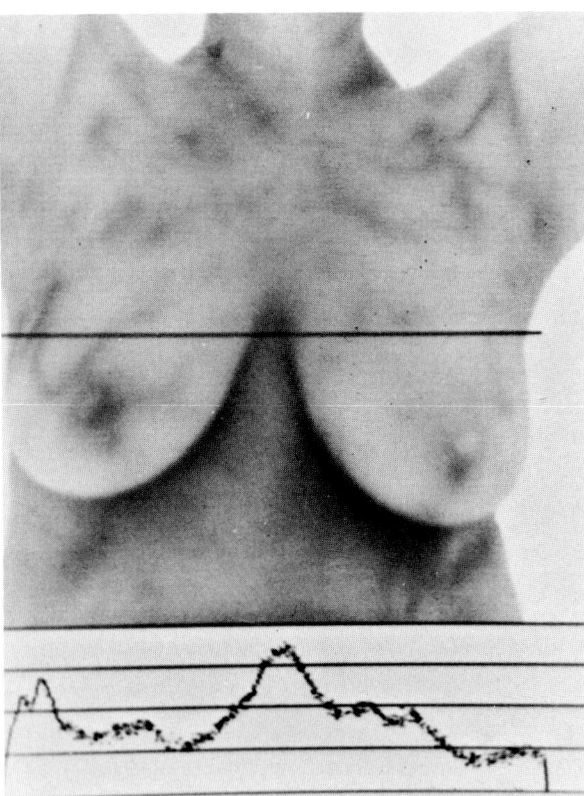

Figure 1-3. Abnormal telethermogram in patient with oat cell carcinoma metastasis to right breast. Anterior telethermographic image shows increased temperature in periareolar region and upper outer quadrant of right breast.

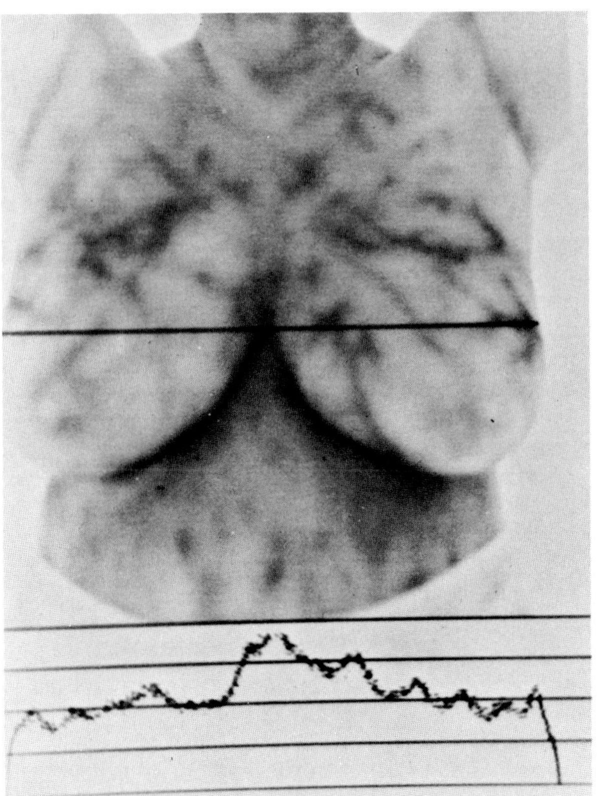

Figure 1-2. Normal telethermogram. Note relative symmetry of venous heat patterns of these normal breasts.

Contact (LCT) Thermography

In contact, liquid-crystal thermography (LCT), a sheet of thin plastic containing heat-sensitive encapsulated liquid cholesterol esters is placed on the breasts. Infrared radiation causes the black cholesteric crystals to change colors, which vary with the infrared energies being emitted from the breast surface. The color image on the plate is photographed while the plate is in contact with the breast (Fig. 1-4).

Projections for contact thermography include anterior and oblique (emphasizing the upper outer quadrant) images of each breast obtained both before and after cooling. Cooling is performed with a hand-held electrical air blower.

Criteria for abnormal contact thermograms are abnormal vascular patterns, "hot spots," and an abnormal "dynamic" response to cooling.[2] The physician-thermographer, rather than a technologist, usually per-

Table 1–1
Telethermography Criteria

A. Normal
B. Suspicious or asymmetric thermogram. Not clearly normal or abnormal. This category should include and be reported if any one of the following are present:
   I. Graphic criteria
      a. Unilateral or asymmetric vascularity with vessels of normal caliber and temperature
      b. Localized rigidity ("edge sign")
   II. Thermal criteria
      a. Unilateral increase in vessel temperature of approximately 2°C or less without increase in vessel number or caliber
      b. Localized (focal) area of increased nonvascular surface temperature of approximately 2°C or less, including the areolar area

   Any two of the above criteria found in one breast should be considered as a clearly abnormal breast thermogram.
C. Abnormal thermogram
   I. Graphic criteria
      a. Marked unilateral increase in vascularity (number), caliber, or configuration of vessels
      b. Diffuse rigidity of contour of the breast
   II. Thermal criteria
      a. Focal increase of approximately 3°C or more including the areolar area
      b. Diffuse regional or quadrant hyperthermia

From Lapayowker MS, Barash I, Byrne R, et al: Criteria for obtaining and interpreting breast thermograms. Cancer 38:1935, 1976. With permission.

forms the examination. Certain vascular patterns are called abnormal even when they are bilaterally symmetrical. The vascular temperature changes, or "dynamics," after cooling are the most important aspect of the examination[20] (Fig. 1-5). Warm or hot areas that are associated with underlying cancer should persist longer during cooling and reappear sooner after cooling than vessels not associated with cancer. These interpretive criteria are extremely subjective. Many physicians who utilize contact thermography believe that certain vascular patterns are indicative of cancer, whereas telethermographers use asymmetry in the infrared emission as the most important determinant of abnormality.

Computed Thermography

In computerized thermography, multiple thermistors are used to detect infrared radiation. The electronic signals are fed to a computer, which utilizes various algorithms to calculate whether the measurements are normal or abnormal. An image of the breast is not usually obtained.

For computerized thermography, the patient is positioned about 1 foot from the detector, with the detector centered at the nipple (Fig. 1-6). The temperature data are instantaneously recorded. Computer analysis of the data takes only several minutes. A computerized unit evaluated at our center contains 64 sensor-mirror elements mounted in an 8 × 8 array. A thermopile is mounted at the focal point of each spherical mirror. The mirrors are coated with acrylic-coated vaporized aluminum and collect the infrared radiation from an area of approximately 1 square inch. Using linear discriminant analysis, which extracts certain features of the thermal pattern and uses them as variables, the thermographic data are processed in an on-line microcomputer. Weighting factors for each feature are then calculated to classify the patients. A small printer records the diagnostic data. Although linear discriminant analysis has previously been used, a template-matching, pattern-recognition technique is undergoing testing.

In contrast to the interpretation of telethermography and contact thermography, interpretation of computerized thermography is entirely objective. Various diagnostic algorithms can be utilized for linear discriminant analysis of the temperature readings. The dividing line between normal and abnormal can be programmed to optimally classify patients.

RESULTS

Because most of the reported investigations on breast thermography have been anecdotal and/or biased, the value of thermography cannot be accurately assessed. Yet, because thermography is rapid, noninvasive, and safe, it was included as a screening modality in the Breast Cancer Detection Demonstration Projects (BCDDP). In the BCDDP, many of the radiologists interpreting thermograms had little or no previous thermographic experience. Continued poor results, with sensitivities of less than 50 percent (even from centers with experienced thermographers) caused the National Cancer Institute to discontinue thermography as a routine breast cancer screening examination. In 1976, the American Thermographic Society and the American College of Radiology jointly declared that thermography was "not an adequate screening method for the detection of breast cancer or other breast disease when used *alone* or with only a physical examination."[16]

In an objective analysis of the role of telethermography in detecting small breast cancers, Moskowitz et al. found that recognized experts could not distinguish women with minimal breast cancer from women without cancer.[15] In a "blind" interpretation test, Threatt et al. found that a group of ten "expert" telethermographers were not able to select women with in situ cancers from the general population.[18] The latter study also showed

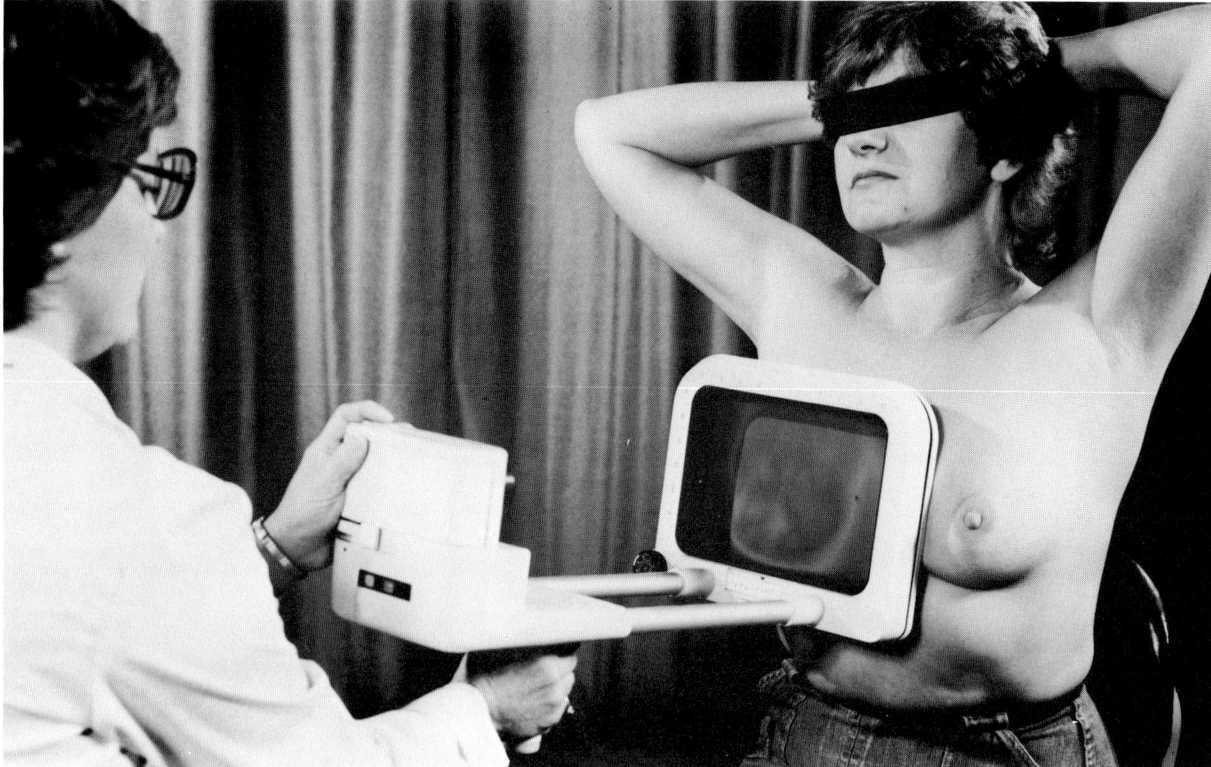

Figure 1-4. Contact plate thermography. Plastic plate embedded with liquid cholesterol esters is placed on breast. Resultant heat patterns (color changes) are recorded on film. Images are obtained both before and after cooling breast.

that the sensitivity of thermography increased directly with the size of the cancer. Because the poorest results occur in those women whose cancers are most amenable to therapy (i.e., those with minimal cancer), thermography appears to have no significant role in breast cancer screening. While thermography has been proposed as an indicator of risk for future development of breast cancer,[3,6] there are presently no objective data to support this contention. Moskowitz, in a recent study, has concluded that thermography has no value as a high-risk indicator.[13]

Thermography has also been proposed as an indicator of prognosis in patients with breast cancer. Williams demonstrated that breast cancer patients with "hot" patterns had a worse prognosis than did those with "cooler" patterns.[21] Gros et al. found the thermogram not only a prognostic index but also an indicator of the treatment that will result in maximum survival.[5] According to Gros et al., surgery alone is recommended for patients with T1, T2, or T3 (TNM system) cancers and mildly abnormal thermographic patterns, whereas surgery plus irradiation is preferred for those patients with similar-stage cancers but a "hot" pattern. According to these authors, thermic abnormalities regress once the cancer has been sterilized, whereas an increase in heat may signal recurrence. Unfortunately, these contentions have not been supported with objective data.

Despite the fact that some investigators advocate biopsy if a pathognomonic pattern is seen in contact (LCT) thermography,[19] neither LCT nor telethermography has yielded objective data to support claims that they can detect small cancers, let alone premalignant mastopathy. Moskowitz et al. reported on an objective investigation revealing that LCT was *not* useful in identifying women with proliferative disorders of the breast, including such premalignant diseases as epithelial and lobular hyperplasia with or without cellular atypia.[14]

Our initial evaluation of a prototype computerized thermographic unit showed sensitivity and specificity of 80 percent.[12] Of the 20 women whose cancers were detected by the computerized unit, however, 80 percent had stage II or greater disease. The usefulness of computerized thermography in detecting early cancers or even proliferative disease thus has yet to be proved.

SUMMARY

Presently, thermography has severe limitations in the detection of breast cancer. It is least reliable in the detection of the small cancers that are most amenable to successful therapy. We feel that thermography is still an

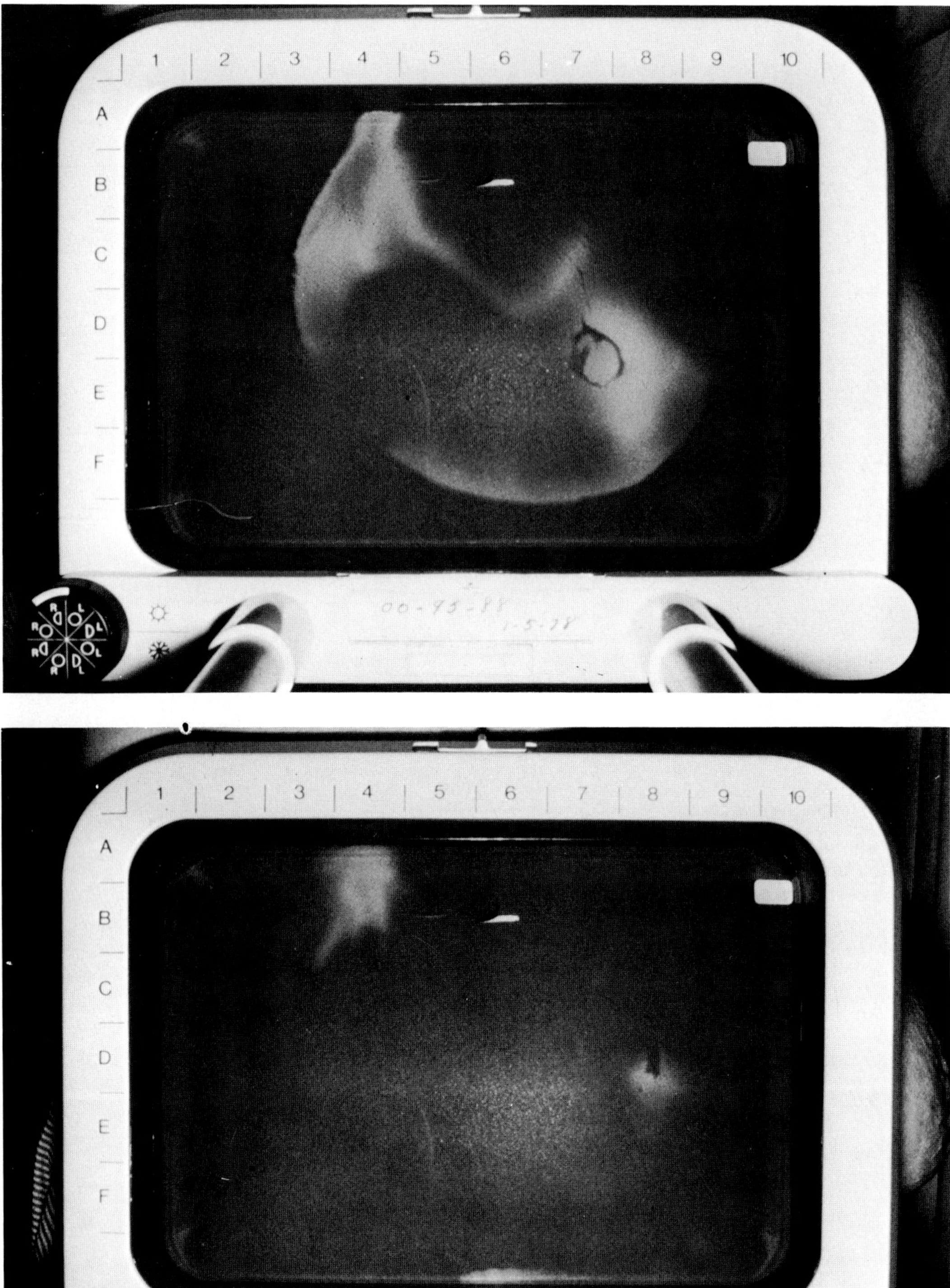

Figure 1-5. Abnormal contact plate thermogram in patient with oat cell carcinoma metastasis to right breast (same patient as in Fig. 1-3). A. Oblique projection of right breast with plate in contact with upper outer quadrant shows abnormal vascular pattern with increased temperature overlying metastatic tumor. B. Plate thermogram following breast cooling. Abnormal vascular pattern and increased heat persist at site of metastatic tumor (arrows).

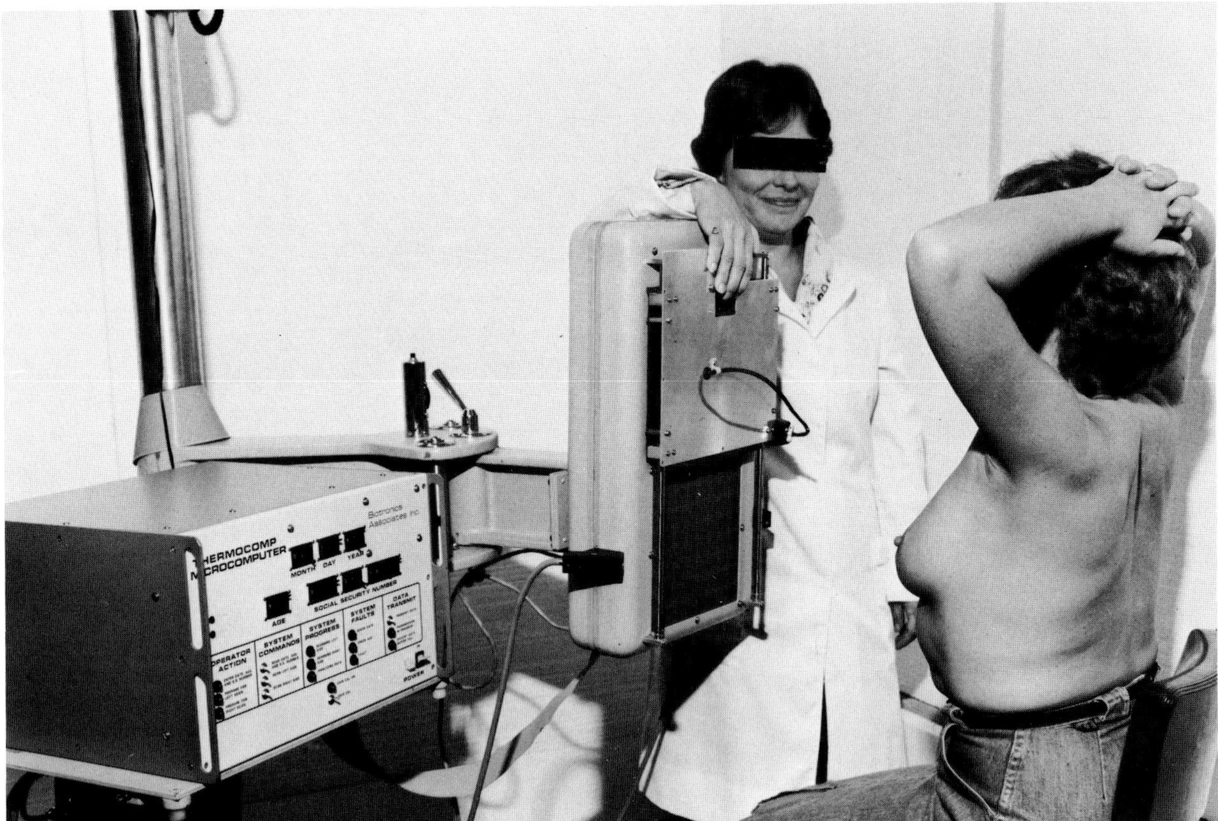

Figure 1-6. Computerized thermography. Array of 64 thermistors is uncovered after patient is properly positioned. Using an algorithm, computer calculates result in several minutes.

investigational tool, to be used in breast cancer screening only when a specific protocol that allows subsequent objective evaluation of results is available. The role of thermography in determining prognosis and treatment of breast cancer patients should continue to be scientifically investigated. It is especially important that additional research be undertaken to determine the nature of tumor thermogenesis.

REFERENCES

1. Amalric R, Spitalier JM, Giraud D, et al: Thermography in diagnosis of breast diseases. In Bibliotheca Radiologica, no. 6, Thermography. Proceedings of the First European Congress, New York, Karger, 1975, pp 65–76
2. Brun del Re R: Thermographic in der Klinik und in der Praxis. Gynakologe 11:14–22, 1976
3. Byrne R: The value of breast thermography as a risk indicator. Acta Thermographica 2:55, 1977
4. Dodd GD, Zermeno A, Wallace JD, et al: Breast thermography: The state of the art. Curr Probl Radiol 3:1–47, 1973
5. Gros C, Gautherie M, Bourjat P: Prognosis and post-therapeutic follow-up of breast cancers by thermography. In Blbliotheca Radiologica, no. 6, Thermography, pp 77–90
6. Hobbins WB: Thermography: Highest risk marker in breast cancer. Acta Thermographica 2:55, 1977
7. Isard HJ: Cancer in the "cold" breast thermogram. AJR 127:793–796, 1976
8. Isard HJ: Thermographic "edge sign" in breast carcinoma. Cancer 30:957–963, 1972
9. Lapayowker MS, Barash I, Byrne R, et al: Criteria for obtaining and interpreting breast thermograms. Cancer 38:1931–1935, 1976
10. Lawson R: Implications of surface temperatures in the diagnosis of breast cancer. Can Med Assoc J 75:309–310, 1956
11. Love TJ: Thermograph as an indicator of blood perfusion. Ann NY Acad Sci 335:429–436, 1980
12. Milbrath JR, Schlager KJ: Direct measurement and on-line automatic interpretation of breast thermographs. In Gray JE, Haus AG, Hende WR, et al. (eds): Application of Optical Instrumentation in Medicine VIII, SPIE Proceedings, vol. 233. Bellingham, WA 1980, pp 282–285
13. Moskowitz M: Thermography: A risk indicator for breast cancer? Results and review of recent literature. J Reprod Med 30(6):451–459, 1985
14. Moskowitz M, Fox SH, Brun del Re R, et al: The potential value of liquid-crystal thermography in detecting significant mastopathy. Radiology 140:659–662, 1981
15. Moskowitz M, Milbrath J, Gartside P, et al: Lack of

efficacy of thermography as a screening tool for minimal and stage I breast cancer. N Engl J Med 295:249–252, 1976

16. Schmidt AM, Whitehorn WV, Martin EW: Thermography restriction. FDA Drug Bull 6:32, 1976
17. Thermography for Breast Cancer Detection. Health Technology Assessment Reports, no. 22. U.S. Department of Health and Human Services, Public Health Service, Office of the Assistant Secretary for Health, 1983
18. Threatt B, Norbeck JM, Ullman NS, et al: Thermography and breast cancer: An analysis of a blind reading. Ann NY Acad Sci 335:501–519, 1980
19. Tricoire J: Personal communication, 1978
20. Tricoire J, Mariel L, Amiel JP, et al: Thermographie en plaque. Presse Med 55:2483–2486, 1970
21. Williams KL: Thermography in the prognosis of breast cancer. In Bibliotheca Radiologica, no. 5, Medical Thermography. Proceedings of Boerhaave Course for Postgraduate Medical Education, New York, Karger, 1969, pp 62–67

Catherine Cole-Beuglet, M.D.

2

Ultrasound

Breast ultrasound and ultrasound mammography are the terms currently given to the evaluation of the mammary gland using ultrasound B-scans. Ultrasound mammography is a direct result of the recent development of specialized equipment to evaluate the large volume of soft tissue comprising the breast.

In England in the 1960s, Wells and Evans proposed the use of a large water bath with transducers at its base.[54] The freely hanging breasts of the prone patient were immersed within the water. The transducers were moved to image the nipple, which could then be used as an anatomical landmark. The water-path technique also allowed the use of large-aperture transducers, which could be focused to a place within the breast for maximum resolution.[27,36] B-scans obtained in this manner could be reproduced on subsequent examinations, and bilaterally symmetrical regions of both breasts could be compared. The use of water between the transducers and skin resolved several of the problems encountered by early investigators in the development of clinical scanning techniques. Prior to the innovation of Wells et al., contact scanning at pre-set intervals over the entire breast was attempted with the patient supine. The results, however, were poor because the breast in the supine position was too mobile on the chest wall.[52]

In Australia in the early 1970s, Kossoff et al. developed the Octoson,* a multipurpose water-path B-scanner, incorporating eight large-aperture 3-MHz transducers.[36] In order to evaluate the potential of B-scanning of the mammary gland, they concurrently developed a special dedicated breast scanner with two transducers mounted in a smaller water bath.[27] In Japan, Wagai et al.[53] and later Kobayashi[30,31] scanned quadrants of the breast with the patient supine. They utilized an enclosed water-path technique to couple sound waves from high-frequency 5-MHz transducers to the skin of the breast. In the United States in the late 1970s, dedicated water-path breast scanners were developed to image the entire mammary gland.

The development of real-time imaging equipment with multiformat imagers has allowed continuous viewing and recording of the images on videotape, videodisc, and/or film disc, with the potential for rapid imaging of the mammary gland and rapid viewing for diagnosis. This is a distinct advance over the earlier techniques of pulsed A-mode and contact B-scan imaging of palpable breast masses.[4,45,52,55] Palpable breast masses nevertheless can still be successfully evaluated with real-time linear and sector B-scan imaging to determine their internal composition.[4,18,44] Since the entire breast is difficult to examine in this manner, the majority of investigators confine their evaluations to the palpable

Work supported in part by National Cancer Institute Grant #1-CB-84273.

* Octoson-Ausonics

BREAST CANCER DETECTION
ISBN 0-8089-1842-7

Table 2-1
Indications for Whole-breast Ultrasound Using Automated Breast Unit

1. Symptomatic patient with a palpable breast mass
2. X-ray mammography shows dense dysplastic breasts
3. Palpable mass in patient under 30 years of age
4. Pregnant patient with breast complaint
5. Recurrent masses in a patient with fibrocystic disease
6. Differentiation of normal breast tissue from a true abnormality
7. Inflammatory breast disease: mastitis, abscess
8. Breast trauma, hematoma, fat necrosis
9. Augmented breast
10. Male breast enlargement or palpable masses
11. Classifying breast parenchymal patterns

mass and, especially, to the differentiation of a cystic from a solid mass.[29,32,51]

PRINCIPLES OF PHYSICS GOVERNING ULTRASOUND

Sound waves in the range above those detectable by the human ear (greater than 20 hertz) are called ultrasound. Pulsed waves from a transducer are directed through the soft tissues of the body with a coupling agent of water, mineral oil, or acoustic gel.

The transducer contains a crystal with piezoelectric characteristics—i.e., the ability to vibrate and emit mechanical sound waves when an electrical current is applied to it. The width of the beam of sound waves is proportional to the diameter of the transducer face and may be focused with an acoustic lens. The focal-depth range of the transducer utilized for ultrasound is expressed in centimeters and is essential information. The object to be studied utilizes the maximum resolution of the system when it is insonated in the focal zone of the transducer. Resolution is measured in the axial direction (parallel to the beam) and in the lateral direction (perpendicular to the beam). When the sound beam encounters an interface with a difference in acoustic impedance, a small portion of the beam will be reflected back to the source, the transducer. This acoustic mechanical wave is again converted into an electrical impulse as it reacts with the piezoelectrice crystal. The information obtained from the reflected sound waves is displayed on a scan convertor for immediate viewing or recording.[37]

METHODOLOGY FOR ULTRASOUND EXAMINATION OF THE BREAST

Patients referred for ultrasound evaluation of the breast are examined clinically by a physician, or a nurse or medical technologist who has been trained in breast physical examination. Sites of mass lesions, other palpable abnormalities, thickening, biopsy scars, and retraction are diagrammed on paper for subsequent correlation with the ultrasound and x-ray mammograms. If a mass lesion is palpable, the site of the mass is outlined with a felt-tip marker pen on the overlying skin. At the time of the physical examination, a history is obtained of past breast diseases in the patient and her family.

Table 2-2
Indications for Localized Breast Ultrasound Using Hand-held High-frequency Transducer

1. Clinical suspicion of an abnormality in a radiographically dense breast
2. Nonpalpable mass detected on an x-ray mammogram
3. Palpable mass for which needle aspiration has failed to produce fluid
4. Pregnant patient with a palpable mass or breast complaint
5. Inflammatory breast disease: mastitis, abscess
6. Breast trauma, hematoma, fat necrosis
7. Breast abnormalities in the postoperative or postirradiation periods
8. Localizing dilated ducts imaged on an x-ray mammogram
9. Palpable mass anterior to an implant for augmentation
10. Male breast or chest wall masses
11. Guiding needle-aspiration biopsy

Automated Whole-Breast Examination

The patient for one type of automated scanner lies supine and a water-filled polyethylene bag is positioned over the area of the breast to be examined. The weight of the water flattens the breast against the anterior chest wall and provides some breast compression and immobilization. Mineral oil or sonic gel couples the polyethylene bag to the skin. The pulsed sound wave from the transducer within the water bag travels through the water and into the breast. Sagittal, transverse, and a combination of both B-scans can be obtained at 1 to 5 mm increments and recorded on a videotape and/or multiformat imager. The indications for automated whole-breast ultrasonography are listed in Table 2-1.

Limited Examination of a Palpable Abnormality

The indications for localized ultrasound of the breast using a hand-held transducer are listed in Table 2-2. For an examination of a palpable abnormality by contact gray scale[52] or real-time water-path B-scanning techniques,[2,21] the patient is placed in a supine oblique position with a pillow or other support under the shoulder of the breast to be examined. With the patient in this

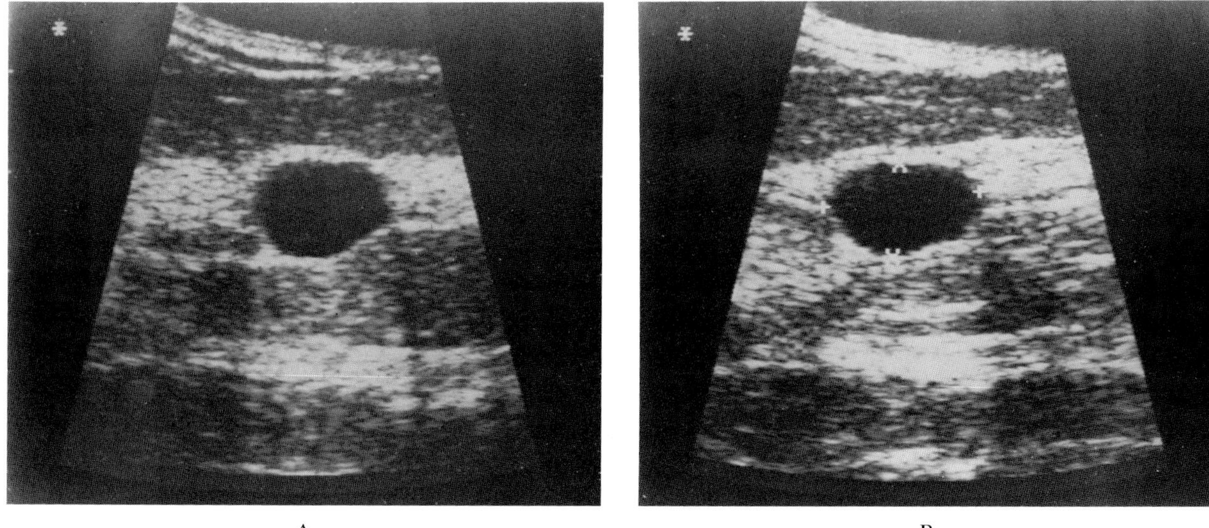

A B

Figure 2-1. Simple cyst. 35-year-old woman with palpable mass. A. Smoothly marginated echo-free cyst exhibits lateral wall shadows and enhanced sound transmission distally. (Hand-held water-delay 7.5 MHz transducer.) B. Application of compression changes shape of cyst (calipers) and narrows the layer of subcutaneous fat.

position, the breast lies naturally flattened over the anterior chest wall. The site of the palpable mass is marked on the overlying skin. If the mass is located in the upper-outer quadrant or axillary tail of the breast, the arm is extented under the patients head to stretch the breast over the thoracic wall. A coupling agent, mineral oil or sonic gel, is applied directly to the skin over the mass. The mass may be immobilized with one hand while the clinician makes sector contact scans over the mass using the other hand. Alternatively, real-time linear array or sector water-path scanners can be placed directly over the mass. The weight of the scanner head results in some compression of the breast tissue against the chest wall and immobilizes the mass. Adipose tissue and cysts are compressible (Fig. 2-1), whereas solid tumors are non-compressible. The use of standard abdominal ultrasound equipment makes the detection of small solid lesions (<1 cm) difficult, especially in the fatty elderly breast. For optimal resolution, medium- and high-frequency transducers (5, 7.5, and 10 MHz) are utilized. The correct transducer is determined by the size and position of the palpable breast mass and the depth of penetration required. The area to be examined will be optimally imaged when it is placed within the focal range of the transducer selected. When the ultrasonic image is examined, the area of the mass is compared with the adjacent glandular tissue to determine whether the mass is fluid-filled or solid. The ultrasound criteria of mass lesions for patients examined in the supine position have been outlined by Kobayshi, and Cole-Beuglet and Beique, using water-path systems.[4,30]

Fleischer et al. reported on 71 symptomatic patients who had xeromammography (XR) and hand-held ultrasound (US) examinations of the breast followed by biopsy. The US examination was performed using hand-held real-time 5- and 6-MHz transducers applied to the area of palpable masses. US demonstrated an accuracy of 96 percent (39/41) in the detection of 41 cysts, XR 69 percent (29/41). For benign solid lesions, US detected 8 of 9 fibroadenomas and XR 7 of 9. Of the 7 carcinomas biopsied, XR detected all 7, whereas US detected 5 of 7. In this small series, the authors found that the combined use of both x-ray and ultrasound of patients with palpable breast masses resulted in greater overall accuracy than if either modality were used alone.[18] Rubin et al., using a hand-held real-time 7.5-MHz transducer, found sonography a useful adjunct to the x-ray mammogram in three groups of patients: (1) patients with dense breasts and localized symptomatology or a suspicious area on x-ray mammograms; (2) patients with nonpalpable abnormalities discovered on x-ray mammogram; and (3) patients with palpable masses considered indeterminate on x-ray mammogram.[47]

The advantages of hand-held high-frequency real-time techniques are: (1) supine position of the patient; (2) improved resolution to 1 mm or less; and (3) the ability to vary the amount of compression to assess tissue compliance and fixation. Ultrasound examination can also be used for guiding needle-aspiration biopsies and localizing dilated ducts in patients with persistent nipple discharge[39,40] (Fig. 2-2).

BREAST ANATOMY

The breast is composed of four major types of tissue: fat, parenchyma (ducts and alveoli), loose connective tissue, and dense connective tissue. The relative amounts of these tissues change according to age and

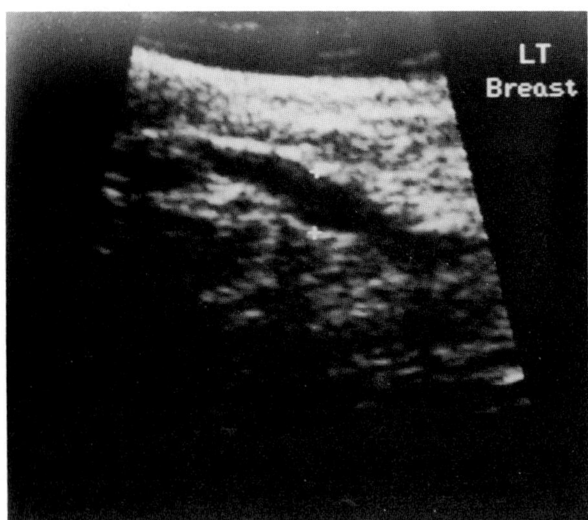

Figure 2-2. Prominent duct in left breast of a 48-year-old woman. Dilated tubular structure 6 mm in diameter (calipers) extends from the nipple radially into the breast parenchyma. Hand-held water-delay 7.5 MHz transducer.

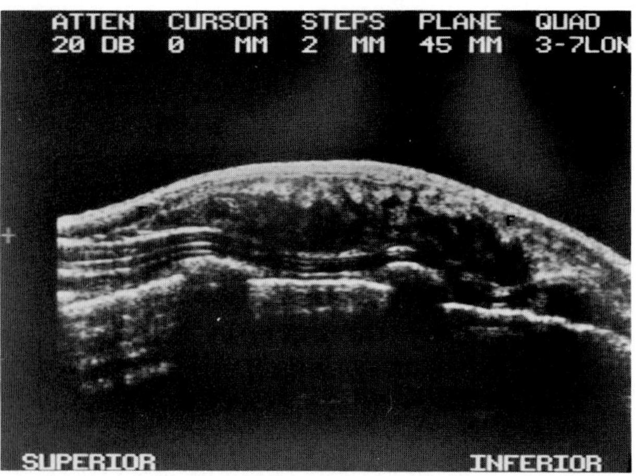

Figure 2-3. Premenopausal breast. Supine 7.5 MHz water-path (longitudinal) B-scan shows intermediate-strength parenchymal (P1) echoes in a homogeneous distribution. The subcutaneous fat layer (F) is narrow. Anterior skin line and the fascia on the pectoralis major muscle are the strongest echo interfaces.

body habitus, resulting in differing sonic attenuation effects. Of the normal anatomical structures, the connective tissue septa of the breast have the highest acoustic impedance. The amplitude of the echo produced by an ultrasound reflection at tissue interfaces is a function of the relative difference in acoustic impedance of the tissues forming the interface. The greatest difference occurs at fat-fibrous connective tissue interfaces, which appear as strong echogenic lines. The fat-parenchyma interfaces, with a smaller difference in acoustic impedance, present as intermediate echo-reflective areas.[3,48]

The angle of incidence of the ultrasonic beam on the reflecting interface is an important factor in the relative echogenicity of the various interfaces within the breast. When perpendicular to the beam, the interfaces appear as bright echogenic lines. When parallel to the beam, the interfaces are imaged poorly or not at all. The fibrous connective tissue septa of the breast are arranged in a radial fashion from the subcutaneous fat to the retromammary fascia. Much of the ultrasonic beam is absorbed and reflected by dense connective tissue, resulting in reduced sound transmission to the deeper areas of the breast. In the free-hanging position, the inferior surface of the breast is more steeply curved than the superior surface. The surface and peripheral breast structures thus may be well imaged, but, because of reflection, absorption, and attentuation, the central structures may be obscured.

In a prone normal B-scan at the nipple level, there is a cone-shaped shadow, the apex of which is directly below the nipple. This shadow differs from nipple shadowing, represented by a narrow, echo-free zone less than 1 cm wide directly below the nipple. Nipple shadowing results from sound absorption by the dense connective tissue stroma of the retroareolar ducts, in combination with reflection and/or refraction from the obliquely oriented sides of the protruding nipple.

In one investigation, cadaver breasts and 20 mastectomy specimens were sectioned in the sagittal plane, and histologic sections of normal and pathologic structures were correlated with the preoperative sagittal B-scan images.[2] This study showed that the normal skin of the breast has a thickness of less than 2 mm. When thickened, the skin is depicted as an increased echo-dense line thicker than 2 mm, and sometimes as thick as 12 mm.[20,35] Occasionally, thickened skin will manifest a narrow echolucent line within its center, giving the appearance of relatively echogenic outer and inner surfaces and a narrow echolucent center.[35]

The subcutaneous fat immediately beneath the skin is clustered in lobules surrounded by connective tissue walls and septa which are usually less than 1 mm thick. Smaller fat lobules occupy the retromammary zone overlying the chest wall muscles. The connective tissue of the subcutaneous septa (Cooper's ligaments) are continuous superficially with the connective tissue of the dermis. The parenchyma is situated between the superficial and deep connective tissue fascial planes. The retromammary zone separates the deep mammary fascia from the fascia overlying the pectoralis major muscle.

The parenchyma is made up of lobules, each of which contains a lactiferous duct. These ducts are usually collapsed in the nonlactating female, but may attain a diameter from 2 to 8 mm at the level of the lactiferous sinuses immediately below the nipple. The deeper lactiferous ducts and their lobular branches

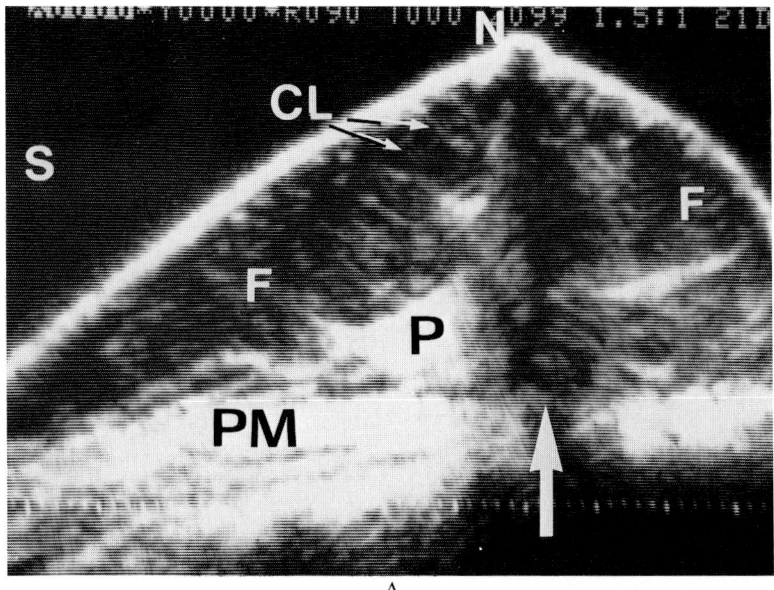

A

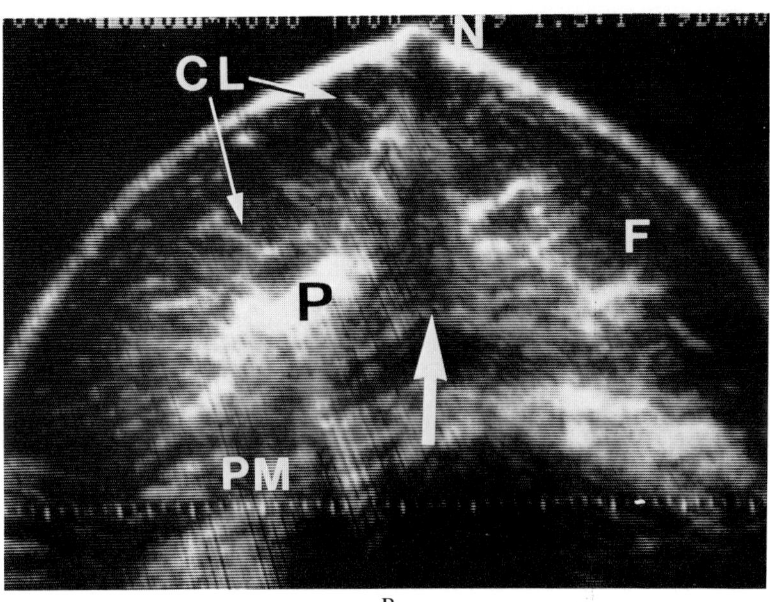

B

Figure 2-4. Normal postmenopausal breast. 55-year-old woman with no breast complaints. A. Sagittal B-scan at nipple level (N). Superior (S) to left. Brightly echogenic skin interface. (F = subcutaneous fat. CL = Cooper's ligaments. P = parenchyma. Arrow, nipple shadow. PM = Pectoralis major muscle.) B. Transverse B-scan at nipple level (N). Lateral to left.

gradually curve radially into a plane paralleling the skin surface. They also enter the connective tissue planes surrounding the parenchyma as well as the connective tissue septa between the fat lobules within the parenchyma. The lobular ducts and terminal alveolar ducts are surrounded by loose intralobular connective tissue. On a B-scan image of a functional breast, the tissues of the parenchyma are manifested as intermediate-strength echoes in a fine homogeneous pattern (Fig. 2-3). In postmenopausal breasts, lobules of fat eventually replace the functioning parenchyma, resulting in images containing round-to-oval areas of low acoustic impedance, with curvilinear lines of dense connective tissue interspersed with Cooper's ligaments (Fig. 2-4).[3,7]

ULTRASOUND PATTERNS OF BREAST PARENCHYMA

Wolfe has correlated the varying x-ray mammographic breast parenchymal patterns with age.[57] Ongoing evaluation of ultrasound mammograms has led us to the recognition of several dominant ultrasound breast patterns based on the arrangement and brightness of the echoes.[46]

In a breast B-scan, the skin line and the fibrous tissue of the retromammary fascia manifest the brightest echoes. Subcutaneous fat is weakly echogenic and interspersed with strongly echogenic Cooper's ligaments. Functional breast parenchyma is intermediate in echogenicity. In the younger patient, it has a fine, uniform "tightly packed" echogenic pattern. Coalescence of these echoes may result in a sheetlike configuration of the glandular tissue extending in a radial fashion from the subareolar area throughout the gland. The subcutaneous and retromammary fat may be 5 mm or less in thickness. In the older patient, fatty replacement of the parenchyma extends into the central core of the breast, and the echo amplitude of the glandular tissue decreases. Oval-to-round areas of weak echogenicity, representing fat lobules, are interspersed between sheetlike areas of higher amplitude parenchymal echoes.[48]

Fluid-filled lactiferous ducts may be imaged as echo-free tubular structures radiating for variable distances from the nipple into the breast parenchyma. The dimensions of these ducts can be measured, and the extent of their penetration into the breast parenchyma recorded. In the majority of women, they are less than 2 mm in width. When the ducts are overdistended with fluid (as in late pregnancy or lactation), their diameter increases. Whereas in x-ray mammograms the visualized ducts comprise the lumen, epithelial lining, and periductal collagen tissue,[57] in ultrasound mammograms, the lumen alone is responsible for the image.

In B-scan, the middle-aged breast may show sheetlike areas of bright echogenic tissues immediately beneath the subcutaneous fat. This tissue has scalloped anterior margins paralleling the skin surface and arching toward the skin where traversed by Cooper's ligaments. The fibrous tissue cap has a cone-shaped or triangular configuration, with the apex beneath the nipple, and may manifest great echo attenuation. The central core of glandular tissue may be echo-free because of considerable overlying fibrous stroma and therefore may not be imaged. In these cases, compressing the breast against the chest wall with a thin sheet of plastic often realigns the dense fibrous tissue so that it becomes incidental to the insonating beam. Rescanning with compression then allows imaging of the central cone of breast tissue previously shadowed by fibrous tissue.[17]

FLUID-FILLED MASSES

Fluid-filled cysts have well-defined smooth margins, echo-free interiors, well-defined posterior walls, and enhanced sound transmission distally (Fig. 2-1).[26] Regardless of sensitivity setting, the central area should remain echo-free. Cysts are generally round or oval, but if multiple, they may manifest a lobulated or septated appearance (Fig. 2-5). Jellins et al., using dedicated breast ultrasound equipment, reported a 98% accuracy rate in the detection of fluid-filled masses within the breast.[26] With the use of high-resolution (7.5- and 10-MHz) transducers, fluid-filled area as small as 2 mm can be detected. Rosner et al. demonstrated a 95 percent accuracy in the detection of cysts, using hand-held high-frequency equipment.[44] Patients with chronic cystic mastitis may occasionally have a cyst with a wall so thick and inflamed as to deflect the needle during an attempted cyst aspiration, giving the clinician the false impression that the mass is solid. The use of ultrasound will readily demonstrate the true cystic nature of such lesions and can be used to monitor aspiration. Chronic fibrocystic disease may result in thickening of the cyst wall. Needle aspiration may lead to a distorted shape of the cyst or to hemorrhage within it, producing internal echoes. The finding of thick septations, internal papillary projections from the cyst wall, and/or echogenic debris within the cyst warrants cytologic and histopathologic investigation, as carcinoma may rarely arise in the wall of a cyst.[43] In these cases, needle aspiration usually yields hemorrhagic fluid containing atypical and/or malignant cells.

Ducts, abscesses, and hematomas may also be fluid-filled. Abscesses are usually periareolar and, when acute and localized, have irregular margins and appear relatively echo-free. Chronic abscesses fill in with weak echoes until they appear solid. This response, consisting of a reduction in diameter and a gradual filling in with echoes, may be observed when the patient receives appropriate antibiotic therapy. An increased thickness and brightness of surrounding Cooper's ligaments may persist for several months after treatment. Thickening and retraction of overlying skin may mark the site of a previous abscess.

Mastitis is a term applied to diffuse inflammation of the breast. It is seen most frequently in the postpartum period, during lactation, or in the perimenopausal period. The inflammation of the breast may be diffuse or localized. When localized, an abscess may occur in the subareolar area. X-ray mammography is difficult to perform and interpret because compression of the breast during the x-ray exposure causes considerable discomfort, leading to poor compression and a resultant poor image, in which the irregular radiodensity of the abscess may mimic carcinoma. On ultrasound, the abscess appears as an irregular, thick-walled, fluid-filled

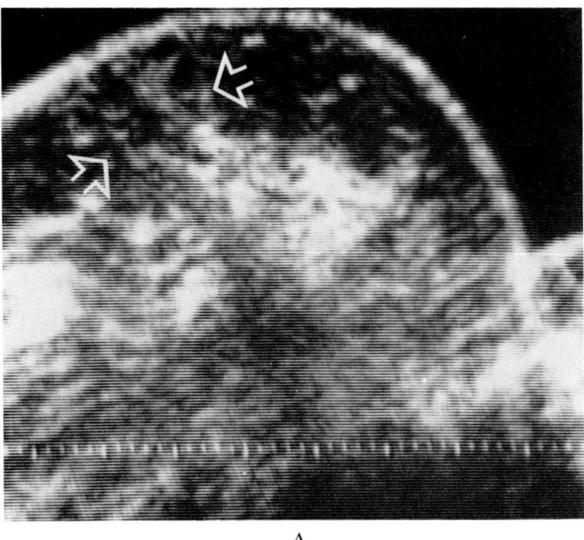

A

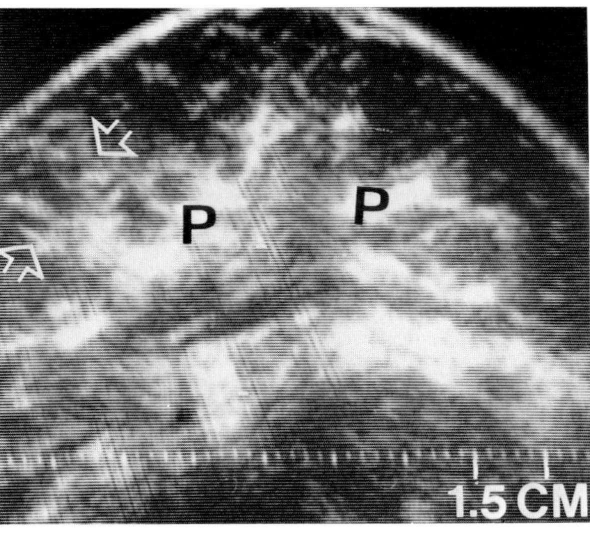

B

Figure 2-5. Lobulated cyst. A. Sagittal B-scan 2 cm lateral to nipple. Cyst (arrow) is echo-free area, 2.5 cm in diameter, with lobulated, smooth margin and enhanced sound transmission posterior to it. (PM = pectoralis major muscle.) B. A-mode histogram superimposed on mass demonstrates echo-free area.

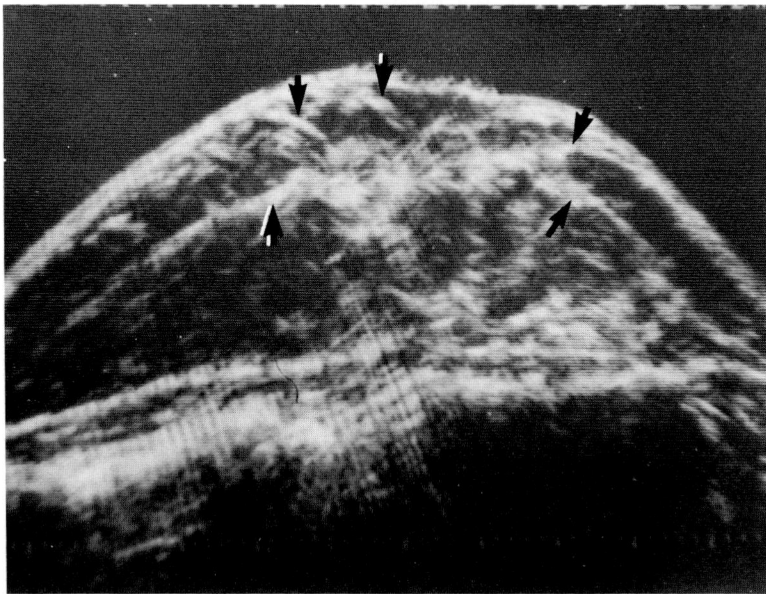

Figure 2-6. Skin retraction and thickened Cooper's ligaments, late signs of infiltrating carcinoma in 55-year-old woman with recent left nipple retraction. Sagittal B-scan just lateral to nipple. Irregular intensity of anterior skin is associated with thickened and retracted Cooper's ligaments (arrows).

region containing weak echogenic debris. During pregnancy, lactation, or in an older women, diffuse inflammation of the breast can occur as a result of rapid growth and lymphangitic spread of an infiltrating duct carcinoma. The resultant inflammatory response has led to the designation "inflammatory carcinoma." Skin thickening, either localized or diffuse, may occur as a result of either inflammation or tumor infiltration.[35] On an ultrasound B-scan, the volume of the affected breast parenchyma is generally increased compared to the contralateral normal breast. The supporting structures of the breast, Cooper's ligaments, and parenchyma may appear altered and displaced. Thickening and retraction of the fibrous connective tissue strands can often be imaged as brightly echogenic curvilinear lines extending to the skin surface (Fig. 2-6).

A hematoma can usually be related to a history of trauma and evidence of overlying skin discoloration. A hematoma may occur following needle aspiration biopsy of a palpable mass (Fig. 2-7). On a B-scan performed within days of the trauma, the area appears as a weakly echogenic region of architectural distortion. One to 3 weeks later, as the hematoma becomes organized, the involved area manifests greater amplitude echoes and thickened Cooper's ligaments. A large hematoma may require many months to resolve. In such cases, sequential B-scans show a gradual decrease in size of the distorted area as well as a decrease in intensity of echo reflections, ultimately returning to a normal pattern.

During pregnancy and lactation, proliferation of terminal ducts within the breast causes increased density on x-ray mammograms and limits x-ray evaluation. However, pregnant or lactating women who develop palpable breast masses or questionable abnormalities are good candidates for ultrasound examination. The

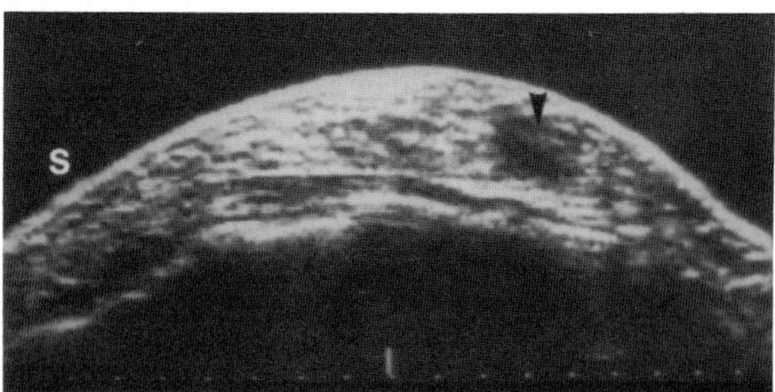

Figure 2-7. Hematoma 6 days after needle aspiration biopsy of suspected mass in lower medial quadrant of right breast in a 48-year-old woman. Longitudinal prone water-bath B-scan shows an irregular-margined hypoechoic area (arrowhead) between the skin and the chest wall muscles, with no significant distal acoustic attenuation.

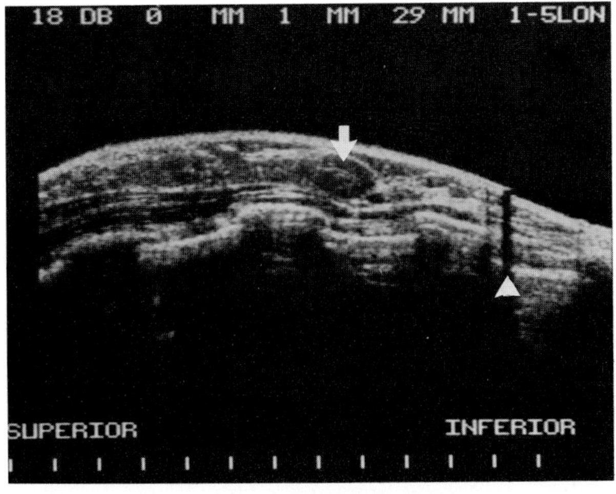

A

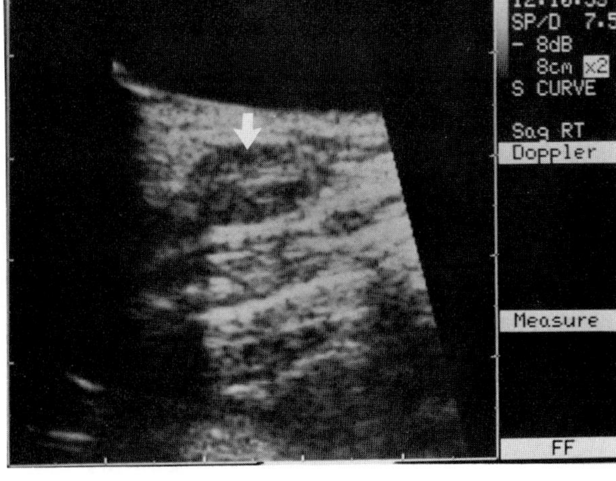

B

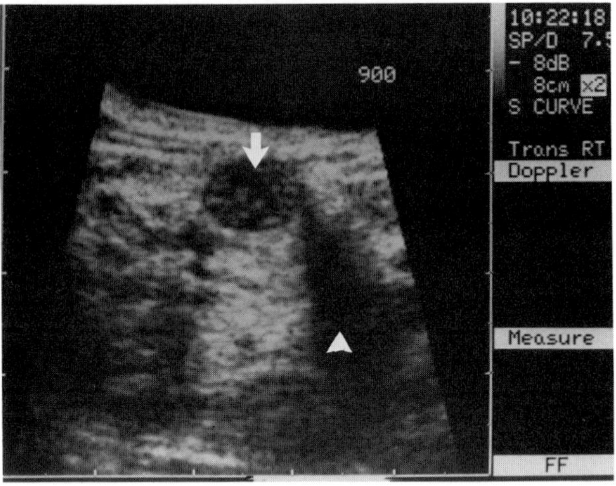

C

Figure 2-8. Fibroadenoma. This 36-year-old woman presented with palpable 1 cm mass at the 9 o'clock position in the right breast. X-ray mammography showed dysplastic breast parenchyma and the mass was not imaged. A. A longitudinal 7.5 MHz supine water-delay sonogram of the right lateral breast shows oval, smooth-margined hypoechoeic mass (arrow) within parenchymal cone. Mass contains weak internal echoes. No acoustic attenuation is noted behind mass. Note strong area of acoustic attenuation from skin surface (arrowhead) due to entrapped air bubble between water-bag membrane and skin. B. A 7.5 MHz hand-held water-delay sagittal sonogram over the palpable mass shows smooth-margined, oval shaped hypoechoeic solid mass (arrow). C. A transverse 7.5 MHz hand-held water-delay sonogram shows scattered variable strength internal echoes within the mass (arrow). Broad right lateral wall shadow is present (arrowhead). Excision biopsy confirmed 1.5 × 1 cm fibroadenoma.

hyperplastic glandular tissue is imaged as uniform fine echoes throughout the gland. There is also a decrease in the amount of adipose tissue that is imaged. In late pregnancy and during lactation, the duct lumens enlarge and may attain a diameter of 6–8 mm, appearing on a B-scan as tubular, branching, echo-free structures radiating from the nipple into the uniformly echogenic breast parenchyma. Fluid-filled masses may represent cysts, abscesses, or galactoceles.

Galactoceles, localized accumulations of milk behind an obstructed duct, may be seen during lactation. On B-scans, the galactocele is a mass with poorly defined margins containing low-level uniform echoes. The high-protein fluid contents of a galactocele are weakly echogenic, in contrast to the echo-free contents of a cyst.

SOLID MASSES

The ability of ultrasound to reveal the nature of breast thickening, hardening, or lumpiness can greatly assist the clinician.[14,15] Although it is useful to ultrasonically distinguish benign from malignant solid masses, the distinction is often impossible. Clinicians therefore generally biopsy any solid mass. When a patient presents with radiographically dense breasts, masses may not be delineated in the x-ray mammogram. Ultrasound mammography, however, can often demonstrate lesions within the uniformly echogenic glandular tissue. In women under 30 years of age, ultrasound is a primary method of imaging palpable masses, as the majority of such women have dense breasts on x-ray mammography, and the palpable mass may not be imaged within the dense glandular tissue.[4,6,8,16,18,19,50] Frazier et al. used whole-breast ultrasonography to evaluate consecutive patients in whom x-ray mammography showed dysplastic breasts. The presence of dysplasia obscured mammographic visualization of the breast parenchyma and the underlying duct structures. In the absence of clustered microcalcifications suggesting malignancy, the dysplastic (DY) pattern on a mammogram made evaluation for malignancy difficult, and produced frequent

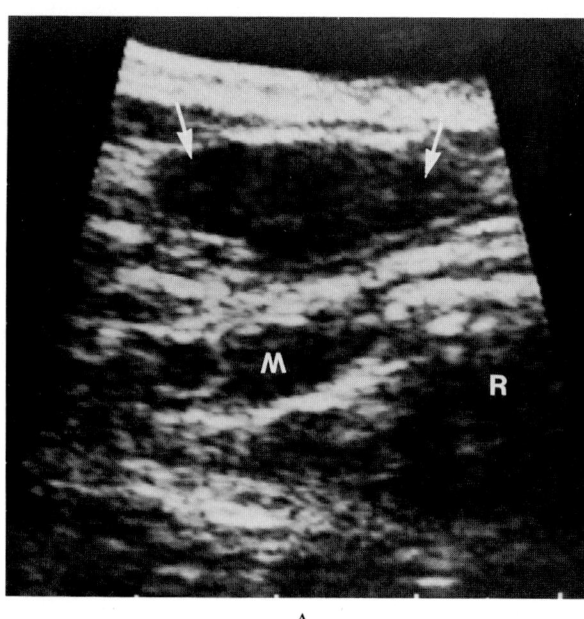

A

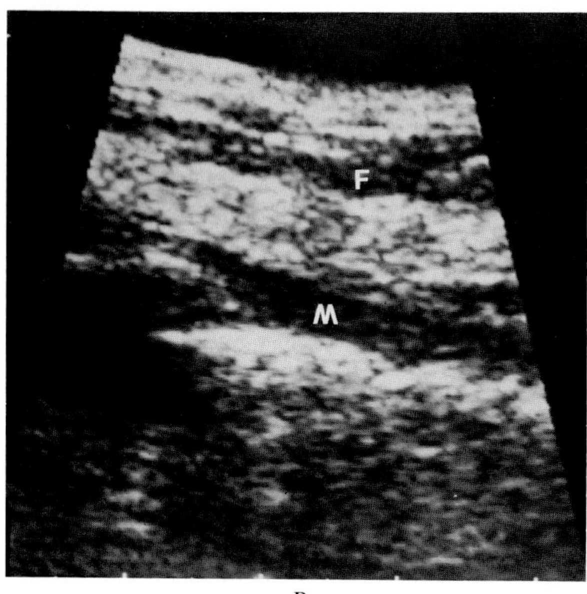

B

Figure 2-9. Fibroadenoma. A. Hand-held water-delay 7.5 MHz transducer over palpable breast mass in 38-year-old woman. Mass (arrows) contains low-level internal echoes, has well-defined lobulated margin, and does not exhibit acoustic attenuation. (M = muscle; R = rib) Excision biopsy confirmed a 2.2 × 1 cm fibroadenoma. B. Longitudinal hand-held B-scan of normal contralateral breast. Note echogenic parenchyma between subcutaneous fat (F) and Pectoralis major muscle (M).

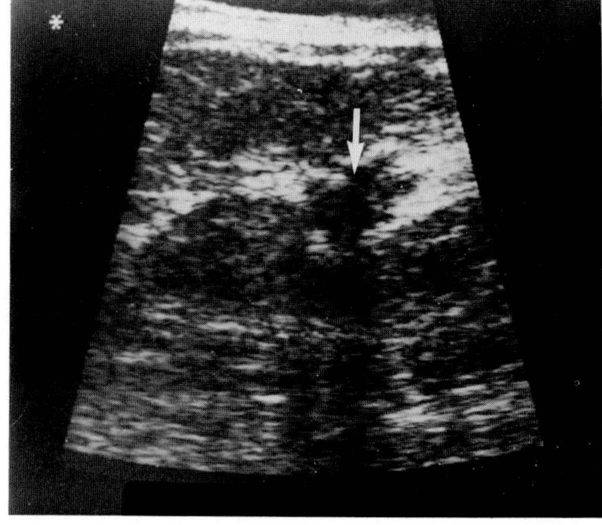

Figure 2-10. Infiltrating duct carcinoma. Hand-held water-delay sector B-scan, 7.5 MHz, shows irregular-marginated mass (arrow) containing weak internal echoes and exhibiting distal acoustic attenuation. Excision biopsy confirmed a 1 cm infiltrating duct carcinoma.

false-negative results. Whole-breast ultrasound detected 3 malignant and 2 suspicious lesions in the 135 patients. Fine-needle aspiration or biopsy confirmed 3 carcinomas and 2 fibroadenomas.[19]

Benign solid masses usually show smooth contour, round-to-oval shape, uniform, weak internal echoes, and well-defined anterior and posterior margins (Figs. 2–8 and 2-9). Acoustic attenuation is moderate, resulting in intermediate-strength echoes beyond the mass.[11,13,23,24,49] Another evaluation of 240 biopsy-confirmed solid breast masses with a dedicated breast scanner yielded 6 cases that exhibited characteristic benign-appearing criteria, but which proved on biopsy to be infiltrating duct carcinomas. For this reason, ultrasound B-scan criteria have been expanded to include as potentially malignant all imaged solid masses.[11,12] Thus, the histopathology of all dominant solid masses much be confirmed by fine-needle aspiration or open-excisional biopsy.

Malignant masses tend to manifest irregular or lobulated contours (Fig. 2-10).[33] From a retrospective review of 117 confirmed breast carcinomas of all histologic types, the majority (77 percent) of malignant solid masses demonstrated an irregular contour and contained weak internal echoes. Some degree of acoustic attenuation was evident in over two-thirds of these tumors (Figs. 2-10, 2-11, and 2-12).[5,12,33,53]

Infiltrating duct carcinomas comprise the majority of infiltrating breast cancers and elicit a desmoplastic reaction as they grow in stellate fashion into the breast parenchyma. For this reason, they are called scirrhous carcinomas. On a B-scan, they image as irregularly

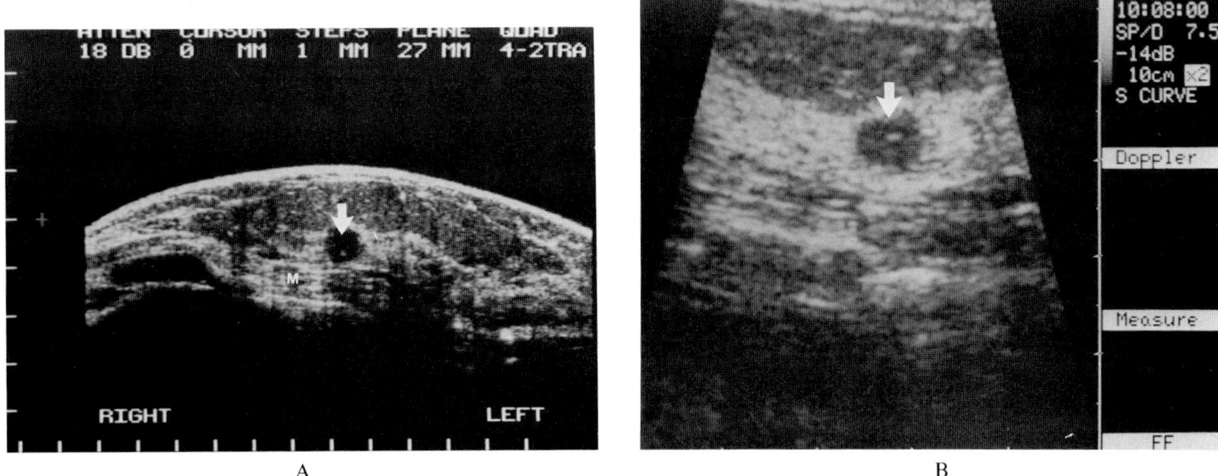

Figure 2-11. Infiltrating duct carcinoma. This 67-year-old woman had screening x-ray mammography that revealed 8 × 9 mm mass in left upper inner quadrant. A. Supine water-path 7.5 MHz transverse B-scan of superomedial aspect of left breast shows mass (arrow) within echogenic parenchyma. Mass has irregular margins and contains variable-strength, weak internal echoes. Some acoustic attenuation distal to mass extends through pectoralis major muscle (M). B. Hand-held 7.5 MHz water-delay longitudinal B-scan over the mass at higher gain setting shows "fill-in" of internal echoes. Biopsy confirmed a 9 mm infiltrating duct carcinoma.

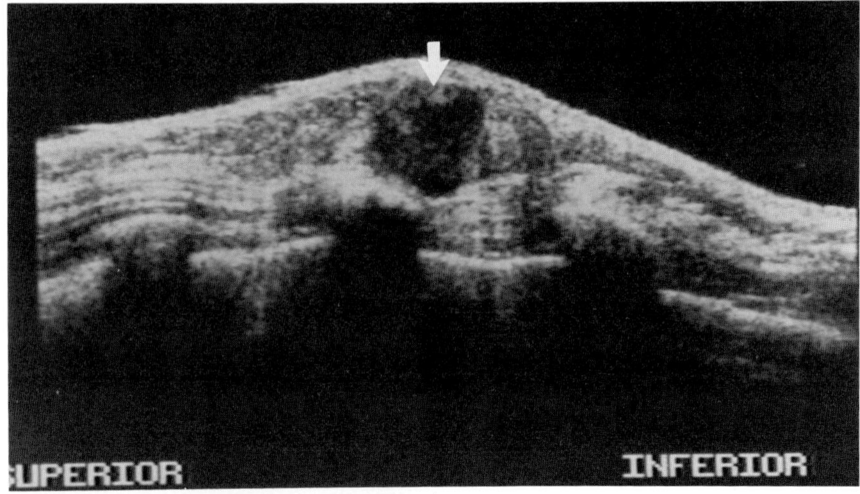

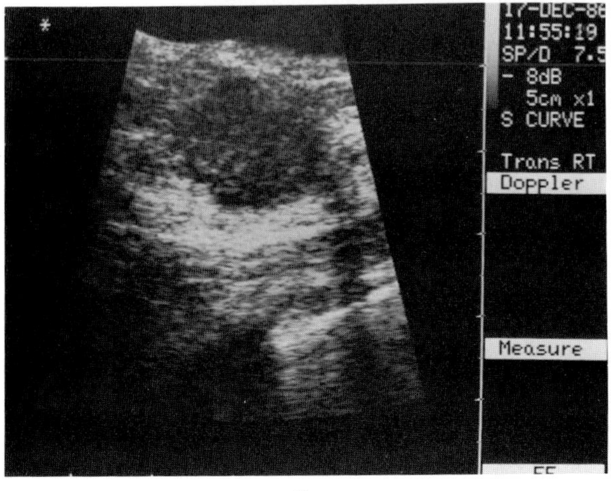

Figure 2-12. Infiltrating duct carcinoma. This 54-year-old woman presented with palpable mass in the right upper outer quadrant. A. 7.5 MHz supine water-path longitudinal B-scan shows a 2 cm irregular-margined solid mass (arrow) that contains variable strength internal echoes. Mass causes skin to bulge anteriorly. B. 7.5 MHz hand-held, water-delay real time transverse B-scan shows anterior skin bulge, slightly thickened skin, and the irregular margins of the mass. Biopsy confirmed infiltrating duct carcinoma.

marginated, variably shaped masses containing weak, nonuniform internal echoes distributed in a heterogeneous fashion. These tumors exhibit moderate-to-great acoustic attenuation, imaged on a B-scan as a central shadow distal to the mass.[1,4,5,12,31,35]

A small percentage of breast carcinomas are primarily cellular, as opposed to the previously described hypocellular carcinomas. Medullary carcinoma is an example of a cellular carcinoma. These generally bulky tumors may have a smooth periphery compared to the stellate periphery of infiltrating duct carcinomas. When imaged on ultrasound, medullary carcinomas have smooth or slightly lobulated margins and contain weak internal echoes. The distribution of the echoes within the mass may be nonhomogeneous. Because the mass does not exhibit significant acoustic attenuation, echoes are usually recorded distal to it.

Besides the aforementioned criteria for distinguishing benign versus malignant solid masses, additional criteria have been encountered in the evaluation of 4000 ultrasound mammograms performed at a university hospital. In premenopausal and postmenopausal women, an area of persistently strong acoustic attenuation sometimes represented an infiltrating carcinoma.[5,12,19] Areas of architectural distortion or areas that appeared different from the normal parenchyma sometimes represented malignancy. Bilateral subareolar asymmetry also indicated malignancy in some cases. Thickened or retracted Cooper's ligament and/or skin thickening in ultrasound images are signs of advanced infiltrating carcinoma (Fig. 2-6). Thickened skin may also be imaged at sites of keloid scar formation and at sites of irradiation following lumpectomy for early carcinoma.[20,34]

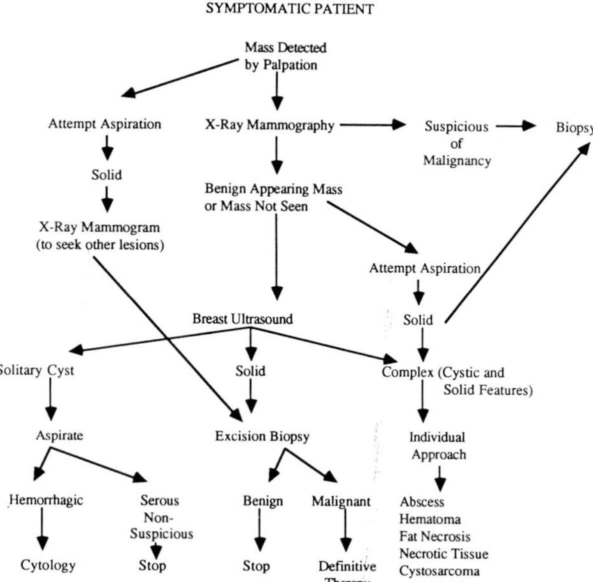

Figure 2-13. Current use of ultrasound mammography.

CALCIFICATIONS

Possible sources of abnormally increased acoustic attenuation include diffuse, dense fibrous connective tissue, biopsy scars, and clustered calcifications.[16,38] The coarse calcifications seen within mature fibroadenomas in x-ray mammograms are imaged on ultrasound B-scans as discrete, bright echoes on their anterior surfaces with acoustic shadowing posteriorly. The use of 7.5- and 10-MHz transducers permits identification of calcifications a few millimeters in diameter. However, ductal microcalcifications and vascular calcifications in the micron-size range are not usually recognized. When they are located within tissue that has a different acoustic impedance than that of the surrounding normal breast tissue (e.g., carcinoma), microcalcifications may rarely be visible as small, brightly echogenic foci with acoustic shadowing distally. Indeed, they may be partly responsible for the great acoustic attenuation observed in some breast cancers.

ADVANTAGES AND LIMITATIONS OF ULTRASOUND MAMMOGRAPHY

The primary attraction of ultrasound mammography is its ability to image the breast repeatedly with no known deleterious effects.[41] In addition, some of the information obtained is unavailable from any other imaging technique. Palpable breast masses can be conclusively determined to be fluid-filled or solid (Fig. 2-13). Whole breast ultrasound permits evaluation of the parenchymal pattern.[46] Data are currently being collected that may enable us to correlate the different ultrasonic parenchymal patterns with risk for breast cancer. Large fatty breasts were initially difficult to examine, but with breast compression this has ceased to be a problem.[17] Since malignant tumors are only weakly echogenic,[1] recognition of the architectural distortion and other subtle parenchymal abnormalities that they may incite has proven useful in distinguishing between fat lobules and small carcinomas.

The major limitation of poor spatial resolution of ultrasound mammograms has been overcome with the recent development of high-frequency transducer systems. Hand-held water-delay linear and sector 7.5- and 10-MHz transducers and higher frequency automated systems now allow resolution in the submillimeter range.[18,47] However, modern x-ray mammograms provide far superior resolution of microcalcifications in the micron range that may be the only sign of early carcinoma. Although ultrasound mammography is not yet suitable as the initial imaging examination for breast cancer screening, the American College of Radiology has recommended its use as an adjunct to x-ray mammography.

Enlargement of the soft tissues in the retroareolar

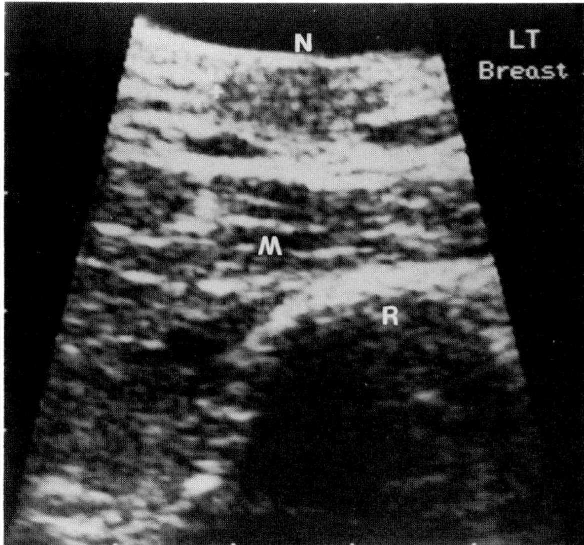

Figure 2-14. Localized gynecomastia. Hand-held sector B-scan over left nipple of 35-year-old man with palpable subareolar nodule. Hypoechoic area beneath nipple (N) represents localized gynecomastia. (R = rib, M = thick pectoralis major muscle). The etiology was chronic marijuana smoking.

region in males may represent proliferation of the secretory ducts. This latter condition is termed gynecomastia,[28,42,56] and can present clinically as a palpable mass. Carcinoma of the male breast may be difficult to differentiate from gynecomastia. X-ray imaging of the soft tissues of the anterior chest wall of the male may be technically difficult.[42] Ultrasound imaging using water-path techniques permits evaluation of the tissues of the anterior chest wall. Both localized and diffuse duct proliferation can be imaged (Figs. 2-14 and 2-15).[9] The criteria for masses are the same as for masses in the female breast.

Augmentation of the female breast may be performed for cosmetic reasons or after subcutaneous mastectomy. Silicone gel prostheses are inserted in the retromammary space for enlargement of small breasts. The breast parenchyma is then located over the surface of the conical prosthesis. Clinical evaluation of the glandular tissue overlying the prosthesis is frequently difficult due to scarring. Scarring occasionally occurs in the tissue immediately adjacent to the envelope of the silicone gel. Nodularity along the incision site may represent scar tissue, granulomas, or unassociated mass lesions. The glandular tissue overlying the prosthesis may be incompletely imaged by x-ray mammography due to superimposition by the excessively radiodense silicone. Ultrasound examination of an augmented breast, however, readily images both the glandular tissue and the prosthesis (Fig. 2-16).[10] Because the speed of sound in silicone is slower than the speed of sound in the parenchyma, the posterior surface of the silicone prosthesis will project posteriorly to the chest wall on a sonogram. This geometric distortion is an

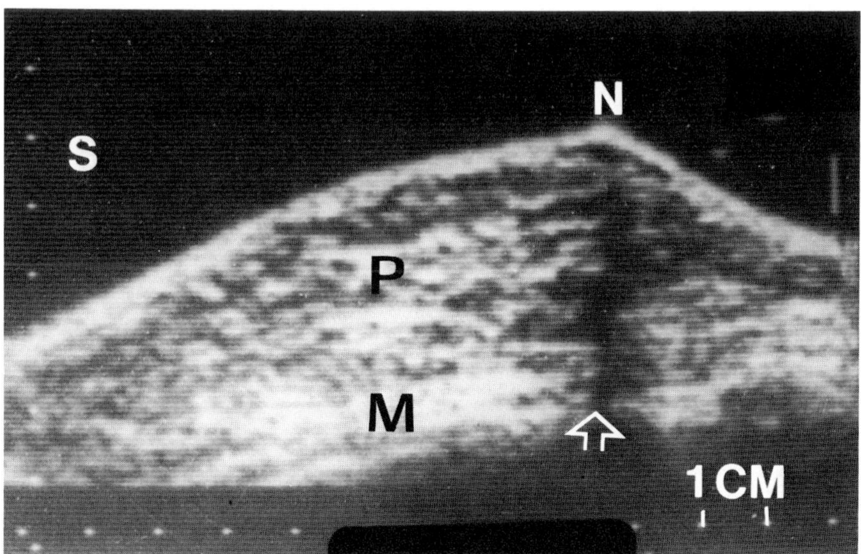

Figure 2-15. Diffuse gynecomastia in 74-year-old man with right breast enlargement. Sagittal B-scan through right nipple (N). Linear echo-free shadow under nipple extends through chest wall (arrow) and represents shadowing from nipple. (P = parenchyma; M = muscle; S = superior.) Patient had liver cirrhosis.

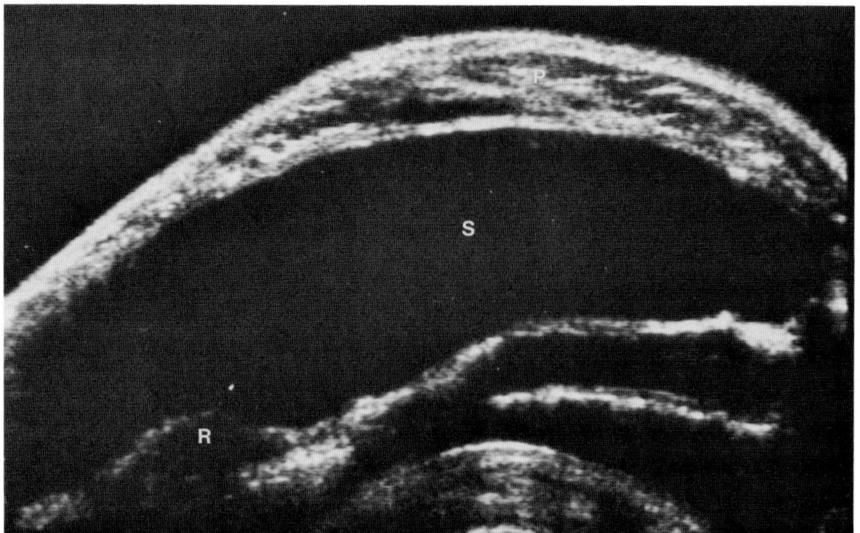

Figure 2-16. Breast augmentation with silicone bag prosthesis. A thin layer of breast parenchyma (P) present anterior to echo-free prosthesis (S). Posterior wall of bag shows artifact due to geometric distortion caused by slower speed of insonating beam in silicone; it appears to project posteriorly into chest wall. R = rib.

artifact that presents no diagnostic problem. Of course, if the prosthesis is saline-filled, there will be no such displacement of its posterior margin. A small percentage of patients develop a hard fibrous capsule around the silicone bag prosthesis. When this occurs, the prosthesis may assume a distorted shape, and a thickened bright line appears at the margin of the flattened or distorted silicone bag.[10]

FUTURE APPLICATIONS

Future applications of ultrasound mammography may include its use as the initial imaging examination. Repeated examinations are possible at any age without known hazard, an important factor for young women in whom x-ray mammography is less accurate than in older women in whom radiation exposure is of greater concern.[22] Combining ultrasound mammography with x-ray mammography increases diagnostic accuracy.[18,19,25]

REFERENCES

1. Calderon C, Vilkomerson D, Mezrich R, et al: Differences in the attenuation of ultrasound by normal, benign, and malignant breast tissue. J Clin Ultrasound 4:249–254, 1976
2. Cole-Beuglet C: Correlation of gross and microscopic anatomy of the breast with its ultrasound appearance. In Telles N (ed): Atlas of Breast Ultrasound. Cleveland, Ohio, Technicare, 1980, pp 49–71
3. Cole-Beuglet C: Ultrasound characteristics of normal breast structures. In Telles N (ed): Atlas of Breast Ultrasound. Cleveland, Ohio, Technicare, 1980, pp 38–48
4. Cole-Beuglet C, Beique RA: Continuous ultrasound B-scanning of palpable breast masses. Radiology 117:123–128, 1975
5. Cole-Beuglet C, Goldberg BB: Ultrasound in the diagnosis of breast cancer. In Goldberg B (ed): Ultrasound in Cancer: Clinics in Diagnostic Ultrasound. New York, Churchill Livingstone, 1981, pp 157–166
6. Cole-Beuglet C, Goldberg B, Kurtz A, et al: Clinical experience using a real-time dedicated breast scanner. AJR 139:905–911, 1982
7. Cole-Beuglet C, Kurtz AB, Rubin CS, et al: Ultrasound Mammography. Radiol Clin North Am 18:133–143, 1980
8. Cole-Beuglet C, Kurtz AB, Rubin CS, et al: Ultrasound mammography: A comparison to x-ray mammography. Radiology 140:693–698, 1981
9. Cole-Beuglet C, Schwartz GF, Kurtz AB, et al: Ultrasound mammography for male breast enlargement. JUM 1:301–305, 1982
10. Cole-Beuglet C, Schwartz GF, Kurtz AB, et al: Ultrasound mammography for the augmented breast. Radiology 146:737–742, 1983
11. Cole-Beuglet C, Soriano RZ, Kurtz AB, et al: Fibroadenoma of the breast: Sonomammography correlated with pathology of 122 patients. AJR 140:369–375, 1983
12. Cole-Beuglet C, Soriano RZ, Kurtz AB, et al: Ultrasound analysis of 104 primary breast carcinomas classified according to histopathologic type. Radiology 147:191–196, 1983
13. Cole-Beuglet C, Soriano RZ, Kurtz AB, et al: Ultrasound, x-ray mammography and histopathology of cystosarcoma phylloides. Radiology 146:481–486, 1983
14. Croll J, Kotevick J, Tabrett M: The diagnosis of benign disease and the exclusion of malignancy in patients with breast symptoms. Semin Ultrasound 3:38–50, 1982

15. Egan RL, Egan KL: Automated water-path full-breast sonography: Correlation with histology of 176 solid lesions. AJR 143:493–499, 1984
16. Egan RL, McSweeney MB, Murphy FB: Breast sonography and the detection of cancer. In Brunner S, Langfeldt B, Andersen PE (eds): Early Detection of Breast Cancer. New York, Springer-Verlag, 1984, pp 90–100
17. Ezo MG: Tissue compression for the optimization of images in water-path breast scanning. Med Ultrasound 5:113–117, 1981
18. Fleischer AC, Muhletaler CA, Reynolds VH, et al: Palpable breast masses: Evaluation by high frequency, hand-held, real-time sonography and xeromammography. Radiology 148:813–817, 1983
19. Frazier TG, Cole-Beuglet C, Kurtz AB, et al: Further evaluation by ultrasound of mammographically determined breast dysplasia. J Surg Oncol 19:69–70, 1982
20. Grant EG, Richardson JD, Citgay OS, et al: Sonography of the breast: Findings following conservative surgery and irradiation for early carcinoma. Radiology 147:532–540, 1983
21. Harper PA, Kelly-Fry E: Ultrasound visualization of the breast in symptomatic patients. Radiology 137:465–470, 1980
22. Harper PA, Kelly-Fry E, Noe JS: Ultrasound breast imaging: The method of choice for examining the young patient. Ultrasound Med Biol 7:231–237, 1981
23. Harper PA, Kelly-Fry E, Noe JS, et al: Ultrasound in the evaluation of solid breast masses. Radiology 146:731–736, 1983
24. Heywang SH, Lipsit ER, Glassman LM, et al: Specificity of ultrasonography in the diagnosis of benign breast masses. J Ultrasound Med 3:453–461, 1984
25. Isard HJ: Other imaging techniques. Cancer 53:658–664, 1984
26. Jellins J, Kossoff G, Reeve TS, et al: Detection and classification of liquid-filled masses in the breast by gray-scale echography. Radiology 125:205–212, 1977
27. Jellins J, Kossoff G, Reeve TS, et al: Ultrasonic gray-scale visualization of breast tissue. Ultrasound Med Biol 1:393–404, 1975
28. Kalischer L, Peyster R: Xerographic manifestations of male breast disease. AJR 125:656–661, 1975
29. Kelly-Fry E: Breast imaging. In Sabaagha RE (ed): Diagnostic Ultrasound Applied to Obstetrics and Gynecology. Hagerstown MD, Harper & Row, 1980, pp 327–350
30. Kobayashi T: Clinical Ultrasound of the Breast. New York, Plenum, 1978
31. Kobayashi T: Diagnostic ultrasound in breast cancer: Analysis of retrotumorous echo patterns correlated with sonic attenuation by cancerous connective tissue. J Clin Ultrasound 7:471–479, 1979
32. Kobayashi T: Gray-scale echography for breast cancer. Radiology 122:207–214, 1977
33. Kobayashi T: Ultrasonic detection of breast cancer. Clin Obstet Gynecol 25:409–423, 1982
34. Kopans DB, Meyer JE, Proppe KH: Double line of skin thickening on sonograms of the breast. Radiology 141:485–487, 1981
35. Kopans DB, Meyer JE, Steinbock RT: Breast cancer: The appearance as delineated by whole breast water-path ultrasound scanning. J Clin Ultrasound 10:313–322, 1982
36. Kossoff G, Carpenter DA, Robinson DE, et al: Octoson: A new rapid general purpose echoscope. In White D, Barnes R (eds): Ultrasound in Medicine (vol. 2). New York, Plenum, 1976, pp 333–339
37. Kossoff G, Garrett WJ, Carpenter DA, et al: Principles and classification of soft tissues by gray-scale echography. Ultrasound Med Biol 2:89–105, 1976
38. Kossoff G, Kelly-Fry E, Jellins J: Average velocity of ultrasound in the human female breast. J Accoust Soc Am 53:1730–1736, 1973
39. Laing FC, Jeffrey RB, Minagi H: Ultrasound localization of occult breast lesions. Radiology 151:795–796, 1984
40. Lees WR: Breast ultrasonography. In Saunders RC (ed): Ultrasound Annual 1982. New York, Raven, 1982, pp 301–326
41. Lele PP: Revue: Safety and potential hazards in the current applications of ultrasound in obstetrics and gynecology. Ultrasound Med Biol 5:307–320, 1979
42. Michels L, Gold R, Arndt R: Radiology of gynecomastia and other disorders of the male breast. Radiology 122:117–122, 1977
43. Reuter K, D'Orsi CJ, Reale F: Intracystic carcinoma of the breast: The role of ultrasonography. Radiology 153:233–234, 1984
44. Rosner D, Weiss L, Norman W: Ultrasonography in the diagnosis of breast disease. J Surg Oncol 14:83–86, 1980
45. Rubin CS, Kurtz AB, Goldberg BB, et al: Ultrasonic examination of the breast. In Marchant DJ, Nyirjesy I (eds): Breast Disease: Proceedings of an International Symposium. New York, Grune & Stratton, 1978, pp 126–135
46. Rubin CS, Kurtz AB, Goldberg BB, et al: Ultrasonic mammographic parenchymal patterns: A preliminary report. Radiology 130:515–517, 1979
47. Rubin E, Miller VE, Berland LL, et al: Hand-held real-time breast sonography. AJR 144:623–627, 1985
48. Schneck CD, Lehman DA: Sonographic anatomy of the breast. Semin Ultrasound 3:13–33, 1982
49. Sickles EA, Filly RA, Callen PW: Benign breast lesions: Ultrasound detection and diagnosis. Radiology 151:467–470, 1984
50. Sickles EA, Filly RA, Callen PW: Breast cancer detection with sonography and mammography: Comparison using state-of-the-art equipment. AJR 140:843–845, 1983
51. Teixidor HS: The use of ultrasonography in the management of masses of the breast. Surg Gynecol Obstet 150:486–490, 1980
52. Teixidor HS, Kazam E: Combined mammographic-sonographic evaluation of breast masses. AJR 128:409–417, 1977
53. Wagai T, Takahashi S, Ohashi H, et al: A trial for quantitative diagnosis of breast tumor by ultrasonotomography. Japan Med Ultrasonics 5:39, 1967
54. Wells PNT, Evans KT: An immersion scanner for two-dimensional ultrasonic examination of the human breast. Ultrasonics 6:220–228, 1968
55. Wild JJ, Reid JM: Further pilot echographic studies of the histologic structure of tumors of the living intact human breast. Am J Pathol 28:839–854, 1952
56. Wilson J, Arman J, MacDonald P: The pathogenesis of gynecomastia. Intern Med 25:1–32, 1980
57. Wolfe JN: Breast parenchymal patterns and their changes with age. Radiology 121:545–552, 1976

Carl J. D'Orsi, M.D.
Royal J. Bartrum, M.D.
Myron M. Moskowitz, M.D.

3

Lightscanning of the Breast

Transillumination of the breast, first reported by Cutler in 1929, was originally limited to direct visualization of the breast in a light-free environment.[3] In the 1960s, Gros et al. introduced photographic recording of the transilluminated breast on color film.[9] In the 1970s, Ohlsson et al. used infrared-sensitive film to enhance diagnostic capability.[13] Currently, video systems are employed that utilize light in the red and near-infrared part of the spectrum[2]; the transmitted light is televised with a red-infrared-sensitive vidicon tube, allowing continuous observation of the examination on a display monitor and recording on videotape or disc.

BASIC PRINCIPLES

The basis of lightscanning is that different tissues have different patterns of light absorption when transilluminated with light in the red and near-infrared portions of the electromagnetic spectrum. When an electromagnetic wave such as light impinges on biologic tissue, two effects occur: scattering and absorption. Scattering and absorption both cause attenuation, so that the wavelengths of light exiting the breast are less than those entering. [17] Light wavelengths ranging from 600 to 1060 nanometers (nm) in the red and near-infrared portion of the spectrum are used for the examination. Wavelengths below 600 nm are very strongly absorbed, producing markedly diminished transmitted light, while wavelengths above 1060 nm are difficult to study due to the sensitivity limitations of detector systems.

The equipment we have been using produces a transmission image of the breast in two separate wavelength bands, one in the red and the other in the near-infrared range. A composite image is reconstructed by a computer. The reconstructed imaged contains two parameters: *luminence* or total light transmission, and *ratio* or the ratio of near-infrared to red transmission (IR/R). It is hoped that specific tissues, e.g., cancerous versus normal, eventually will be found to have specific transmission signatures. Although further experimentation into the interaction of light and biologic tissue is warranted, preliminary findings are available for review.

It has been shown that adipose tissue manifests greater transmission in the red region than does glandular or cancerous tissue. Transmission of light in the red/near-infrared region is strongly inhibited by hemoglobin. Thus, although experimentally there is little difference in tissue transmittance between glandular and malignant tissue per se, *in vivo* carcinoma in most instances yields a lower transmission than does glandular tissue due to the higher hemoglobin content of carcinoma. However, the decreased transmission is not specific for cancer, but merely reflects the increased blood flow and hemoglobin content of carcinoma.[5]

BREAST CANCER DETECTION
ISBN 0-8089-1842-7

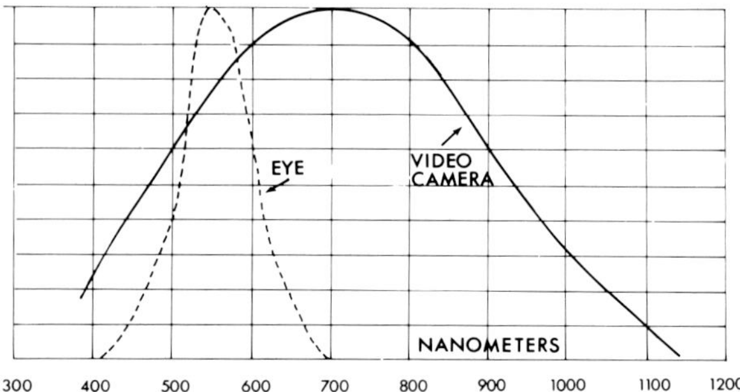

Figure 3-1. Operating range for video camera. Spectrum of wavelengths ranges from 400 to 1100 nanometers with peak at 700 nm (red-orange). Compared to human eye, camera has greater depth of sensitivity. (Modified from Merrit CRB, Sullivan MA, Segaloff A, et al: Real-time transillumination lightscanning of the breast. RadioGraphics 4:991, 1984.)

DESIGN AND OPERATION OF A CLINICAL LIGHTSCANNING INSTRUMENT

Lightscanning instruments employ a tungsten light source that produces a broad-spectrum white light that is then modified by rapidly rotating filters to a predominately red and near-infrared output. This narrowed spectrum of light is carried to the breast via fiberoptic bundles terminating in a wand that is positioned against the breast. A specially modified video camera sensitive to wavelengths in the red and near-infrared range records transmission data from the opposite surface of the breast (Fig. 3-1). These analog video signals are then passed through an analog-to-digital converter and stored in digital format in a 512 × 256 × 256 matrix similar to those of computed tomography or magnetic resonance imaging. The total light transmission values, one for red and one for near-infrared, of each pixel are averaged, producing the luminence parameter that is then displayed on a television monitor in shades of gray (Fig. 3-2). The ratio parameter, established by dividing the red transmission into the near-infrared, is displayed in a color-coded format (Fig. 3-3). Ratios with values greater than one are assigned colors in the blue family, while those under one are allotted colors in the red family. A ratio of one is white, and therefore yields no color (Fig. 3-4). Several display programs are available. A black-and-white program is used to display luminence information alone. Combined luminence and differential transmission information is displayed with varying contrast in color-coded programs.

Several factors may act to inhibit the identification of an abnormality. The most important of these that affects lesional definition is the penumbra effect. For example, the shadow produced by a hand placed in a beam of light becomes sharper the closer the hand is moved toward the surface on which the shadow is projected. Thus if we consider a pinpoint-sized source that produces a beam of light, which then passes through a nonscattering medium and strikes an object that absorbs all of the light, the resultant shadow will be larger the further the absorber is from the projection surface, while still maintaining a relatively sharp margin (Fig. 3-5). However, if the light source is larger than a pin-point and/or passes through a diffusing medium such as the breast, a penumbra effect is encountered. This means that the further the shadowing object is from its projection surface, the more diffuse is its shadow, the less is its contrast, and the more indistinct is its margin. The penumbra effect can be diminished by placing the light-absorbing surface as close as possible to the surface through which the light exits (Fig. 3-6).

A lightscan requires extensive operator input, attention to technique, and proper machine preparation. Six views of each breast are obtained as the breast is compressed (Fig. 3-7). This permits all of the glandular tissue to be evaluated and decreases the thickness of the breast, thereby bringing shadowing objects closer to the projection surface, in order to minimize the penumbra effect. The actual amount of transilluminating and exiting light for both wavelength bands is available for each pixel (Fig. 3-8). Normally these amounts should be approximately equal for equivalent views of each breast.

THE NORMAL BREAST AND BENIGN DISORDERS

Since most judgments concerning the presence or absence of breast disease in images rely on a comparison of similar views of each breast, the lightscanning unit is equipped with a split-screen monitor to simultaneously view mirror images of both breasts. Normal breasts tend to appear bilaterally symmetrical in comparable views recorded either in the black-and-white mode or with the various color sequences (Fig. 3-9).* The veins are clearly visible due to their superficial location and hemoglobin content, and appear black in the black-and-white program and blue-black in the color program. Because the veins of normal breasts may be bilaterally asymmetric in their distribution and depth, asymmetry is not a reliable clue to underlying cancer (Fig. 3-10).

After the instrument is properly balanced for each patient, the color program reveals an approximately symmetrical distribution of reds and blues in both breasts. Deviation from this symmetrical pattern, either in luminence or color, is an indication of possible malignancy. The subareolar region contains an abun-

* Figures 3-9 through 3-22 are color plates placed between text pages 174 and 175.

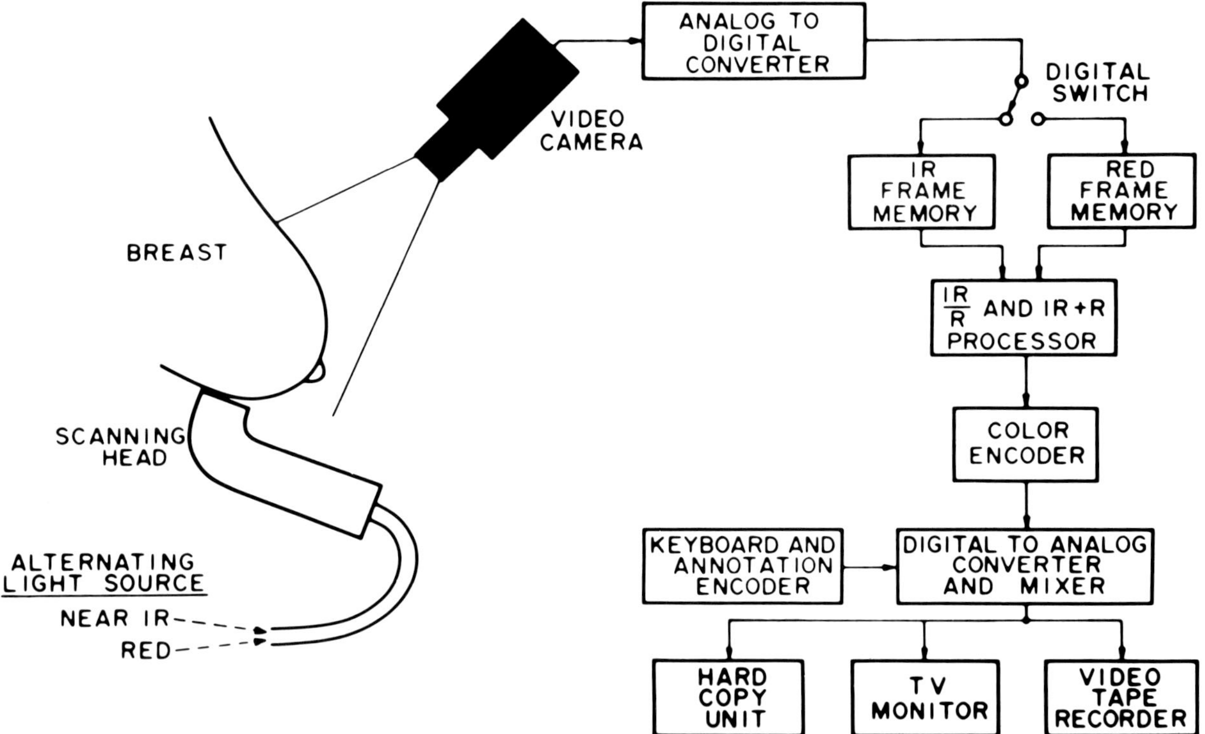

Figure 3-2. Operation of clinical lightscanning unit. (Modified from Merritt CRB, Sullivan MA, Segaloff A, et al: Real-time transillumination lightscanning of the breast. RadioGraphics 4:991, 1984.)

dance of vascular and ductal structures in a confined area, and often produces shades of blue to black (Fig. 3-11).

The features of fibrocystic change are variable. Mild change is indistinguishable from the normal, while severe change may result in multiple areas of increased luminence. Macrocyst formation, because of its increased luminence, tends to produce a colorless area that often stands out from the surrounding breast tissue (Fig. 3-12).[10,16,18] Fibroadenomas vary in appearance, from a mass indistinguishable from adjacent normal tissue to a mass with sharply decreased luminence and a high infrared-to-red ratio mimicking carcinoma.

CANCER

Lightscan criteria for cancer may conveniently be divided into direct and indirect signs (Table 3-1). Direct signs relate to a malignant mass, while indirect signs relate to changes in structures adjacent to a cancer, such as vessels, parenchyma, and skin. The most important and consistent sign of cancer is increased light absorption. The resultant decrease in luminence can be seen with all display programs, but is best appreciated in the black-white mode. The enhanced absorption may be focal, regional, or total.[6,11] Focal absorption is a function of the malignant mass itself (Fig. 3-13). At times, and for reasons not completely understood, a malignant

Figure 3-3. Pixel parameters. Each pixel contains luminence and ratio information. (IR = infrared; R = red.)

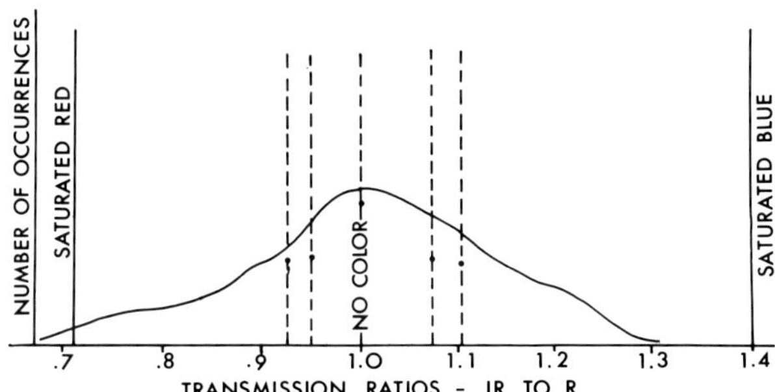

Figure 3-4. Color code map. Colors are assigned according to value of transmitted near-infrared light divided by transmitted red light (IR/R).

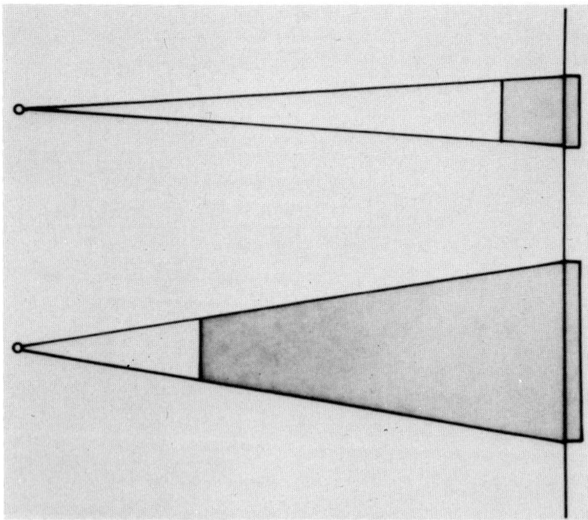

Figure 3-5. Penumbra effect. A pinpoint source of light will progressively magnify the shadow of a light-absorbing object the farther it is from the projection surface, but the shadow will retain a relatively sharp margin.

mass may diminish light transmittance regionally or throughout the breast (Fig. 3-14). This is understandable with a large infiltrating carcinoma, a comedocarcinoma that involves the entire ductal network of a breast, diffuse carcinomatosis, or inflammatory carcinoma. However, the phenomenon may also be seen in association with cancer that does not involve the entire breast or even a quadrant of it.

Opinion differs as to the importance of indirect signs. Ohlsson[13] and Carlsen[2] believe that indirect signs serve as important aids in finding cancer, but our experience regarding their usefulness has been much less favorable. In general, when these signs coexist with the direct sign of increased absorption, the confidence level for the presence of cancer is highest. If the indirect signs are present alone, however, their specificity is greatly dimished. Asymmetry, which is easily ascertained utilizing a split screen, is an extremely important factor to consider when evaluating both direct and indirect signs (Fig. 3-15). Any change on serial examinations is also significant, and increases the probability of cancer (Fig. 3-16).

Various combinations of direct and indirect signs may occur. The greatest weight for a diagnosis of cancer is given to an aggregation of an absorption abnormality, IR/R ratio abnormality, and asymmetric vascularity (Fig. 3-17). Of least significance is an isolated indirect sign.

There are certain pitfalls in evaluating breast lightscans. Since the presence of increased amounts of hemoglobin, whether associated with cancer or not, produces a decrease in light transmittance, the bleeding that may follow biopsy or needle aspiration, or that leads to hemorrhage into a cyst, duplicates the findings associated with cancer (Fig. 3-18). Increased light absorption may be present for 4–6 weeks following needle aspiration. This diagnostic pitfall may be eliminated by obtaining an appropriate history and by performing follow-up scans. The subareolar region is normally vascular and therefore manifests increased light absorption, a finding that should not be misinterpreted as an abnormality. Papillomas, common benign tumors within the major subareolar ducts, are also vascular and may yield lightscan findings indistinguishable from those of cancer (Fig. 3-19).

A biopsy scar has a typical appearance of a line of increased or decreased absorption (Fig. 3-20). Small, highly absorptive rounded foci representing skin moles or nevi are often encountered and do not present a diagnostic problem (Fig. 3-21).

One final caution relates to portions of the breast that are particularly difficult to examine with lightscanning. The region close to the chest wall is particularly treacherous. In Sickles's series, four of seven carcinomas greater than 2 cm in diameter and not detectable by lightscanning were located close to the chest wall.[14] We have found that a meticulous technique is required to adequately examine this region.

Of additional interest is the use of lightscanning for the pathologic evaluation of specimens. Carcinoma in these specimens frequently produces focal absorption or a color shift toward the blue range (Fig. 3-22). This

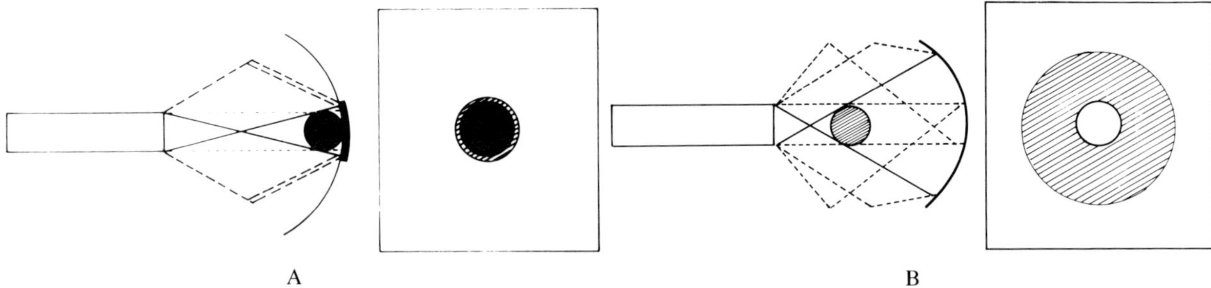

Figure 3-6. Penumbra effect. A. When diffuse light source produces shadow from light-scattering medium, its margins are fairly well maintained when object is close to projection surface, resulting in minimal penumbra. B. When same object is farther from projection surface, larger penumbra is produced.

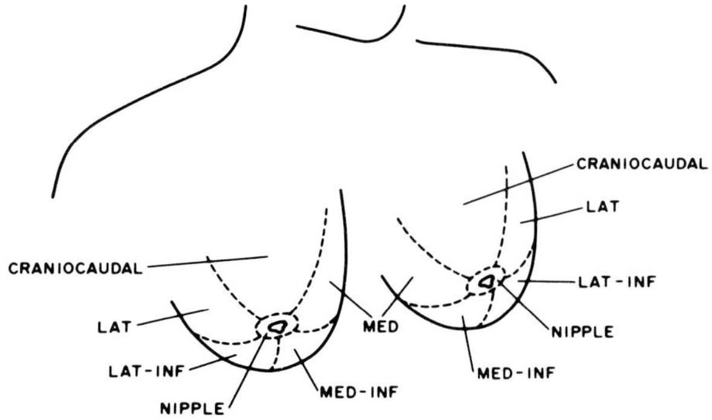

Figure 3-7. Standard views for breast examination.

may assume importance as the clinician attempts to ascertain whether a malignant mass has been included in the specimen. Such information may be difficult to obtain with specimen radiography, particularly if the carcinoma is embedded in dense parenchymal tissue and is uncalcified. Specimen scanning may also aid in ascertaining the dimensions of the cancer for staging.

EFFICACY FOR CANCER DETECTION

Since the advent of modern lightscanning, articles have compared its merits relative to those of x-ray mammography and sonography for breast cancer detection.[1,4,7,8,11,12,14,15] These studies (Table 3-2) have engendered feelings ranging from enthusiastic support for those investigators who suggest that lightscanning has a diagnostic capability similar to that of mammography, to unbridled pessimism. Although it is difficult to come to any concrete conclusions regarding breast lightscanning based on these relatively few published studies, a brief discussion of their design may help us to understand the great disparity in their results, and the ensuing confusion about the efficacy of lightscanning.

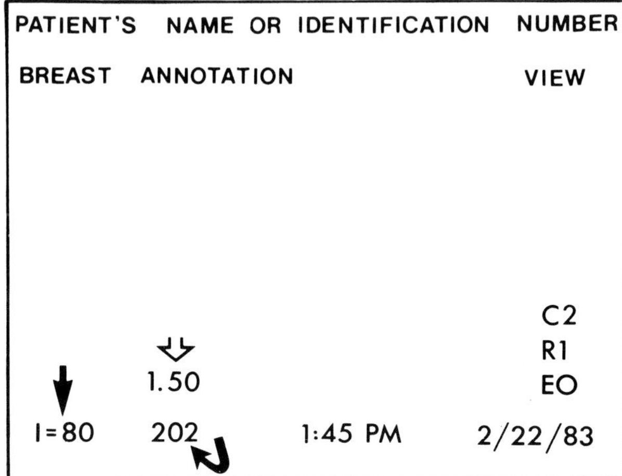

Figure 3-8. Unit annotation. Light intensity (straight arrow), amount of red and infrared light transmitted or luminence (curved arrow), and balance between reds and blues (hollow arrow) are presented at lower left in relative units.

One obvious factor that may explain divergent results pertains to differing equipment and techniques. The equipment in these studies varied from monochromatic, ''in-house'' produced instruments to color-coded commercial units. The significance of the varying equipment is unknown, but it does introduce a significant bias.

The lightscanning technique is one of the most operator-dependent in all diagnostic imaging. In the published investigations, the examinations were performed by individuals with varying degrees of expertise. Physicians performed the examination in most of the studies[6,14,15]; however, in one feasibility study all examinations were carried out by radiologic technologists trained in the technique,[1] while in another study both physicians and technologists were used.[11]

The amount of clinical information provided to the lightscan readers differed among the studies. Some authors interpreted the lightscans with full knowledge of the mammographic findings.[6,14] Others interpreted the lightscans in a blinded fashion.[11,14] Some studies at-

Table 3-1
Transillumination Criteria for Malignancy

I. Direct signs
   A. focal absorption
   B. regional absorption
   C. overall absorption

II. Indirect signs
   A. focal or regional asymmetric color change
   B. vascular asymmetry
   C. vessel clustering
   D. abrupt vessel caliber change
   E. skin retraction
   F. interval change between lightscan examinations

COLOR PLATE LEGENDS

Figure 3-9. Normal examinations. A. Superior view of each breast in color mode. Note bilaterally symmetric distribution of veins. B. Lateral view in color mode demonstrates color balance and bilateral venous symmetry.

Figure 3-10. Normal venous structure. Color mode. Superior surface view illustrates absorption by veins. Sharp margins of veins are due to their superficial position. Asymmetrical venous distribution alone, as in this case, does not imply underlying abnormality.

Figure 3-11. Subareolar region. Color program demonstrating range of blue often exhibited in subareolar portion of breast.

Figure 3-12. Macrocyst. Superior view in color program of area of increased luminence (arrows) typical for benign macrocyst formation.

Figure 3-13. Focal absorption. A. Split screen, black-and-white mode. Area of bilaterally asymmetric focal absorption suspicious for malignancy (arrow). B. Same case presented in color mode.

Figure 3-14. Regional and total absorption. Black-and-white (A) and color (B) modes. Regional absorption (arrows) shown in lateral view on split-screen display, highly suggestive of carcinoma. C. Superior view, color mode. Total light absorption on right, secondary to inflammatory carcinoma.

Figure 3-15. Asymmetry. A. Black-and-white program. Lateral view of asymmetric cluster of veins (arrow) and focal absorption (arrowheads). B. Color program. Superior view discloses venous enlargement (hollow arrow) and focal absorption (arrow). C. Color program. Lateral view reveals unbalanced area of transmission (arrow). As an isolated finding it is not as significant as increased absorption.

Figure 3-16. Serial absorption change. A. Single lateral view, color mode, of vague area of regional absorption (arrow). B. Two-month follow-up illustrates increase in absorption. Carcinoma.

Figure 3-17. Direct and indirect signs of cancer. A. Black-and-white views of superior surface of both breasts disclose focal absorption (arrowhead) and vessel enlargement on left (arrow). Compare to normal contralateral vessel (hollow arrow). B. Color mode. Lateral view on left reveals focal absorption (hollow arrow), shift to blue range (solid arrow), and vascular asymmetry (arrowhead). This constellation of findings is highly suspicious for malignancy.

Figure 3-18. Effects of hemorrhage. A. Color mode. Superior surface view discloses two large regions of light absorption with coalescence (arrows). Patient had two needle aspirations several days previously. B. Follow-up scan reveals marked regression of absorption (arrows). C. Large round area of absorption (arrow) represents hemorrhagic cyst.

Figure 3-19. Papilloma. Prominent asymmetric diminution in light transmittance (arrow) in subareolar region, indistinguishable from malignancy.

Figure 3-20. Biopsy scars. Linear focus of faint absorption (arrows) on superior surface of breast, color mode.

Figure 3-21. Skin nevi. Rounded, sharply etched, light-absorptive foci on superior surface view, color program.

Figure 3-22. Breast specimen lightscan. Carcinoma produces highly absorptive region with strands representing tumor infiltration (hollow arrow). Adjacent region of dense fibrosis (arrow) depicted in blue.

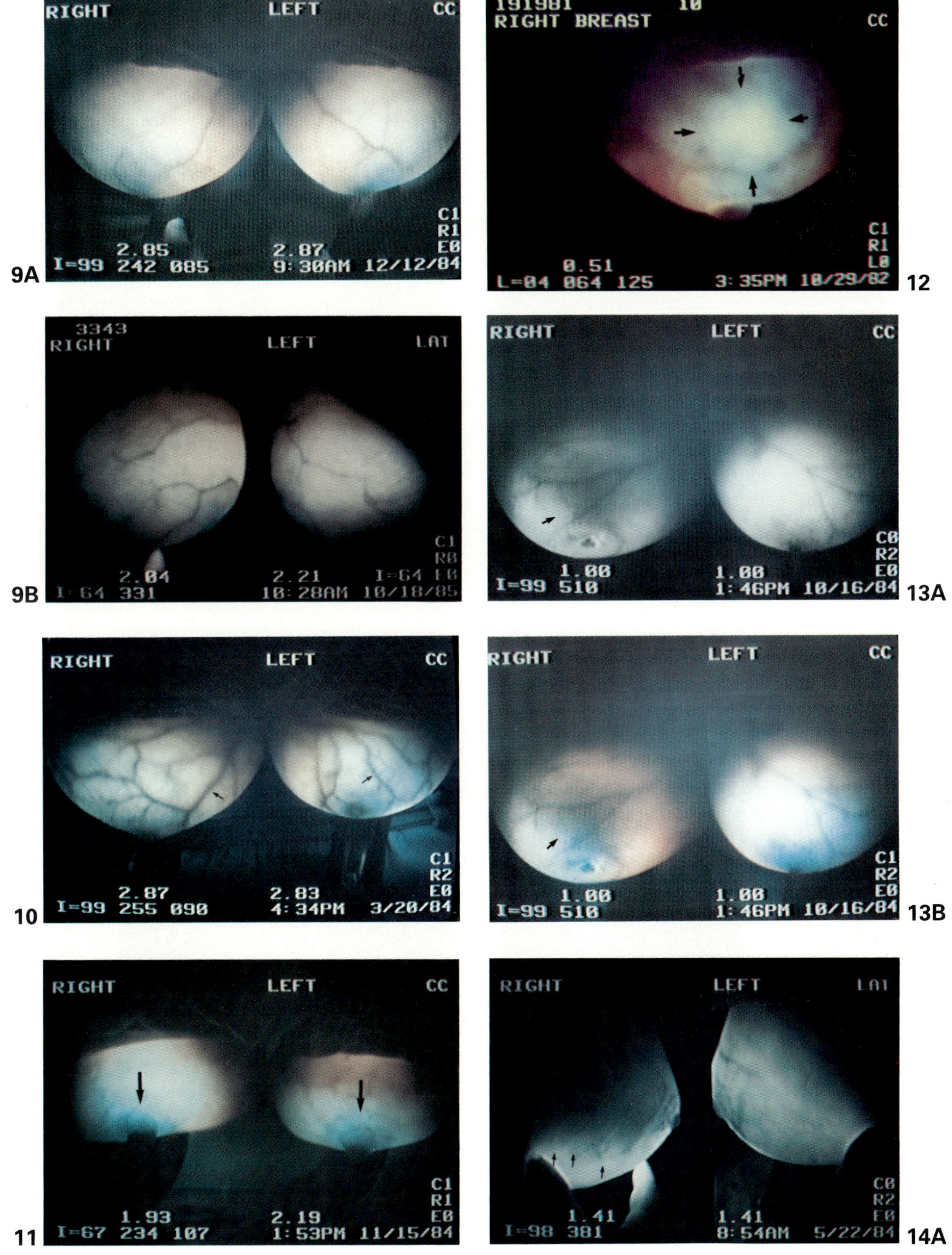

9A

12

9B

13A

10

13B

11

14A

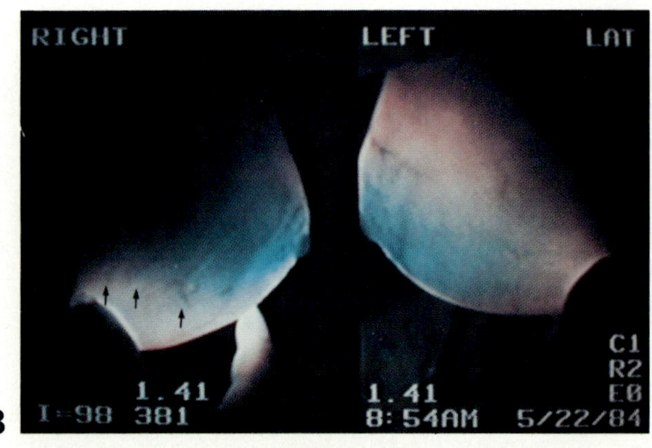

14B

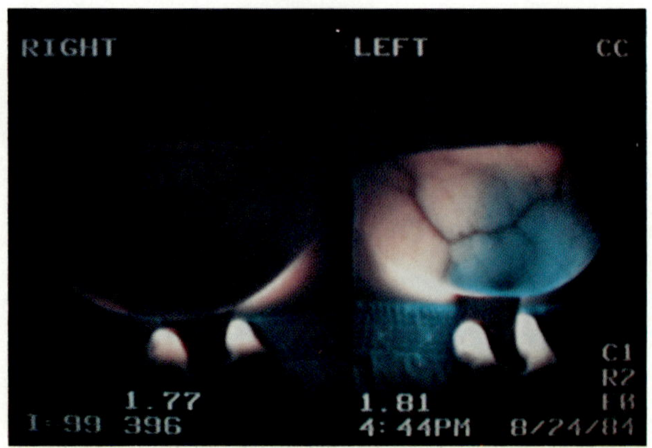

14C

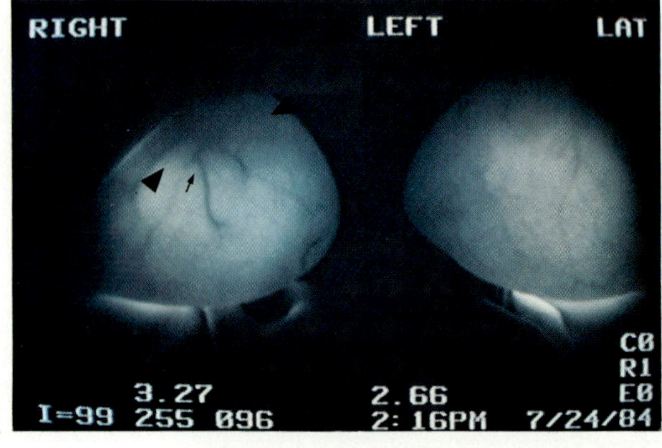

15A

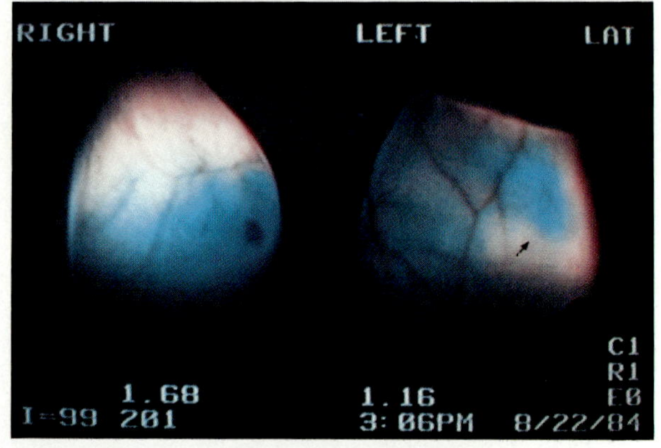

15C

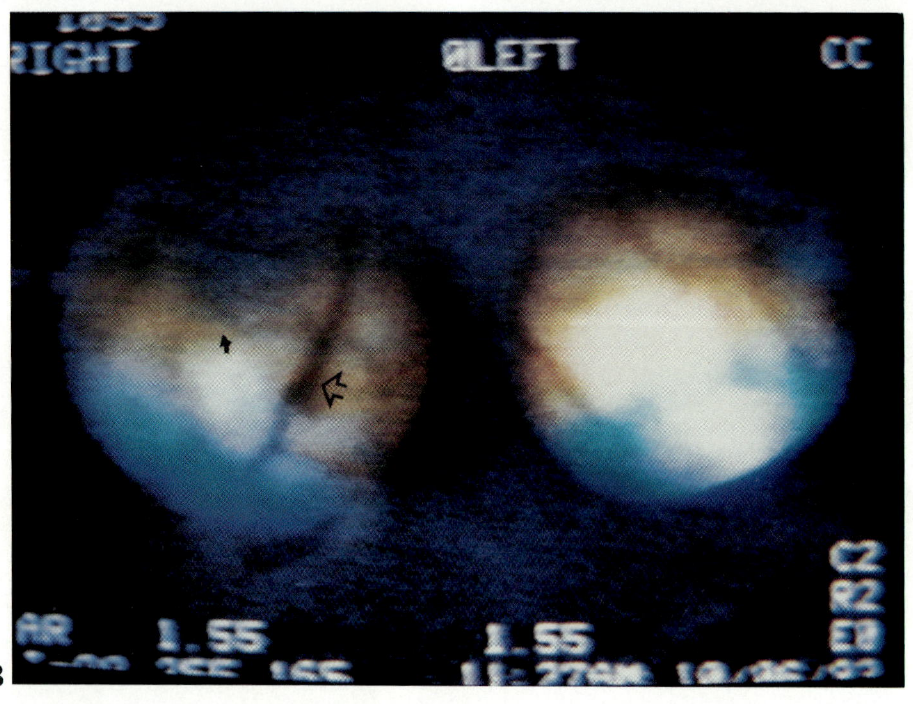

15B

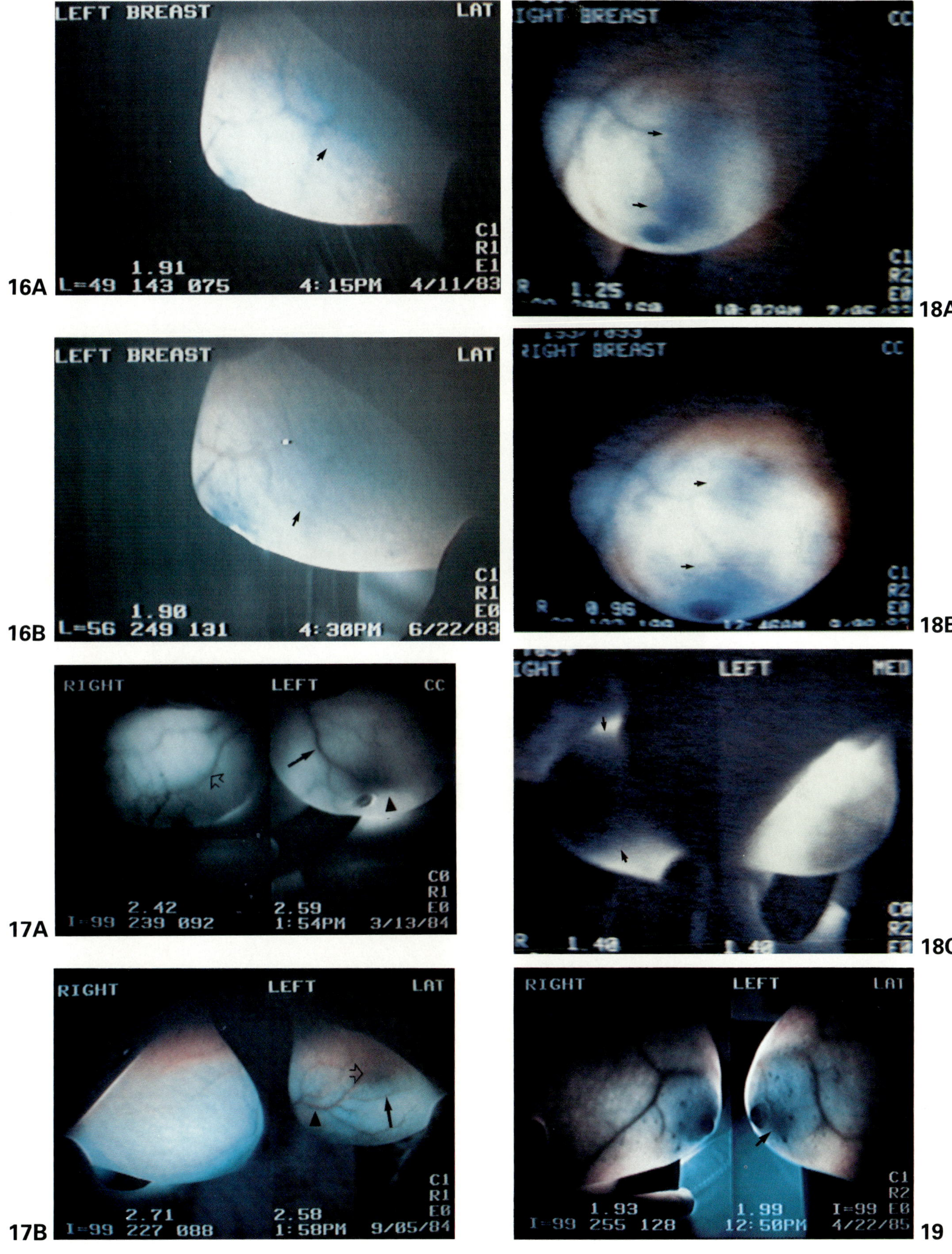

16A

16B

17A

17B

18A

18B

18C

19

20

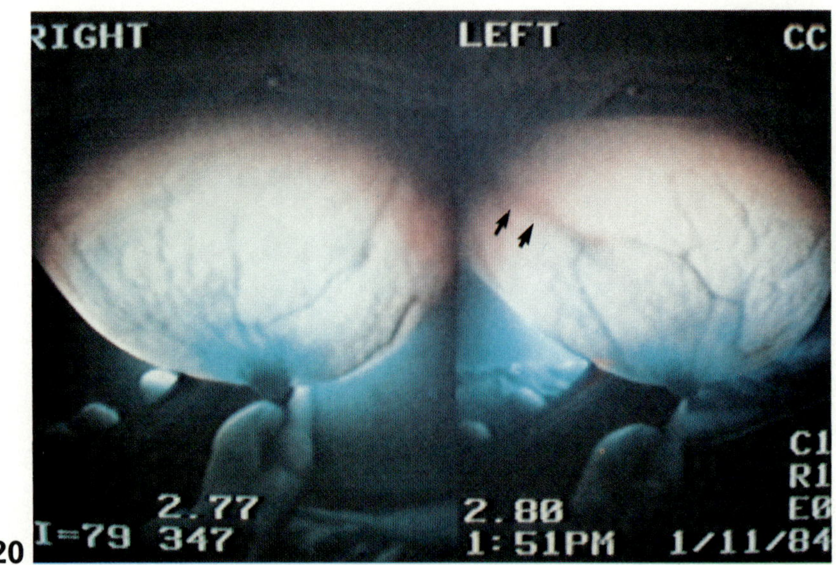
RIGHT
LEFT
CC
C1
R1
E0
2.77
2.80
I=79 347
1:51PM 1/11/84

21

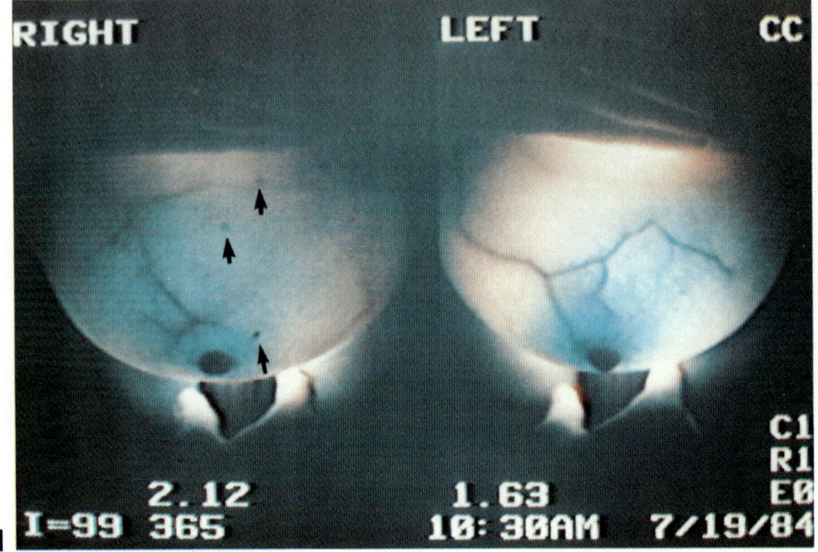
RIGHT
LEFT
CC
C1
R1
E0
2.12
1.63
I=99 365
10:30AM 7/19/84

22

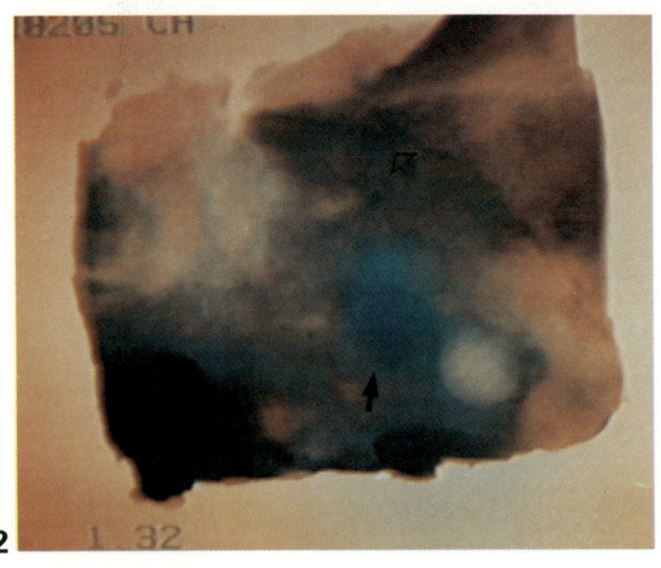
1.32

Table 3-2
Published Reports on Lightscanning

Author	Number of Cancers	Tumor >1 cm or Palpable Masses %	Lightscan Sensitivity %	Lightscan Specificity %	Lightscan + Predictive Value %	Lightscan − Predictive Value %
Wallberg et al.[15]	110	79 Palpable masses	85	91	86	90
Bartrum et al.[1]	33	73 Palpable masses	76	83	12	99
Marshall et al.[11]	34	57 Palpable masses	77	95	—	—
Drexler et al.[4]	26	62 Palpable masses	58	94	—	—
Sickles[14]	83	63 Palpable masses	43	—	—	—
Geslien et al.[8]	33	67 Palpable masses	58	—	—	—
Greene et al.[12]	46	76 Palpable masses	98	79	—	—
Merritt et al.[7]	63	72 Tumors >1 cm	77	83	—	—

tempted both blinded and nonblinded reading.[1] One would expect that knowledge of mammographic data would yield a higher sensitivity for lightscan interpretations than the sensitivity of those evaluated in a blinded manner. Interestingly, most of the studies in which the lightscans were read with full knowledge of mammographic results were among the lowest in sensitivity. Bartrum et al., however, showed a difference in sensitivity between blinded and nonblinded readings, with the former at 76 percent and the latter at 94 percent.[1]

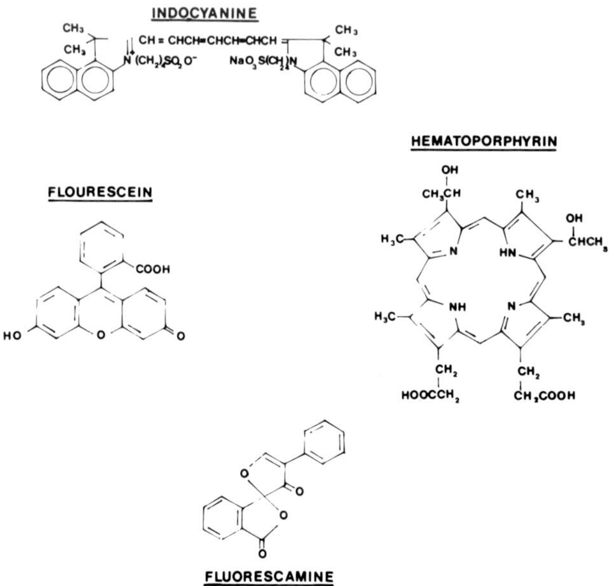

Figure 3-23. Light-sensitive compounds.

Analysis of the literature suggests that most investigators introduced an understandable bias into their research: The mammographic findings usually determined whether or not a patient was to be biopsied; lightscanning played a purely adjunctive role. The fact that a patient with a positive lightscan and a negative mammogram did not go to biopsy tended to decrease the sensitivity of lightscanning and increase the sensitivity of mammography. Geslien et al., however, reported 11 patients with persistently positive lightscans and negative mammograms who came to biopsy,[6] two of whom had carcinoma. Marshall et al. attempted to correct for this bias by calculating "best case" and "worst case" statistics.[11] The "best case" group was composed of all patients with positive lightscans and/or mammograms and who were presumed to have cancer. The "worst case" scenario was composed of 30 nonbiopsied patients with positive lightscans and three with "positive" mammograms, all presumed free of cancer. In the "worst case" setting, the sensitivity and specificity of lightscanning was 76.5 and 95.8 percent, respectively, while in the "best case" scenario it was 87.5 and 98.8 percent, respectively.

The sizes of the detected carcinomas was an issue addressed in several of the studies. Size is an important consideration in ascertaining the efficacy of lightscanning for screening, since most cancers so discovered should be less than 1 cm in diameter. Bartrum et al. found the sensitivity diminished to 44 percent for lesions under 1 cm.[1] Sickles found a sensitivity of 19 percent when only masses under 1 cm were considered.[14] Drexler et al. studied 20 carcinomas under 2 cm and found that lightscanning detected 11 and mammography 19.[4] In the series of Geslien et al., the overall sensitivity

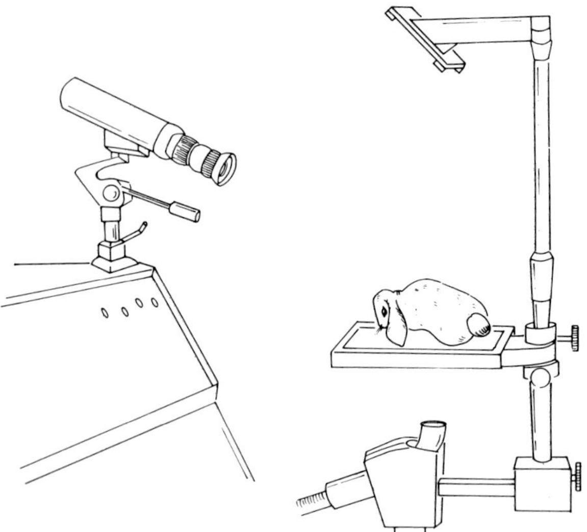

Figure 3-24. Set-up for investigation of *in vivo* contrast enhancement with indocyanine.

was reduced from 58 to 30 percent for carcinomas under 1 cm.[6] The study of Greene et al. is the only one in which a possible screening role for lightscanning is suggested by a sensitivity of 98 percent,[8] but the reason for their success is not immediately clear. Thus, as would be expected, in most of the aforementioned studies the size of the cancer was the most important factor in its detection. Lightscanning had relatively poor sensitivity for cancers under 1 cm.

An intriguing concept is the possible utility of lightscanning as an adjunct to physical examination, and for examining breasts with mammographic evidence of the most risky parenchymal patterns according to Wolfe.[19] Table 3-2 shows that the detection rates of tumors, either palpable and/or greater than 1 cm, range from 57 to 79 percent. This may indicate that screening for asymptomatic cancer is still not vigorously employed, and that the majority that are detected are palpable. If lightscanning were able to characterize palpable masses as suspicious or benign, it might contribute to clinical management. Even were this possible, however, mammography would still be necessary in order to exclude tumor multicentricity and bilaterality, conditions that obviate therapy directed toward breast preservation. The sensitivity for mammography is lowest for dense, dysplastic breasts, (Wolfe's categories P2 and DY).[19] In the series of Merritt et al., 66 percent of patients manifested P2 or DY patterns,[12] which may explain the relatively low mammographic sensitivity of 76 percent, while the lightscan sensitivity was 77 percent. It must be stressed that we do not yet know if the lightscan will benefit patients with P2 or DY parenchymal patterns.

What conclusions can be formed regarding the efficacy of breast lightscanning? One point clearly made in almost all lightscanning articles concerns the relationship between the size of the cancer and its detectability. Since sensitivity is markedly diminished for masses under 1 cm, it is clear that, at the current state of the science, lightscanning should not be used as a screening procedure. Its adjunctive role to mammography deserves further investigation. The diversity of results found in the literature underscores the need for a rigidly controlled three-phase evaluation: Phase one defines the technique and the diagnostic criteria; phase two is a blinded study to determine the value of the procedure in isolation; while phase three is a clinical evaluation in a large number of institutions to ensure that the technique and results are reproduceable. Any diagnostic examination that requires extensive physician time and that can be successfully performed by only a few select individ-

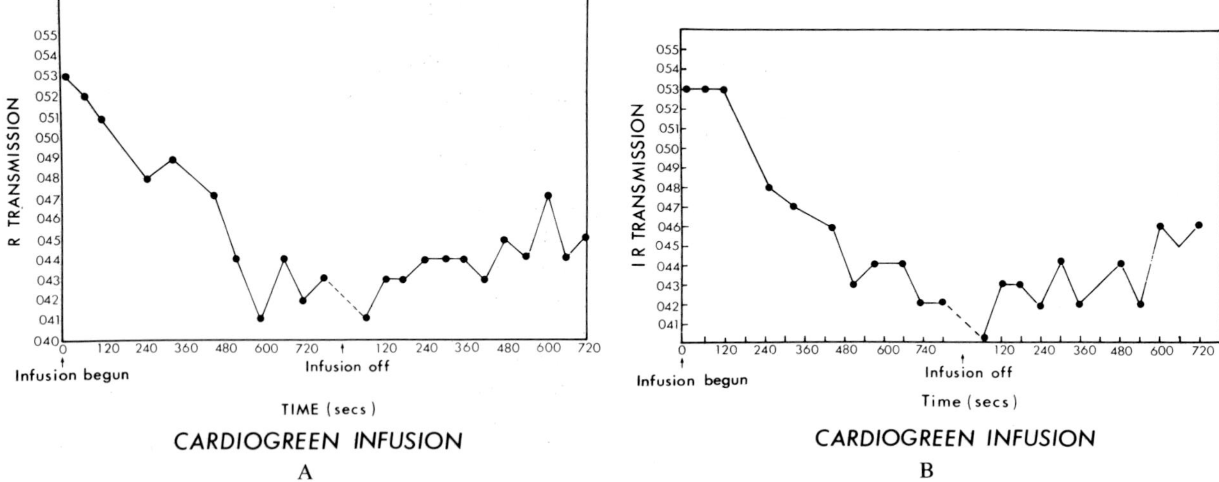

Figure 3-25. Transmission data with indocyanine (cardiogreen) infusion. A. Red transmission values (R) in relative units versus time in seconds. B. Near-infrared transmission values (IR).

uals is useless as a screening test and is severely compromised as an adjunctive test.

CONTRAST ENHANCEMENT

Many diagnostic imaging examinations employ contrast agents, and it is likely that contrast agents may eventually prove useful for lightscanning. Several compounds absorb and/or are excited by light of certain wavelengths and emit light of other wavelengths. Some of these are already being used on an experimental basis in lightscanning. After investigating indocyanine green, fluorescein, hematoporphyrin, and fluorescamine, we decided to evaluate indocyanine more fully because of its high absorption of the wavelengths used for clinical lightscanning (Fig. 3-23).

Initial *in vivo* tests of indocyanine (cardiogreen) were performed on a rabbit ear isolated on an opaque glass surface. A light probe was placed a fixed distance below the ear and a vidicon camera focused on the ear (Fig. 3-24). Readings for luminence and IR/R ratio transmission were taken at three sites on the ear and averaged. An infusion of indocyanine at a dosage following the manufacturer's recommended guidelines for humans and adjusted for the weight of the rabbit was begun, and readings over the three sites were taken for a total of 750 seconds. The infusion was discontinued, and readings were taken for an additional 720 seconds. While the differences were small, there was a definite decrease in the transmission of light in the ear in both the red and near infrared ranges after the start of the infusion. Light transmission gradually returned to preinfusion levels after the infusion was stopped (Fig. 3-25). While this work is preliminary, it suggests that the infusion of indocyanine green during breast lightscanning may enhance the light-absorptive properties of cancer to allow it to be better delineated. Further animal and clinical work in this direction is planned.

In the days before ultrasound, if a physician desired information regarding the possible solid or cystic nature of a breast mass, he or she directed a beam from a source of bright light through the mass. The total investment in equipment was small. The lightscanning equipment of today is costly. Does it provide proportionally more information? Additional investigations with well-controlled studies will, it is to be hoped, provide the answer.

REFERENCES

1. Bartrum RJ Jr, Crow HC: Transillumination lightscanning to diagnose breast cancer; a feasibility study. AJR 142:409–414, 1984
2. Carlsen EN: Transillumination lightscanning. Diagn Imaging 4:28–33, 1982 (April)
3. Cutler M: Transillumination as an aid to diagnosis of breast lesions. Surg Gynecol Obstet 48:721–727, 1929
4. Drexler B, Davis JL, Schofield G: Diaphanography in the diagnosis of breast cancer. Radiology 157:41–44, 1985
5. Ertefai S, Profio AE: Spectral transmittance and contrast in breast diaphanography. Med Phys 12:393–400, 1985
6. Geslien GE, Fisher JR, DeLaney C: Transillumination in breast cancer detection: screening failures and potential. AJR 144:619–622, 1985
7. Girolamo RF, Leis HP: Diaphanography. A fourth dimension in diagnosis of breast cancer. Breast 8:16, 1982
8. Greene FL, Hicks C, Eddy V, Davis C: Mammography, sonomammography, and diaphanography (Lightscanning). Am Surg 51:58–60, 1985
9. Gros M, Quenneville Y, Hummel Y: Diaphanologie mammaire. J Radiol Electrol Med Nucl 53:297–302, 1972
10. Isard HJ: Other imaging techniques. Cancer 53:658–664, 1984
11. Marshall V, Williams DC, Smith KD: Diaphanography as a means of detecting breast cancer. Radiology 150:339–343, 1984
12. Merritt CRB, Sullivan MA, Segaloff A, McKinnon WP: Real-time transillumination light scanning of the breast. RadioGraphics 4:989–1009, 1984
13. Ohlsson B, Gundersen J, Nilsson DM: Diaphanography: a method for the evaluation of the female breast. World J Surg 4:701–705, 1980
14. Sickles EA: Breast cancer detection with transillumination and mammography. AJR 142:841–844, 1984
15. Wallberg H, Alveryd A, Bergvall U, et al.: Diaphanography in breast carcinoma. Correlation with clinical examination, mammography, cytology and histology. Acta Radiol [Diagn] (Stockh) 26:33–44, 1985
16. Wallberg H, Alveryd A, Nasiell K, et al.: Diaphanography in benign breast disorders. Correlation with clinical examination, mammography, cytology and histology. Acta Radiol [Diagn] (Stockh) 26:129–136, 1985
17. Watmough DJ: Diaphanography. Mechanism responsible for the images. Acta Radiol Oncol 21:11–15, 1982
18. Watmough DJ: Transillumination of breast tissues: Factors governing optimal imaging of lesions. Radiology 147:89–92, 1983
19. Wolfe JN: Breast patterns as an index of risk for developing breast cancer. AJR 126:1130–1139, 1976

Franklin S. Alcorn, M.D.

4

Magnetic Resonance Imaging

The capability of x-ray mammography to detect early cancer is well known. The potential for magnetic resonance imaging (MRI) in this endeavor has excited considerable interest. Although unable to image microcalcifications, MRI shows promise for enhancing the delineation of other signs of cancer, particularly in the radiographically dense breast. MRI of the breast, while currently considered experimental, may eventually disclose as-yet-unrecognized signs or signatures of malignancy that are unique to this imaging modality.

THE PHYSICS OF MR IMAGING

A brief discussion of the physics of MRI should prove helpful in providing insight into this new and exciting imaging technique that produces multisectional images without the use of ionizing radiation.

The charged muclei of certain atoms, e.g., hydrogen, phosphorus-31, sodium-23, possess an inherent rotation or spin. This results in the production of dipoles that allow the atoms to behave as tiny bar magnets. The nuclei exhibit random motion as a result of the attracting and repelling forces between them in their magnetic milieu. The hydrogen atom or proton contained in body water behaves in this way, and is the atom used in the production of MR images. The nuclei, when placed in a strong, static magnetic field, B_0, align themselves with the long axis of the field in a uniform order rather than in the disarray of random movement. It is convenient to consider the direction of the force about the static magnetic field in terms of a three-dimensional Cartesian coordinate system. The Z axis lies along the bore of the magnet. The X and Y axes are in the transverse plane, at right angles to the Z axis. The protons of a patient lying the long axis of a large radiofrequency coil will be aligned parallel to the Z or long axis.

In addition to the alignment of the spinning protons in relation to the applied magnetic field, the atoms slowly gyrate or circle around their rotational axis so as to circumscribe the base of a cone. This movement is termed precession, and is similar to the wobble of a spinning top as it loses rotational speed in the earth's gravitational field. There is a characteristic time constant for the precessional frequency of each nucleus. When a radio frequency (RF) signal pulse produces a magnetic field, and the RF corresponds to the frequency of the precession of the proton, a moment of magnetization is produced at a distance and angle from the Z axis. If the magnetic force is of sufficient amplitude and duration, the magnetic vector from the precessing proton is directed away from the Z axis toward the X-Y plane. When the magnetic force is discontinued, the protons will tend to realign themselves with the Z axis. The process of realignment releases the energy required

BREAST CANCER DETECTION
ISBN 0-8089-1842-7

to alter the orientation of the protons with the Z axis. The energy takes the form of radio waves. The return of the magnetic vector from the X-Y plane toward the Z axis, with resultant loss of energy, is known as longitudinal relaxation. This event occurs exponentially with a time known as T_1. The energy released provides the basis for the formation of the MR image.

Another nuclear interaction occurs with a resultant loss of energy from the same vector in the X-Y axis. In this event, the magnetic vector M_x, M_y loses phase coherence along the X-Y axis. The dephasing results in a diminution of the MR signal and a consequent loss of energy in this plane. The loss of energy is in the form of radio waves. The process is known as transverse relaxation, and its exponential time constant is T_2.

Longitudinal and transverse relaxation are the result of two different nuclear interactions. These fundamentally important events in signal decay occur simultaneously and are characterized by their time constants, T_1 and T_2. It is these events that make MR imaging potentially more useful than computed tomography (CT) in the characterization of body tissues. The differences between longitudinal and transverse relaxation are graphically represented in Fig. 4-1.

It should be kept in mind that these relaxation events occur immediately following the cessation of impulses generated by the RF surface coil. By carefully selecting pulse sequences, it is possible to produce easily recognizable and anatomically accurate images of different body tissues. The sequences commonly used today in routine clinical work are spin-echo and inversion recovery. A standard nomenclature has been adopted to describe these pulse sequences. In Fig. 4-2, the two pulse sequences are 90° and 180°. The 90° RF pulse alters the moment of the magnetic vector 90° from the Z to the X-Y axis. The 180° pulse is used primarily to return signal coherence to the rapidly dephasing vector in the X-Y axis, with a resultant increase in the amplitude of the signal. In Fig. 4-2, all of the imaging pulse techniques are a series of 90° and 180° pulses followed by an interval of time. This interval allows the signal to reach its maximum amplitude and permits the system to recover to the point where a new signal can be initiated. The echo time (TE) is the period between the origin of the 90° pulse and the peak amplitude of the detectable echo signal. The repetition time (TR) represents the period from the beginning of one pulse sequence to the beginning of the next. Images produced by pulse sequences with a short TE and a short TR maximize differences in signal intensity from tissues with dissimilar T_1, and are therefore referred to as T_1-weighted images. Images produced by pulse sequences in which the TE and TR are appreciably longer will produce images that emphasize differences in signal intensity as a result of dissimilarities in T_2, and are therefore known as T_2-weighted images. Multiple spin-echoes can be produced by additional 180° pulses following the basic sequence. Thus, the operator, by manipulation of the TE and TR, produces the T_1- or T_2-weighted images that determine image contrast and, in effect, tissue characterization. The spin-echo techniques are the ones most commonly used in breast imaging.

Inversion recovery (IR) techniques that produce highly T_1-weighted images are also of value. In the IR sequence, the initial RF pulse is 180°. This pulse inverts the spin vector to a minus Z axis. The second RF pulse is a 90° pulse that may be shortly followed by another 180° rephasing pulse. This creates an especially effective T_1 signal with a widened range of contrast or signal intensities. The IR sequence is of value in extending the contrast range beyond that of spin-echo techniques.

At this point, a few remarks are in order regarding the factors influencing the blackness and whiteness of the MR image. In MRI, signals of greater amplitude are usually displayed as white, whereas those of lesser amplitude are black. The tissues comprising the breast, i.e., fat, epithelial, and fibrous connective tissues, possess differing relaxation times. The T_1, T_2, and mobile proton density of each tissue, the type of RF pulse sequence, and the pulse timing combine to determine the degree of whiteness or blackness of different parts of the image. The aforementioned tissues of the breast are listed in order of the decreasing intensity of their spin-echo signals. Fat presents as a high-intensity signal on both T_1- and T_2-weighted images because fat has a short T_1 and a long T_2. Most anatomic areas of interest can be identified by their morphology, which is generally similar and often identical to that seen on x-ray mammograms. A change in signal intensity, in response to manipulation of RF pulse sequences, provides an additional parameter of tissue identification. This unique aspect of MRI has stimulated much of the research in that imaging modality.

As previously mentioned, T_1 or longitudinal relaxation is an exponentially increasing curve that characterizes recovery of magnetization along the Z axis. Tissue which has a short T_1, e.g., fat, appears white when a T_1-weighted pulse is applied. Conversely, tissue with a long T_1 emits a weak signal and appears black, as does tissue with a low mobile proton density. T_2 relaxation is an exponentially decreasing decay of magnetization that results from dephasing in the X-Y axis. Tissues with a long T_2, e.g., those that contain abundant water, possess protons that dephase slowly. When influenced by a T_2-weighted pulse sequence, water will also be imaged in white. Tissues that dephase repidly emit a signal of lesser amplitude and are gray-to-black. Repetitive pulse sequences are required for images to maintain signal intensity and contrast range, and to accomplish adequate spatial encoding. Repetition times must be carefully chosen in order to avoid undue loss of contrast. Obviously, a trade-off exists between signal intensity and contrast. Further and more detailed information on the basic physics of MR imaging and pulse sequence selection may be found among the references to this chapter.[11–13,16]

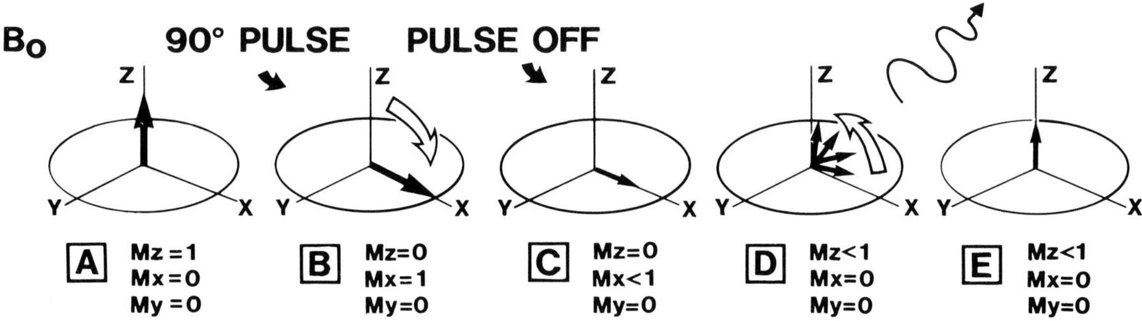

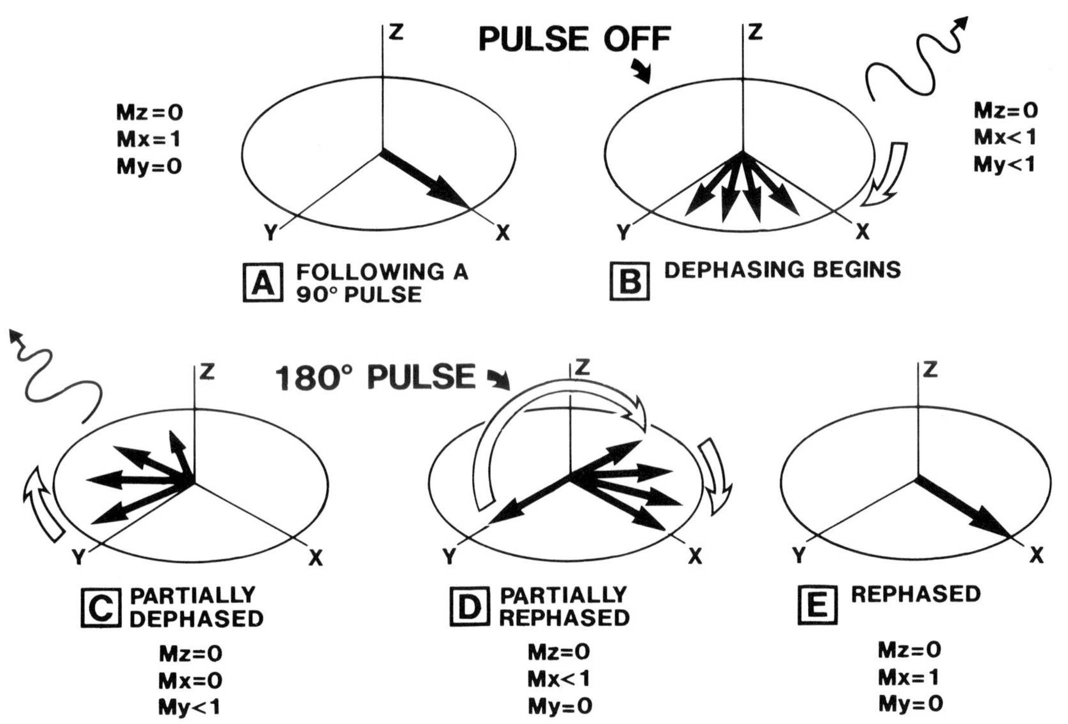

Figure 4-1. Longitudinal and transverse relaxation. M_z, M_x, and M_y represent relative strength of magnetic vector in relation to its changing direction and phase. (Adapted from NMR—A perspective on Imaging. Milwaukee, General Electric Company, 1982, p. 8.)

IMAGE PRODUCTION

Although x-ray mammography is currently the most effective imaging method for the evaluation of breast disease, MRI was recognized early in its development as a potential tool for cancer detection.[5] Early efforts utilizing desk-top laboratory MRI instruments for *in vitro* studies of breast tissue were encouraging, and the availability of large magnets for clinical studies was followed by *in vivo* investigation of a wide range of breast pathology. The appeal of MRI lies not only in its use of electromagnetic fields rather than ionizing radia-

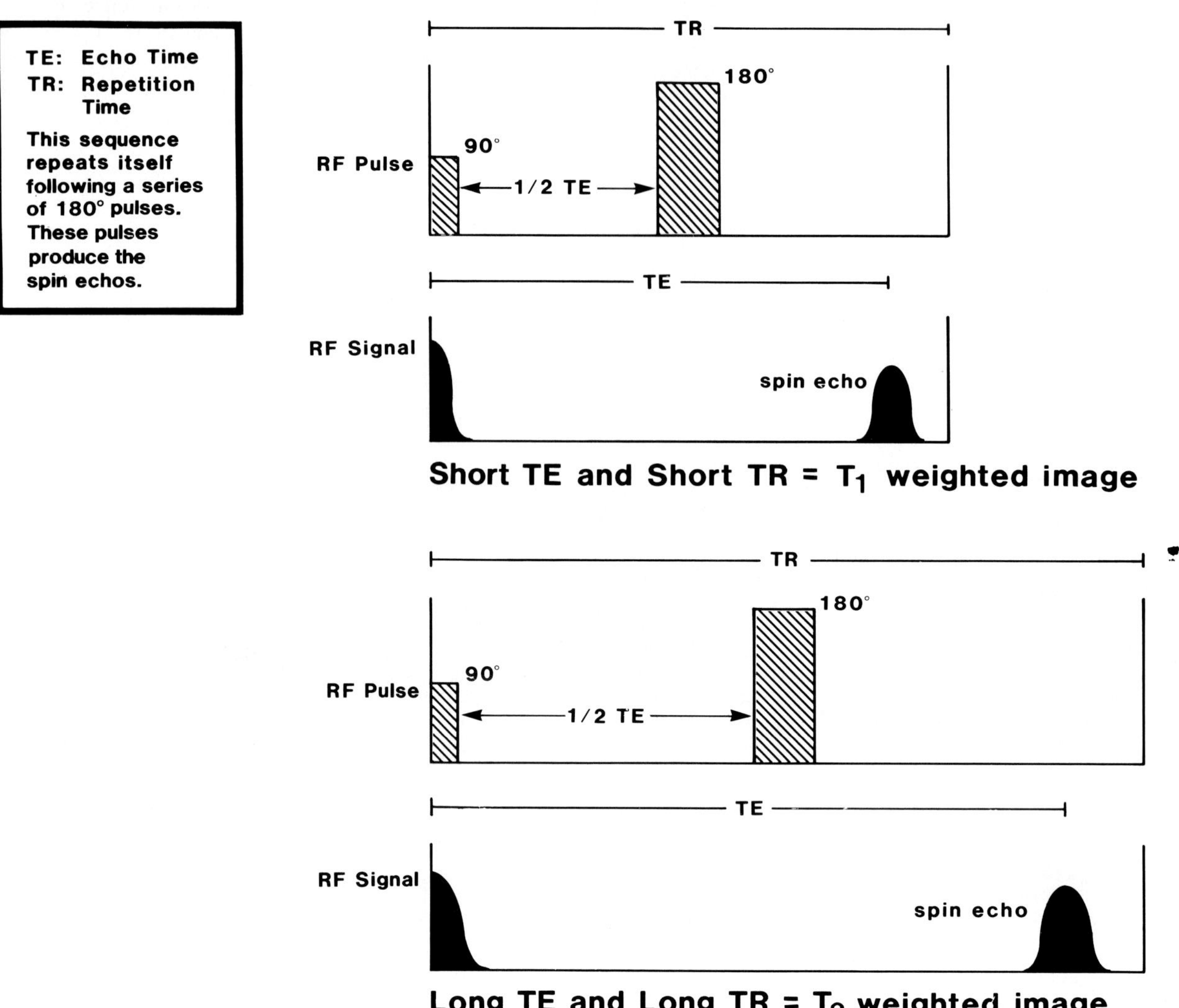

Figure 4-2. Pulse sequences used to produce T_1- and T_2-weighted images. (Adapted from Pavlicek W, Modic M, Weinstein M: Pulse sequence and significance. RadioGraphics 4:52, 1984.)

tion, but also in the fact that it enables differentiation between the basic tissues comprising the breast, e.g., fat, parenchymal tissue, blood vessels, and connective tissue. Additionally, it permits multiple sections of the breast to be obtained in multiple planes. These features, accompanied by the lack of apparent adverse effects of MRI, and by its extraordinary degree of success in imaging the brain and spinal cord, led to its use in preliminary studies of the breast by a number of investigators.[2,8,14]

Although no two investigators or study groups perform MRI of the breast with the same technique, they all exclude from study patients with cardiac pacemakers or metallic clips in the head or heart. Many investigators utilize dedicated breast surface coils. The use of these coils as transmitters and/or receivers of the RF pulse improves the inadequate spatial resolution that results when body coils are used for breast imaging. Surface coils have a much higher sensitivity than do body coils. The increased signal enhances the signal-to-noise ratio, which in turn results in improved resolution and the production of thinner sections. Although most breast surface coils permit the study of one breast at a time, coils have been developed that permit bilateral simultaneous images, allowing a considerable saving in data acquisition time and permitting a comparison of one breast with the other.[17] However, the bilateral images may be degraded by artifactual distortion from contiguous breast surfaces.[10]

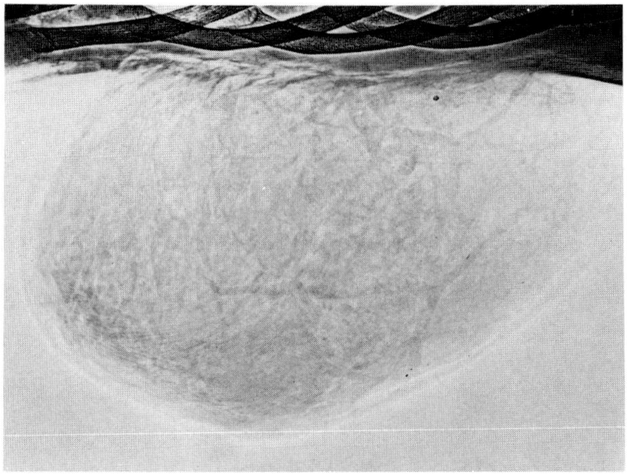

A

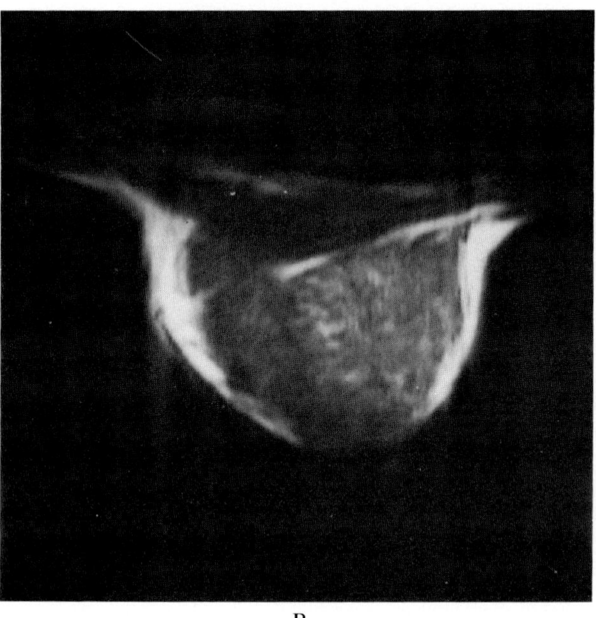

B

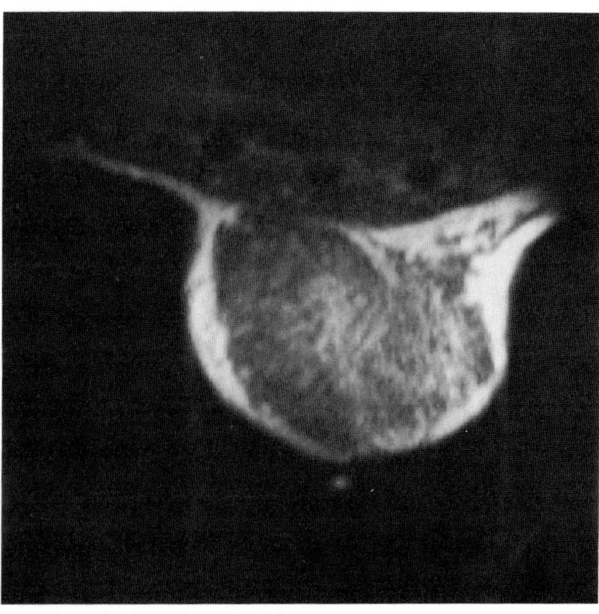

C

Figure 4-3. In this illustration and those that follow, the mammogram has been oriented so as to match the orientation of the MR images. Normal dense breast of young woman. A. Xeromammogram. B. T_1-weighted MR image (TE 30 msec; TR 530 msec). Gray-to-black almost homogeneous breast parenchyma is surrounded by layer of high-intensity subcutaneous fat. C. T_2-weighted MR image (TE 90 msec; TR 2090 msec). Note influence of T_2 on breast parenchyma, where white linear shadows are more apparent than on T_1-weighted image.

MR IMAGES

Investigators agree that both T_1- and T_2-weighted spin-echo pulse sequences are necessary for the most effective study of breast lesions. In surveying the breast, we employ a series of sagittal sections at 1-cm intervals, utilizing T_1- and T_2-weighted images. Additional 5-mm contiguous sagittal sections of the area of interest are often obtained for more detailed information. Occasionally, supplemental sections are acquired in the coronal or axial plane for more precise localization of pathology. Multi-echo sequences, as well as inversion recovery sequences, are also available. Although skin, fat, parenchyma, muscle, veins, and connective tissue are imaged with MR techniques, calcifications are not.

Normal Breast

The appearance of three normal breasts on xeromammography and MR are presented for comparison in Figs. 4-3 through 4-5. The breasts vary in radiographic density depending upon the degree of replacement of parenchymal tissue by fat. Fig. 4-3 shows the breast of a young woman in her late 20s. Physical examination and xeromammography were within normal limits. On the mammogram, the parenchyma occupies most of the breast, resulting in a radiographically dense appearance. There is little subcutaneous fat. The MR image presented in Fig. 4-3B is T_1-weighted. The subcutaneous fat is white as a result of its high-intensity T_1 signal. The breast parenchyma, of low signal intensity, is gray-to-

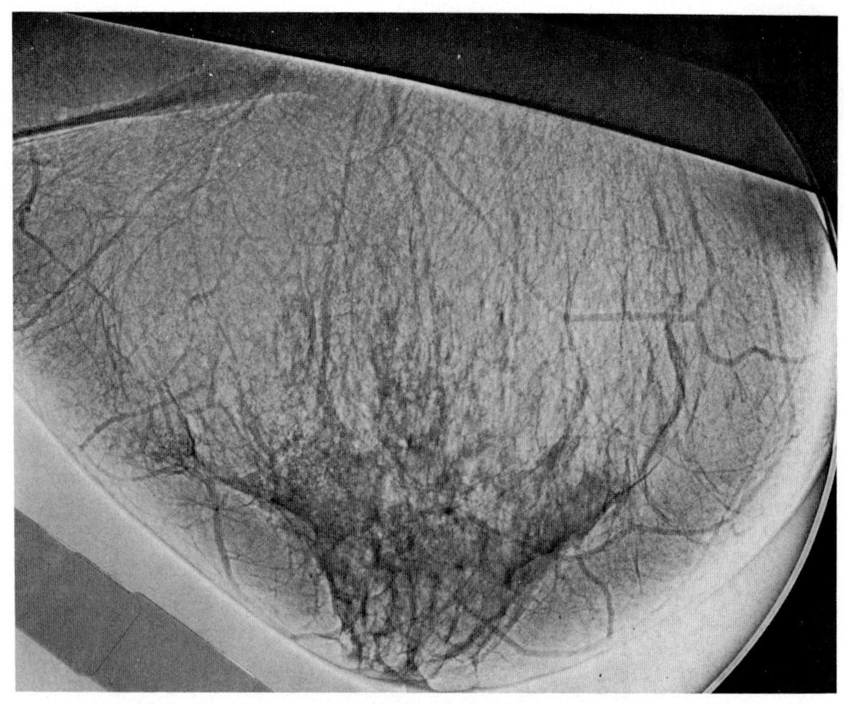

A

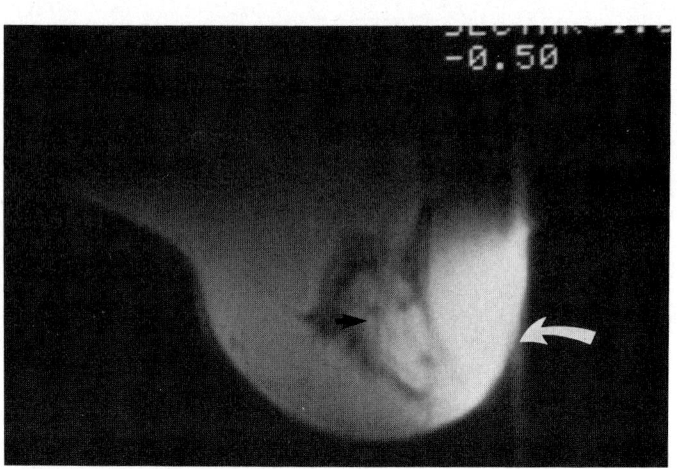

B

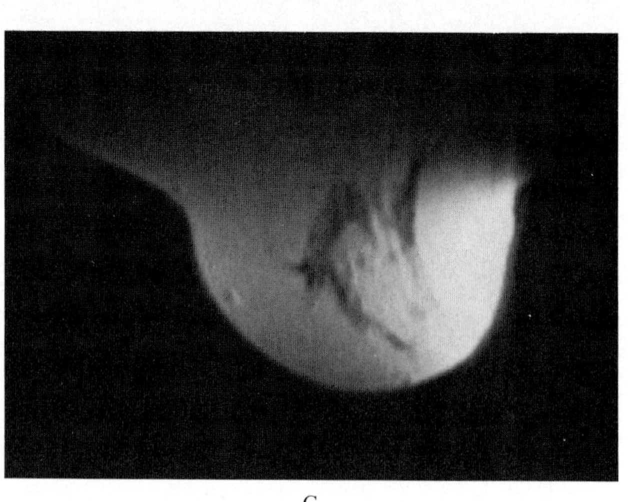

C

Figure 4-4. Postmenopausal breast of intermediate density. A. Xeromammogram. Residual parenchyma is present in subareolar area. Remainder of breast is fat. B. T_1-weighted MR image (TE 30 msec; TR 530 msec). Residual ductal and parenchymal tissues contain high-intensity material (black arrow), in all likelihood fat, clearly shown on both T_1- and T_2-weighted images. Inferior aspect of breast on T_1- and T_2-weighted images (white arrow) displays diffuse increase in signal intensity, an artifact that results from compression of breast by surface coil. C. T_2-weighted MR image (TE 90 msec; TR 2090 msec). Fat has high-intensity signal and fibrous tissue low-intensity signal on both T_1- and T_2-weighted images.

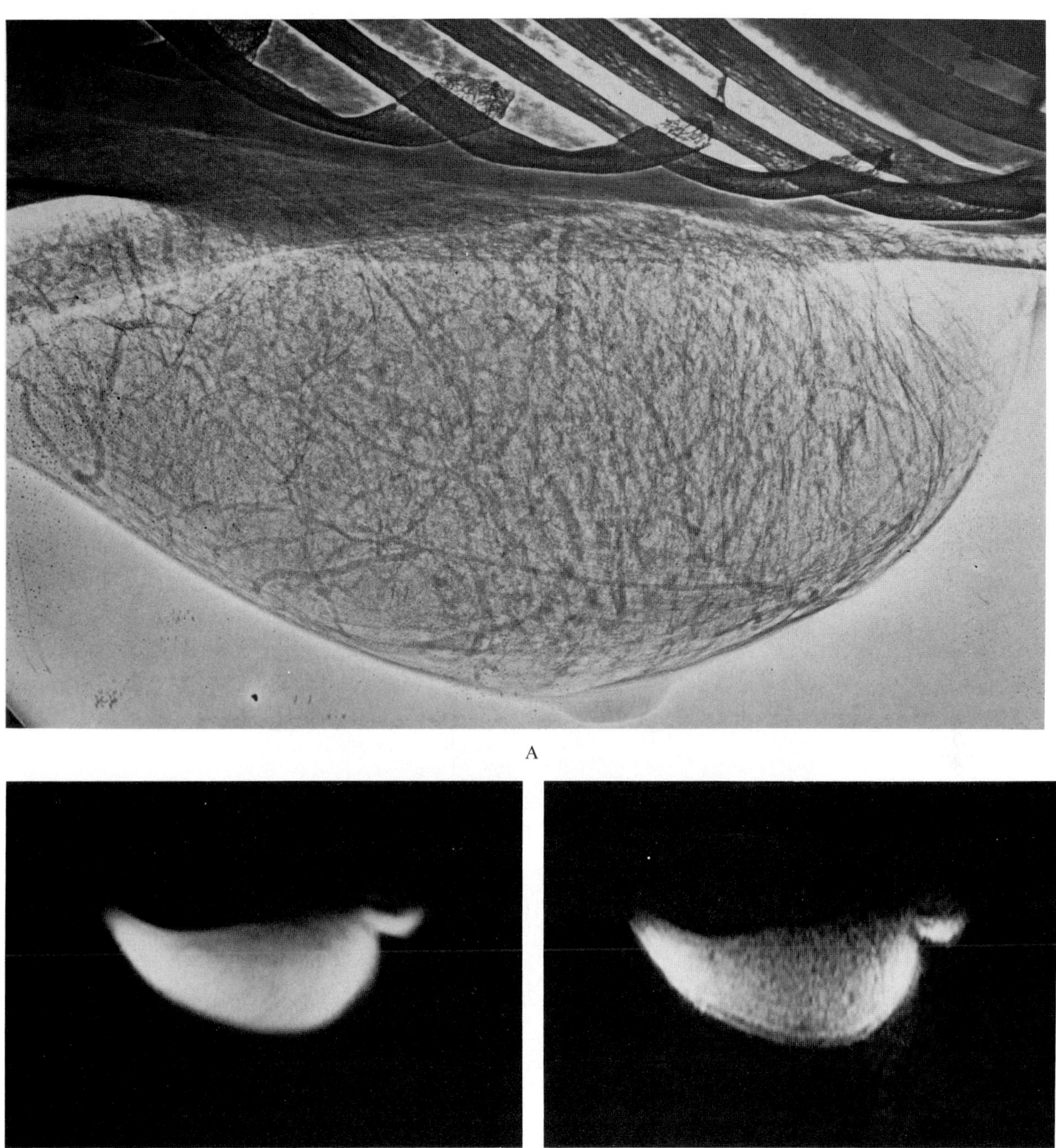

Figure 4-5. Predominantly fatty breast of 70-year-old woman. A. Xeromammogram. B. T_1-weighted MR image (TE 30 msec; TR 530 msec). Uniformly high-intensity T_1 signal predominates in fatty breast. C. T_2-weighted MR image (TE 120 msec; TR 2120 msec). Minute difference in signal intensity occurs between T_1- and T_2-weighted images.

black. Some of the high-intensity linear signals within the parenchyma are presumed to represent ducts containing high-intensity lipid material. Other high-intensity signals may represent a linear arrangement of interductal fat. Fig. 4-3C was produced with T_2 weighting. The parenchyma is less homogeneous as a result of more linear T_2-weighted high-signal elements. The appearance of the parenchyma or background stroma is quite similar on the T_1- and T_2-weighted images.

The breast xeromammogram in Fig. 4-4A depicts the breast of an older woman, and is predominantly fatty, with a few residual parenchymal elements. In the MR images (Figs. 4-4B and 4-4C), the residual lobular and ductal elements appear as low-intensity linear densities corresponding to those on the mammogram. There is little difference in the appearance of these tissue elements in the T_1- (Fig. 4-4B) and T_2- (Fig. 4-4C) weighted images. The slight increase in signal intensity in the T_2-weighted image is probably the result of the predominance of the T_2 effect of the fat that has replaced the parenchyma.

Fig. 4-5A represents a xeromammogram of the breast of a 70-year-old woman in which the parenchymal elements have been replaced entirely by fat. The T_1-weighted MR image in Fig. 4-5B is homogeneous in appearance, similar to the mammogram. Because the breast is comprised entirely of fat, an intense signal is produced on both T_1- and T_2-weighted images. In the T_2-weighted image (Fig. 4-5C), the mottled appearance of the parenchymal signal is the result of a decrease in the signal-to-noise ratio, and results from the prolonged TR interval.

Benign Disease

Fibrocystic change consists primarily of fibrous tissue proliferation, cyst formation, lobular and ductal epithelial changes with resultant ductal prominence. On MRI, cysts and ductal prominence are easily recognized with T_1 and T_2 pulse sequences. Fibrous tissue, however, is difficult to differentiate from normal parenchyma on the basis of morphology or signal intensity. Because of their long T_1 and short T_2 relaxation times, both normal parenchyma and fibrous tissue emit a low-intensity signal. Fibrous tissue, however, is easily discernible in a breast that is predominantly fatty.

Fig. 4-6 shows the change in signal intensity that evolves from T_1- to T_2-weighted images in a breast with diffuse fibrocystic change. In the T_1-weighted image (Fig. 4-6B), the breast parenchyma produces an almost uniformly low-intensity signal. Occasional areas of interspersed high signal intensity probably represent fat. The appearance of the parenchyma is not significantly different from that of the dense but normal breast tissue shown in Fig. 4-3. In the T_2-weighted image (Fig. 4-6C), more high-intensity tissue elements are present. The change in appearance results not only from the T_2-weighted pulse sequence, but also reflects the fact that the section is not precisely equivalent to that of the T_1-weighted image.

Cysts are the most easily recognizable components of fibrocystic change. Cysts tend to be discrete, noncalcified masses on MR images as well as on mammograms. Their low signal intensity on T_1-weighted images increases to an easily recognizable high-intensity signal on T_2-weighted images. The shift in signal intensity represents the most reliable MR clue to the tissue characterization of masses. This sign permits the determination with a high degree of certainty that a mass, even one partially obscured by surrounding fibrous tissue, is cystic and not solid. This sign can be seen even with cysts less than 1 cm in diameter. The sign also holds true in large, dense breasts, and provides a means of identifying small cysts in clinical situations in which the usefulness of ultrasound and mammography may be compromised. In Fig. 4-7A, the xeromammography fails to reveal the presence of any masses. On the T_1-weighted image in Fig. 4-7B, no masses are apparent because of their low signal intensity in relation to that of the surrounding parenchyma. In the T_2-weighted image in Fig. 4-7C, at least two cysts and perhaps a third smaller cyst are obvious because of their high-intensity signal. This dramatic augmentation in signal intensity is the result of the ample "free water" content of cysts.

Fibroadenomas are identifiable on mammograms as sharply marginated, bosselated masses, sometimes containing coarse calcifications. While this is particularly true in the fatty breast (Fig. 4-8A), it is much less so in the dense breast, especially if the fibroadenoma is without calcifications. On MR images, fibroadenomas emit a very low signal intensity on T_1-weighted images (Fig. 4-8B). Depending upon the proportion of fibrous to fatty tissue, the signal intensity of fibroadenomas increases nonhomogeneously on T_2-weighted images (Fig. 4-8C).

Malignant Lesions

The morphology of carcinomas that manifest themselves as masses are the same on MR images as on mammograms. Their characteristic spiculated, irregular, or infiltrating borders are well known to mammographers. However, carcinomas that are characterized not by a mass but primarily by amorphous areas of increased density without calcifications are not as easily recognized either on mammograms or on MR images. This is particularly true of smaller lesions when they are surrounded by dense fibrous or parenchymal tissue. Carcinomas characterized only by clustered calcifications on mammograms may not be detected by MRI. As described above, cysts are easily differentiated from malignant masses by a shift in signal intensity between T_1- and T_2-weighted images. Fibroadenomas may exhibit the same mammographic characteristics as well-circumscribed carcinomas and, when composed predominantly of high-density tissue, their range of signal intensity is similar to that of carcinoma on T_1- and sometimes T_2-weighted images.

Most carcinomas have a relatively long longitudinal

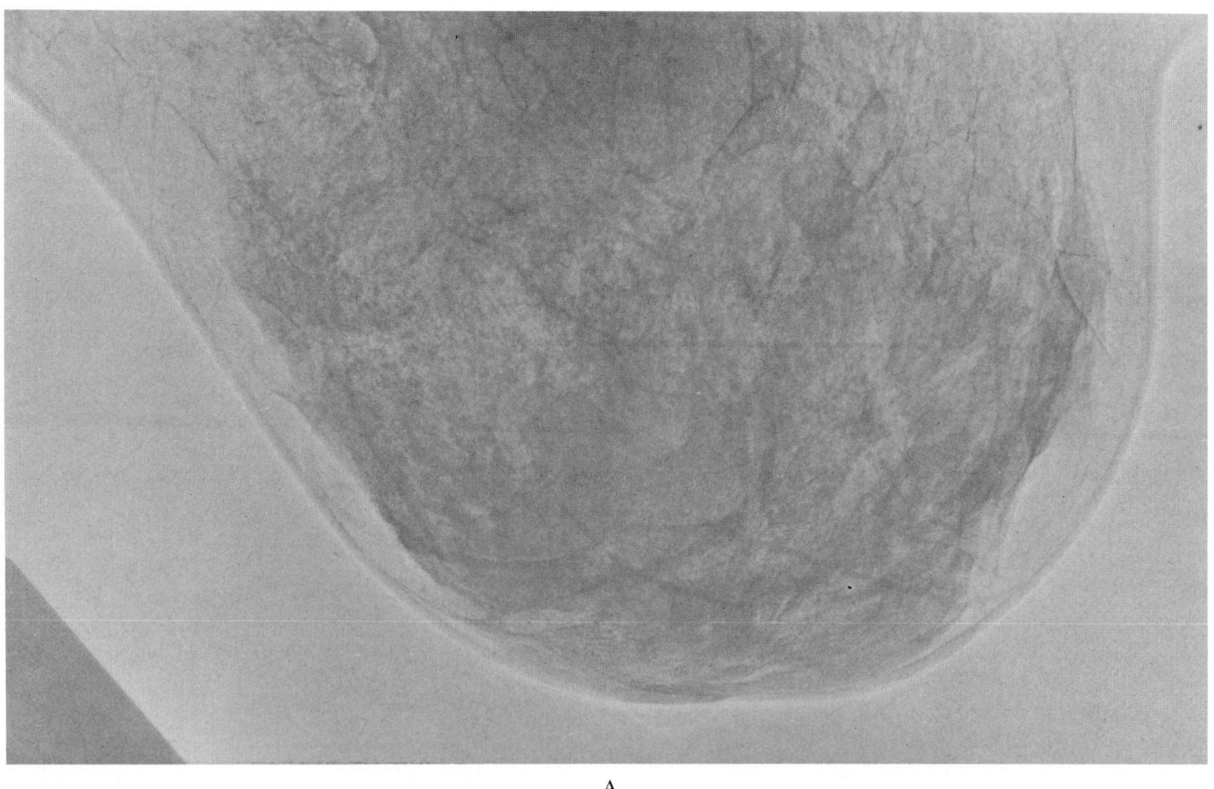

A

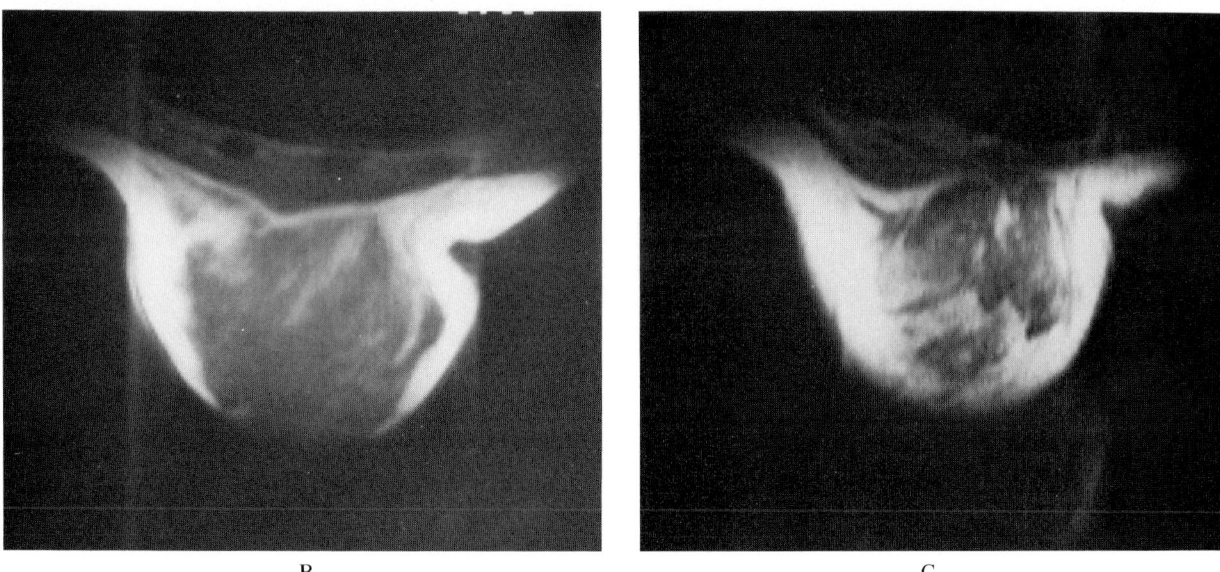

B C

Figure 4-6. Breast manifesting diffuse fibrocystic change. A. Xeromammogram. B. T_1-weighted MR image (TE 30 msec; TR 530 msec). Breast parenchyma is comprised primarily of low-intensity fibrous tissue. C. T_2-weighted MR image (TE 120 msec; TR 2120 msec). Appearance of parenchyma is similar to that on T_1-weighted image.

relaxation time, with a low signal intensity on T_1-weighted images. Their detection is easier when the surrounding parenchyma is fatty rather than dense. It should be kept in mind that, with the exception of cysts, most breast masses are composed of an admixture of tissues. Malignant masses may contain widely varying amounts of cancer cells, fat, fibrous tissue, and ductal ti ssue, and each tissue component has a unique T_2 relaxation time. This accounts for the mixture of signal intensities seen on T_2-weighted images. Generally, the signal intensity of carcinoma is somewhat greater on T_2- than on T_1-weighted images. Changes in signal intensity

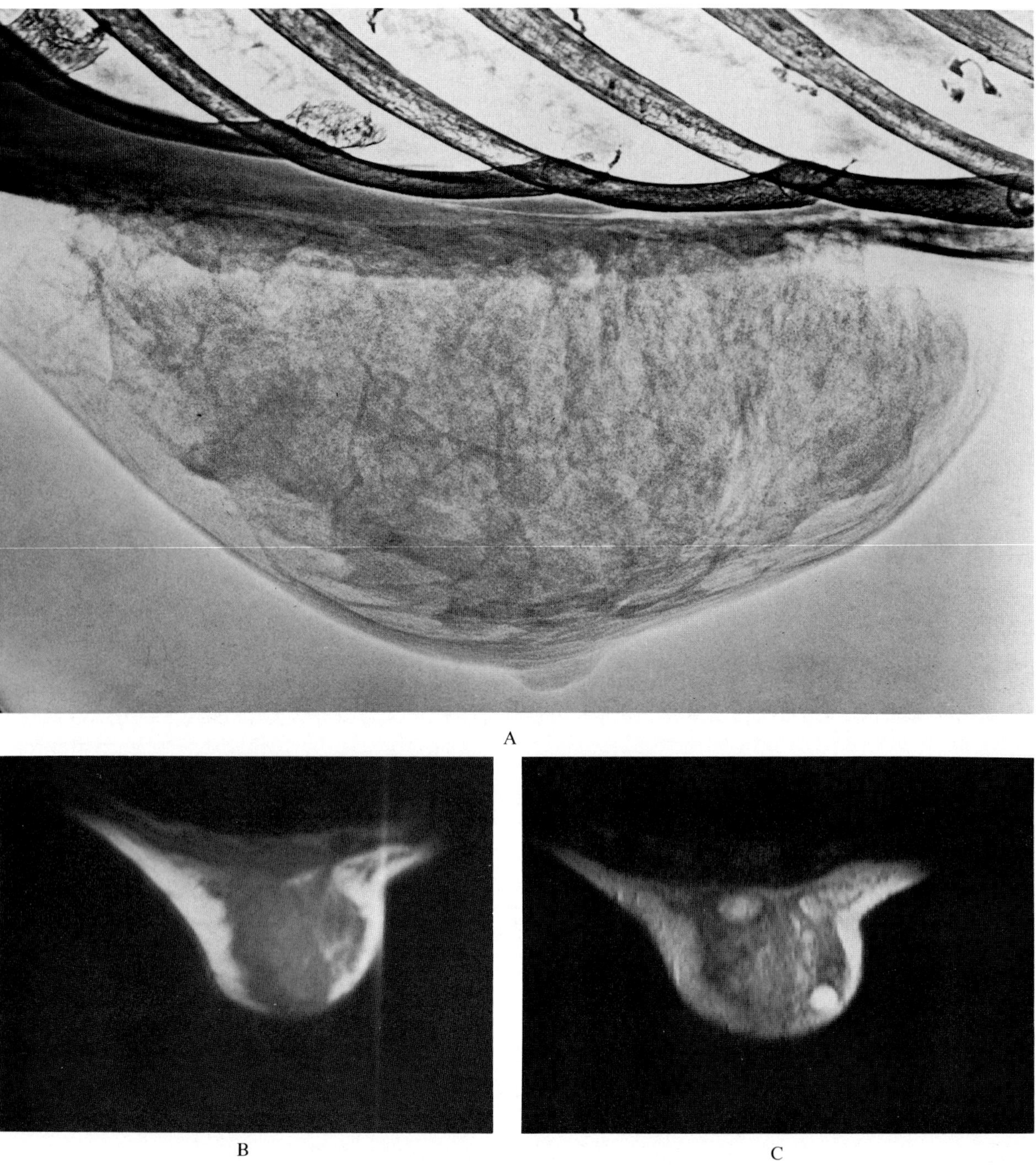

A

B

C

Figure 4-7. Cysts in breast comprised of dense parenchyma A. Xeromammogram. A mass is not identified. B. T_1-weighted MR image (TE 30 msec; TR 530 msec). Parenchyma is almost uniformly dense. No masses are identified. C. T_2-weighted image (TE 90 msec; TR 2090 msec). Note two, and possibly a third, smoothly marginated masses of high signal intensity, appearance typical of cysts.

Figure 4-8. Fibroadenoma. A. Observe small radiodense mass (arrow) in inferior aspect of breast on xeromammogram. Morphologically, this could be carcinoma with well-circumscribed borders, solitary cyst, or fibroadenoma. B. T_1-weighted image (TE 30 msec; TR 530 msec). Observe low, homogeneous signal intensity of mass noted on mammogram. The low-intensity linear cleft adjacent to mass is pressure artifact from surface coil (arrow). C. T_2-weighted MR image (TE 90 msec; TR 2090 msec). Note lack of change in signal intensity between T_1- and T_2-weighted images. Mass was fibroadenoma, comprised almost entirely of dense fibrous tissue.

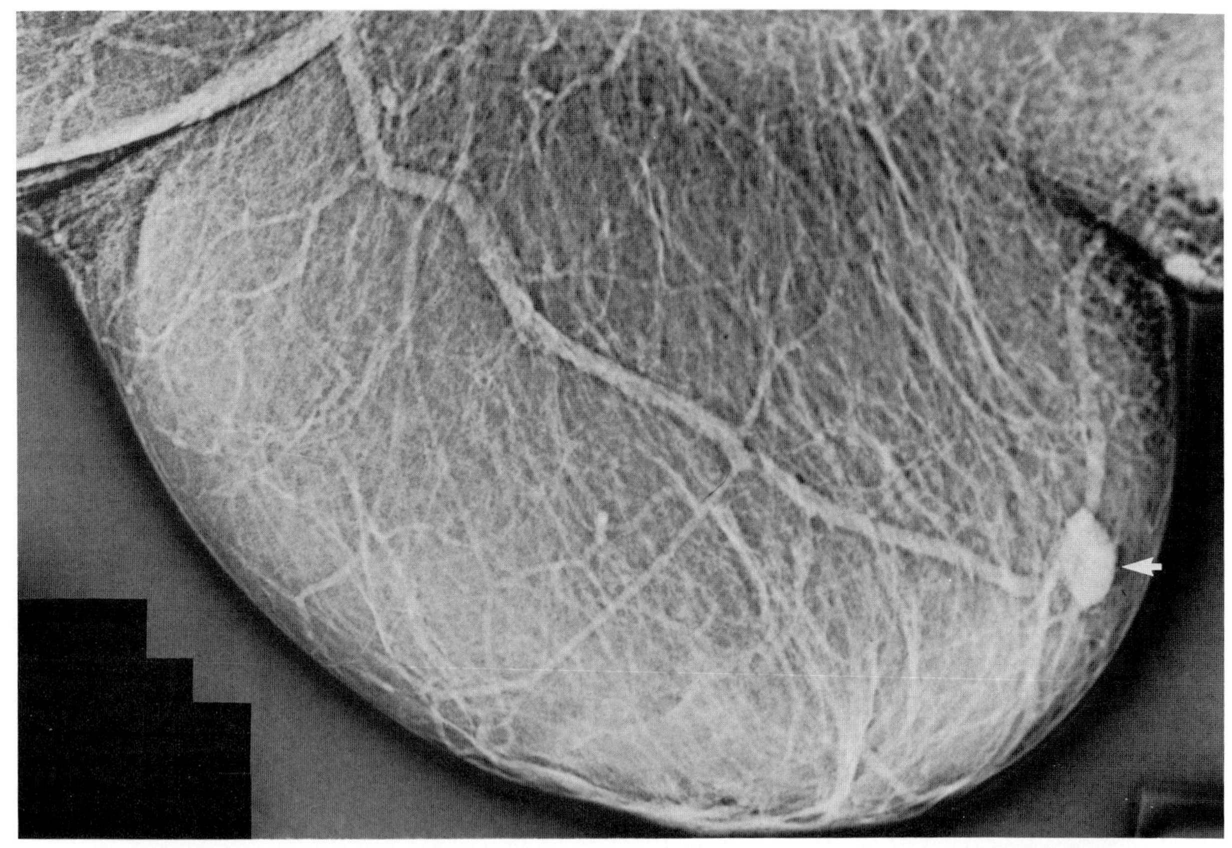

A

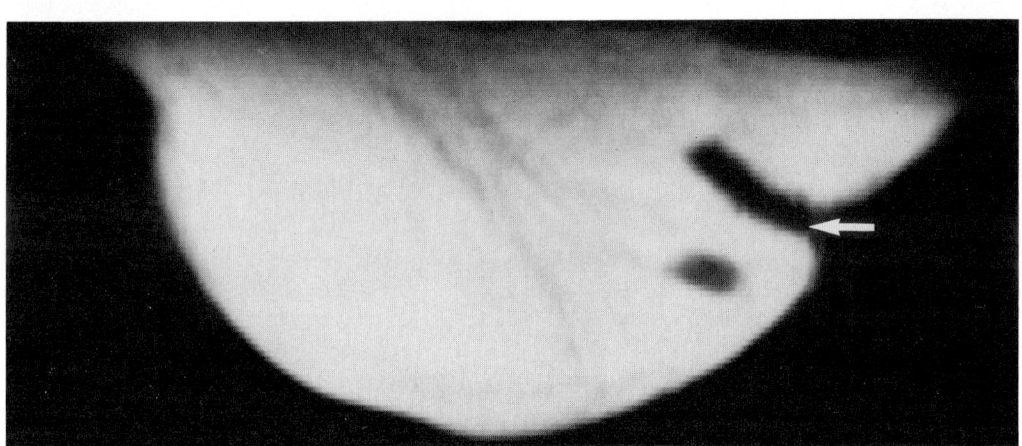

B

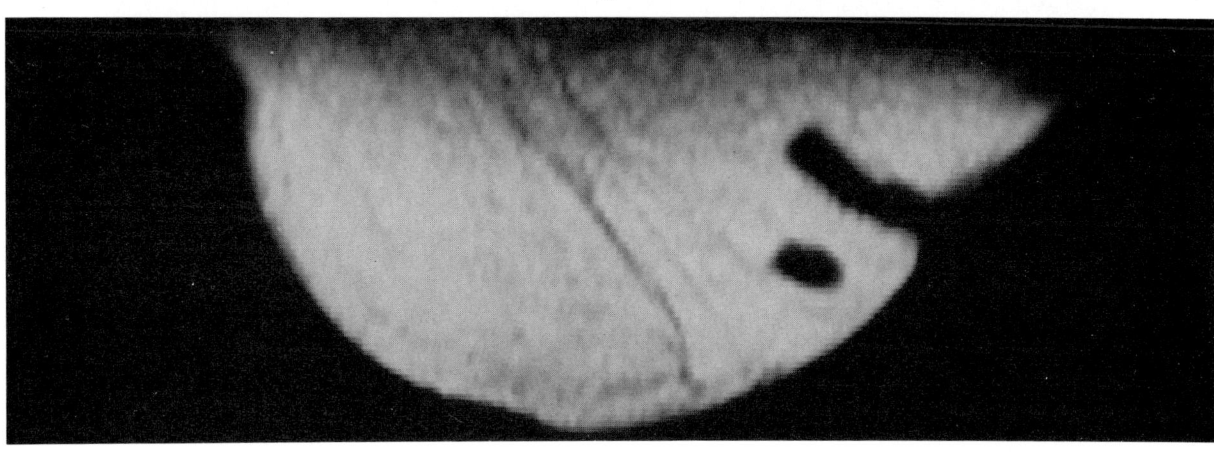

C

as well as morphology are also influenced by partial volume averaging. Larger carcinomas can therefore be identified with more assurance than smaller ones.

Fig. 4-9A reveals a spiculated mass in the tail of the breast on xeromammography. On the T_1-weighted image (Fig. 4-9B), the carcinoma is easily recognizable by its spiculated morphology. The signal is mixed but of low intensity. On the T_2-weighted image (Fig. 4-9C), the mass exhibits a mixed signal intensity approaching that of the surrounding fat. The signal shift between T_1- and T_2-weighted images is not of sufficient amplitude for the carcinoma to be confused with a cyst. However, fibroadenomas of mixed composition could exhibit a signal shift between T_1- and T_2-weighted images similar to that of carcinoma. Clearly, the morphology of a mass contributes significantly to its diagnosis.

Fig. 4-10A shows a xeromammogram depicting a small carcinoma. On the T_1-weighted image (Fig. 4-10B), a small focus of low signal intensity corresponds in location to the lesion seen on the mammogram. There is relatively little change in signal intensity on the T_2-weighted image (Fig. 4-10C) compared to the T_1-weighted image because of a partial volume effect relating to the small size of the tumor, in addition to the effect caused by the increased noise on the T_2-weighted image. It is apparent that, in the preceding case (Fig. 4-9), the shift in signal intensity contributes more to the diagnosis of the mass than it does in this case.

An interesting example of tissue characterization is seen in Fig. 4-11. The mammograms reveal a mass in the upper-outer quadrant of the breast in cephalocaudal (Fig. 4-11A) and mediolateral (Fig. 4-11B) projections. The mass, smoothly marginated anteriorly and noncalcified, could represent a cyst or fibroadenoma. The area immediately posterior to the mass contains clustered punctate microcalcifications suggestive of coexistent carcinoma. The T_1-weighted image (Fig. 4-11C) reveals that the breast parenchyma produces a mixture of signal intensities. The radiographically benign mass is not identified. There is no difference in signal intensity to indicate the presence of a more posteriorly located carcinoma as opposed to the nonmalignant surrounding tissue. The T_2-weighted image (Fig. 4-11D) discloses a smoothly marginated density of very high and homogeneous signal intensity at the site of the mammographic mass, obviously representing a cyst. The area immediately surrounding and posterior to the cyst reveals no signal change to suggest the existence of a carcinoma. At surgery, a cyst was discovered, and, immediately posterior to it, a carcinoma. This case demonstrates the ability of MRI to depict benign pathology, and yet fail to detect a more important adjacent carcinoma.

POTENTIAL USEFULNESS OF BREAST MRI FOR SCREENING

The four As denoting the requirements of a successful screening modality are: accessibility, acceptability, accuracy, and affordability.

MRI has not yet become generally accessible. The scarcity of MRI installations must be compared to the large number of patients who require screening for breast cancer. Examination time on existing MR installations is heavily and justifiably utilized by patients with central nervous system problems, since the sensitivity and specificity of MRI for cerebral and spinal cord pathology exceed its capability in other parts of the body.

The potential acceptability by patients of MRI as compared to x-ray mammography is questionable. Although MRI does not require ionizing radiation, it presents certain deterrents not shared by mammography: the patient is required to lie in the prone position for 30–60 minutes, depending upon the extent of data acquisition required; the breast is placed in a dependent position within a cylindrical dedicated radiofrequency coil which itself may be uncomfortable; and the patient is encased within the bore of a large cylindrical magnet which, for many patients, produces claustrophobia. Thus, although the absence of ionizing radiation is welcome, the general level of acceptance of MRI in asymptomatic patients presenting themselves for breast cancer screening is not likely to be enthusiastic.

The accuracy of MRI in the detection of asymptomatic, subclinical breast cancer presents additional difficulties. Most carcinomas are recognized on the basis of morphologic features rather than differences in signal intensity from that of benign lesions. This leads to problems in detecting minimal cancer in the dense breast. The failure to detect small cancers may arise from the high degree of similarity between the tissue signatures of carcinoma on one hand, and of benign lesions and nonadipose parenchyma on the other, as well as from the partial volume effect. Most importantly, the detection of malignant calcifications, a key feature of x-ray mammography, is not possible with MRI.

Finally, the cost and affordability factor of MRI constitutes a significant drawback to its widespread use. This would hold true were all of the preceding requirements for screening satisfactorily met. The initial cost of equipment, the large amount of physician, engineering, and technologist time, and a relatively slow through-put time per patient contribute to the high cost of the examination. Potential technical advances, especially those relating to simultaneous acquisition of data on contiguous slices of from 5 to 10 mm, and simultaneous acquisition of T_1 and T_2 images, would significantly lower the through-put time. While the development of a small dedicated primary magnet would lower the initial cost of equipment, it probably would not affect operational costs to a significant degree.

At this time, MRI cannot compete with x-ray mammography in any of the above mentioned categories. It is time consuming, expensive, and not sufficiently specific for the detection of small breast cancers to replace the time-honored methods of detection in use

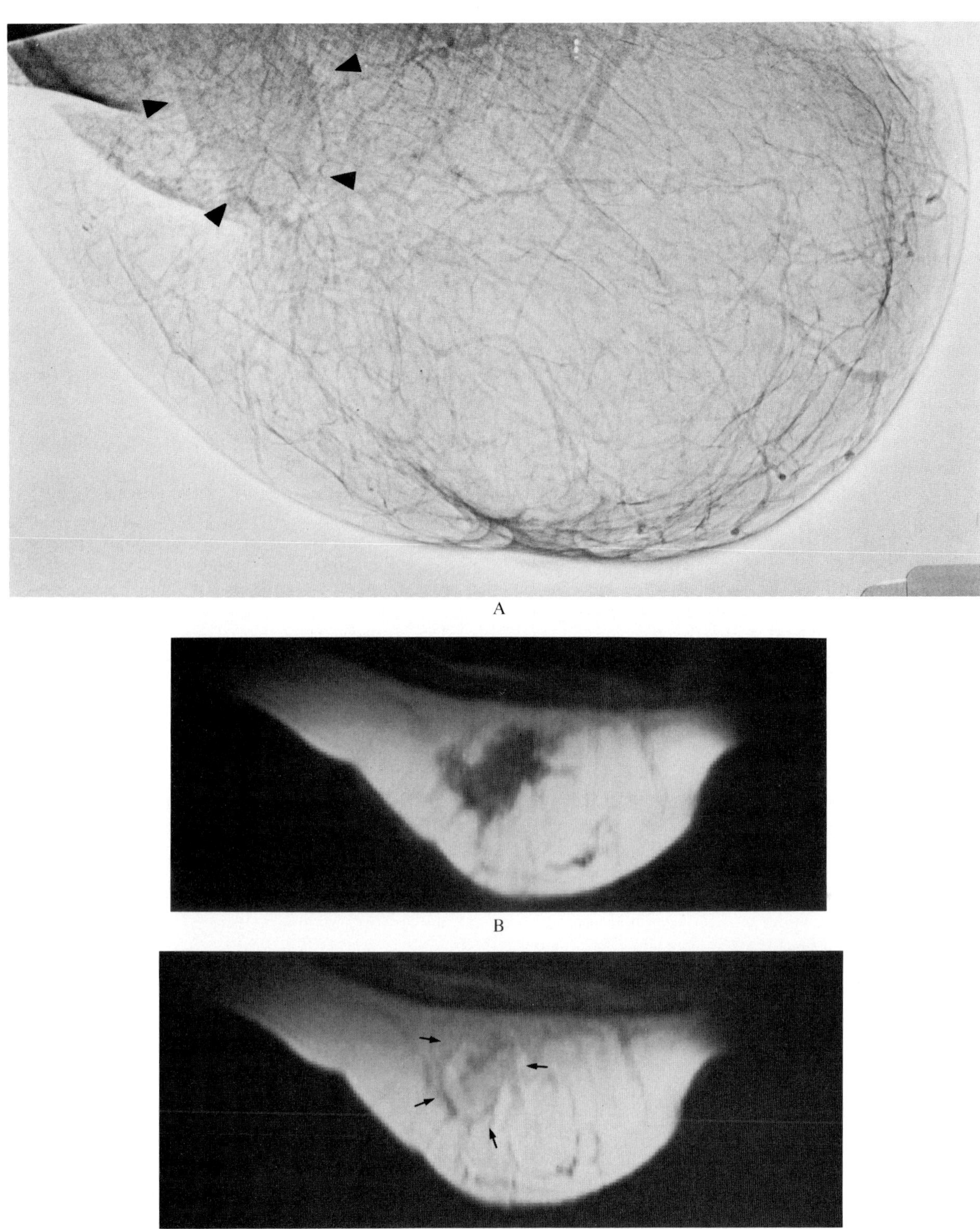

Figure 4-9. Carcinoma. A. Xeromammogram reveals spiculated mass in tail of breast (arrowheads). B. T_1-weighted MR image (TE 30 msec; TR 530 msec). Mass is of low signal intensity. C. T_2-weighted MR image (TE 90 msec; TR 2090 msec). Increase of mixed signal intensity from T_1- to T_2-weighted images (arrows) often characterizes malignant neoplasms.

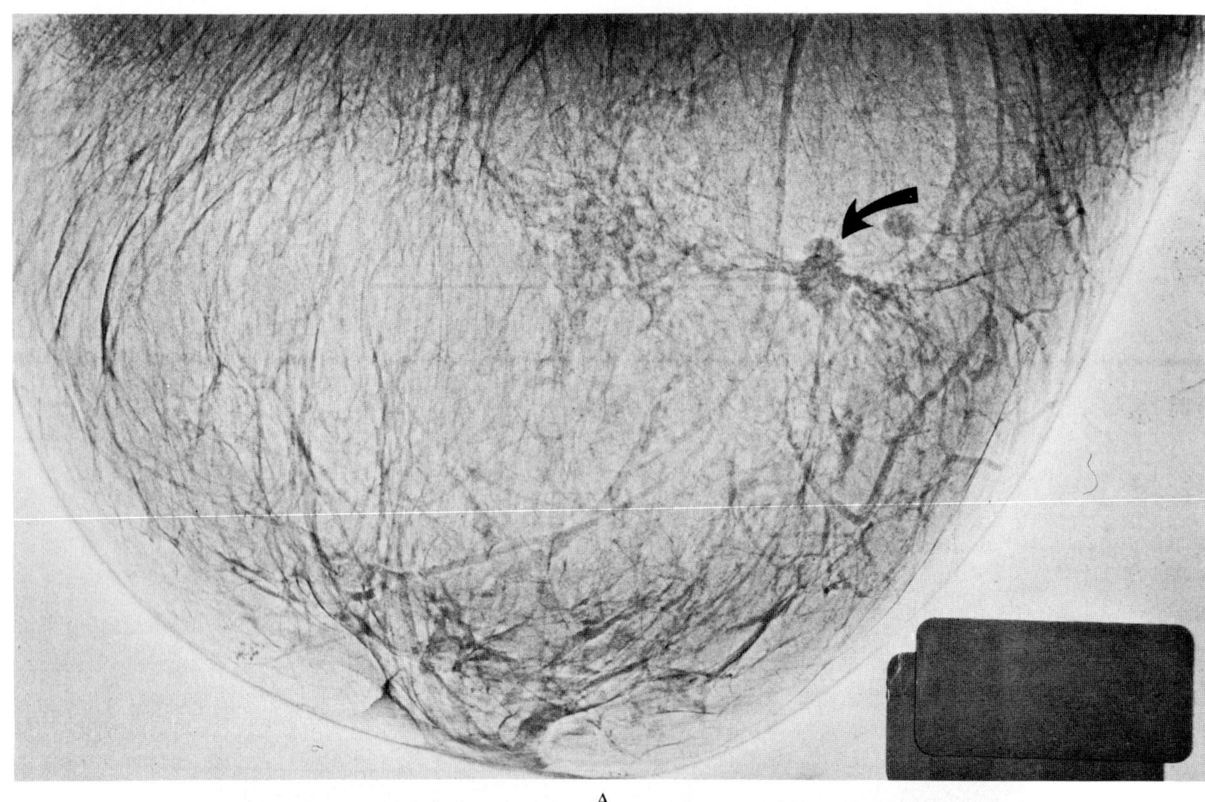

A

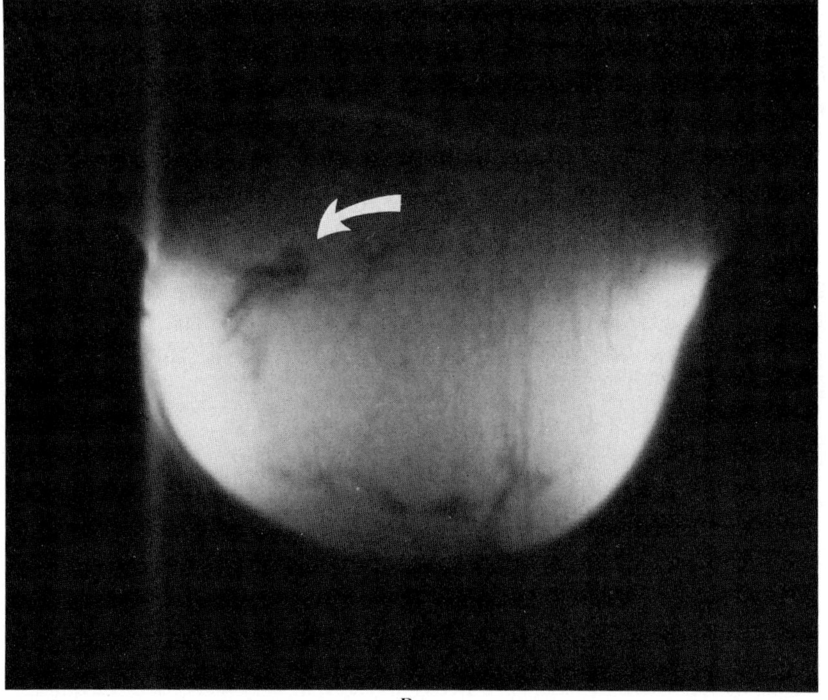

B

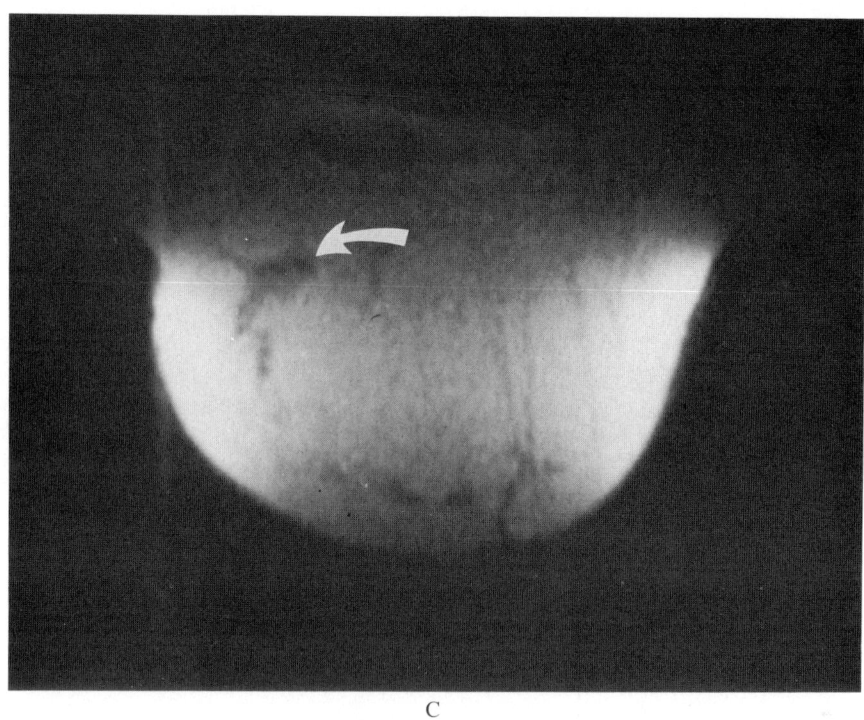

C

Figure 4-10. Carcinoma of breast in elderly woman. A. Xeromammogram discloses 8 mm carcinoma (arrow). B. T_1-weighted MR image (TE 30 msec; TR 530 msec). Carcinoma (white arrow) shown as mass of mixed low-intensity signals. A few low-intensity linear signals are seen extending outward from mass. Appearance and signal intensity of lesion is not sufficiently specific for diagnosis. C. T_2-weighted image (TE 90 msec; TR 2090 msec). Carcinoma (white arrow) shows modest increase in signal intensity compared to T_1 image. Morphologic and signal intensity characteristics are insufficient to permit specific diagnosis. The diagnosis of minimal cancer such as this remains difficult, even when lesion is surrounded by high-intensity fat.

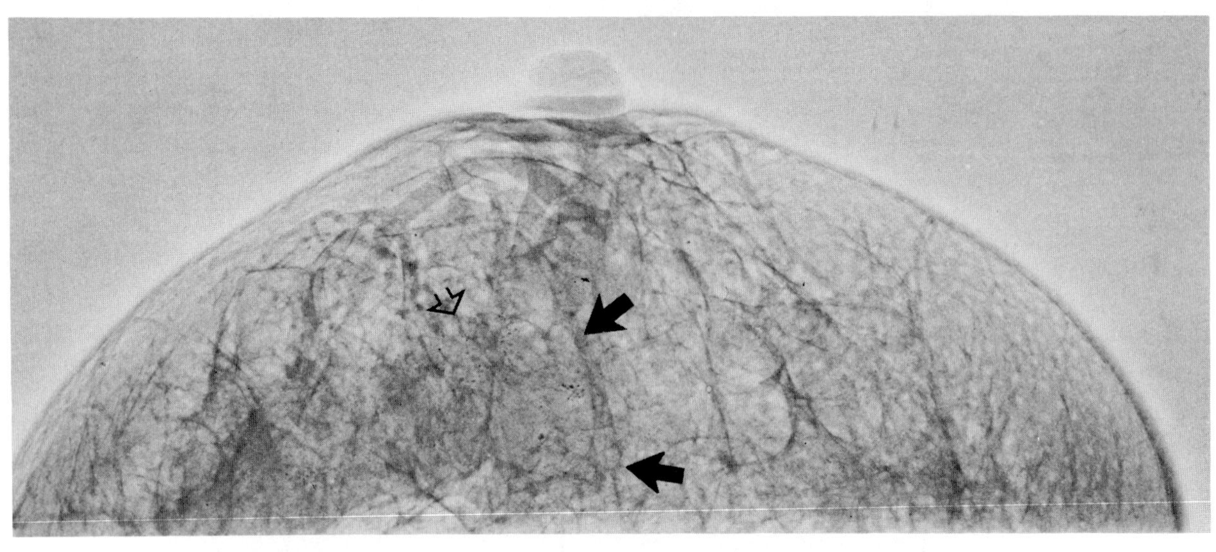

A

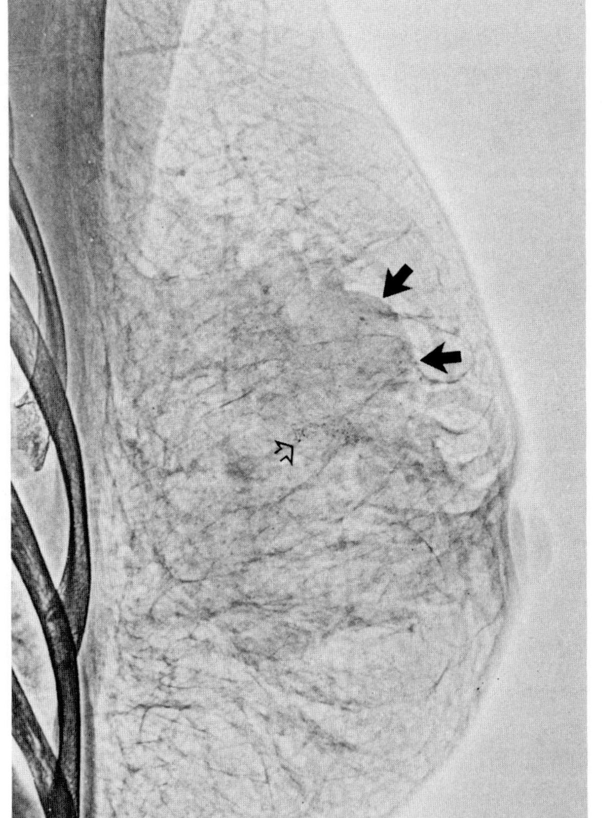

B

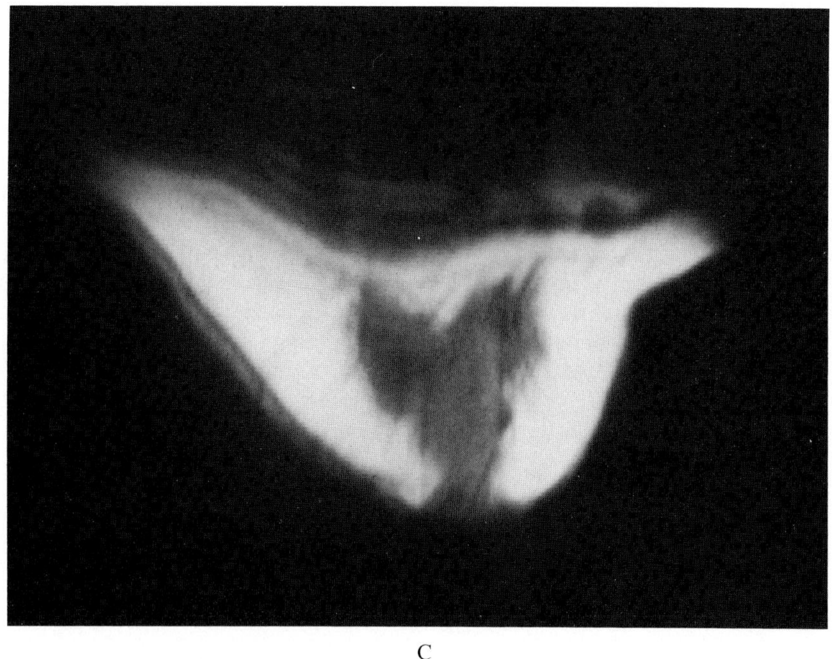

C

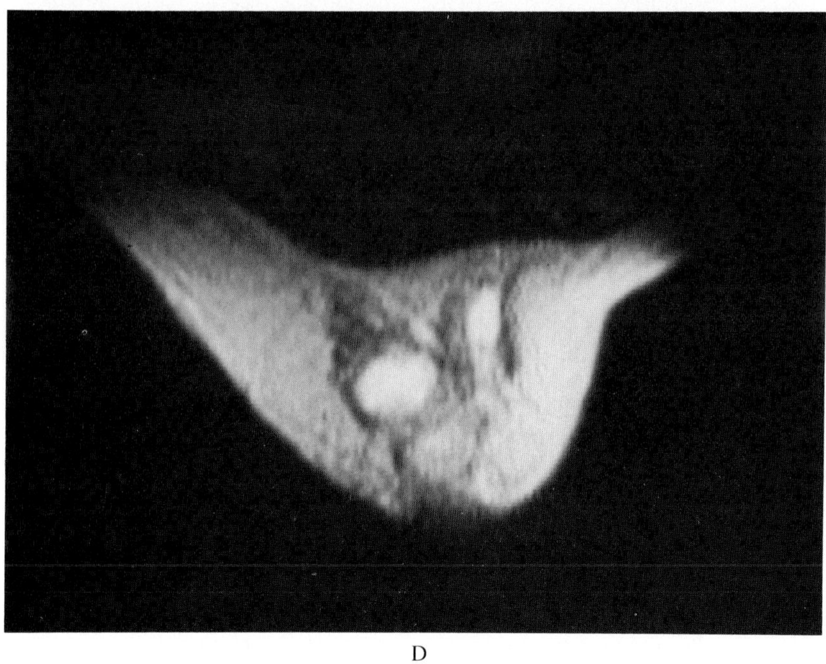

D

Figure 4-11. Carcinoma. Cephalocaudal (A) and Mediolateral (B) xeromammograms of breast with palpable mass in upper-outer quadrant (solid arrows). Cluster of suspicious calcifications resides nearby (open arrow). C. T_1-weighted MR image (TE 30 msec; TR 530 msec). Corresponding area of interest is represented by nonspecific area of low signal intensity. Neither the mass nor area of suspected malignancy can be confidently identified. D. T_2-weighted MR image (TE 120 msec; TR 2120 msec). Area of high signal intensity represents cyst. Adjacent carcinoma, suspected from calcifications in xeromammograms, is not depicted in T_1- or T_2-weighted images.

at the present time. It is thus unlikely in the forseeable future that MRI will become a practical screening modality for the detection of breast cancer. It is more promising for specific clinical situation in which x-ray mammography is inadequate. Small malignant lesions immediately adjacent to the chest wall have always posed a problem in mammographic cancer detection and, especially, in localization for biopsy. With the patient in the prone position and the breast dependent in the surface coil, the breast parenchyma falls away from the chest wall, providing better visualization of the base of the breast, particularly in the sagittal projection, and, to a lesser extent, in the axial and coronal projections. Utilizing a combination of these projections, it is possible to delineate and localize posteriorly located lesions, even those that have invaded the chest wall. This capability is not shared by x-ray mammography to as great an extent.

It is in evaluation of the dense breast that MR imaging may make its most important contribution. Carcinomas are easy to detect by x-ray mammography, as well as MRI, when the breast is comprised of fatty tissue. Both modalities, however, encounter difficulty in detecting carcinomas that are 5 mm or less in diameter and surrounded by dense parenchyma. This is true not only of women with fibrocystic change but also of relatively young women whose breasts are comprised primarily of functional parenchyma. Not only are the calculated T_1 and T_2 values and the relative signal intensities of many benign and malignant masses similar to each other, but the T_1 and T_2 values of the surrounding dense parenchyma are similar to those of malignant disease.[6,9] If a carcinoma is small and the breast dense, detection, much less tissue characterization, is difficult if not impossible. Observed T_1 and T_2 values may be calculated, but this is a lengthy process, and for very small lesions the partial volume effect and the relatively small number of pixels available for sampling tend to lead to unreliable data.[1] These calculations are also of questionable value because of the nonhomogeneous content of parenchyma, fibroadenomas, and carcinomas. Fatty, fibrous, and ductal tissues may all be present in a malignant mass, resulting in a wide range of relaxation times. For MRI of the breast to be of practical value in everyday clinical practice, a method must be found to significantly increase the signal intensity of carcinoma over that of the surrounding breast parenchyma and, it is to be hoped, significantly above those of benign lesions. Moreover, the resultant difference in signal intensities must be readily apparent to the examining radiologist. Excessive dependence upon time-consuming calculations of T_1 and T_2 relaxation times will likely prove inefficient.

The development of suitable paramagnetic contrast agents may provide a solution to the problem of lack of specificity. Paramagnetic substances are for the most part metallic ions, such as those of copper, chromium, iron, magnesium, and gadolinium, with strong magnetic moments. These ions align themselves with the protons in the Z axis of a static magnetic field. When they are present in sufficient concentration in the body, they produce a local magnetic field, shortening the T_1 and T_2 relaxation times, and increasing signal intensity. The effect is greatest upon the adjacent hydrogen nuclei, producing a phenomenon described as "proton relaxation enhancement." *In vitro* and animal studies have been performed using a number of these agents, and gadolinium chelate (DTPA) has been successfully used in humans. The substance is given intravenously and distributed throughout the vascular system, to be excreted unchanged through the urinary tract. Following the injection of gadolinium DTAP, the altered signals are best seen on the inversion recovery pulse sequence. The effect of paramagnetic agents is complex and depends upon the agent, dose, pharmacokinetics of the tissue being studied, size of the lesion, and pulse sequence used to produce the image.[3,4,15]

The practical value of paramagnetic substances to MRI of the breast remains to be determined. A recent study has demonstrated an increase in the signal intensity of small masses following intravenous administration of gadolinium chelate. In this small series of cases, the sensitivity of this method for cancer was 100 percent, but its specificity was low. Fibroadenomas exhibited a similar increase in signal intensity.[7] Although additional work must be directed toward improving specificity, the absence of a heightened signal intensity following administration of gadolinium chelate might provide inferential evidence excluding malignant pathology in a patient with an equivocal x-ray mammogram, possibly avoiding the necessity for biopsy.

The optimal pulse sequences following the administration of paramagnetic substances may not be the same as those used without them. Excessively high levels of contrast enhancement may lead to decreased definition, and may prove paradoxically defeating, especially for small lesions. It must still be shown that paramagnetic substances can be safely administered in sufficient concentrations to permit the detection of small carcinomas in dense breasts.

SUMMARY

MRI of the breast is still in an early, experimental phase. The considerable degree of overlap in T_1 relaxation times between cancer and benign lesions is one of the greatest impediments to its success. Future research must be directed toward enhancing the MR signal so as to permit reliable detection and characterization of abnormal tissues and lesions. Development of a safe and effective paramagnetic substance to increase the difference between T_1 relaxation times of benign and malignant lesions could lead to the widespread clinical use of MRI of the breast. Technical improvements directed toward the reduction of the time needed for image acquisition can be expected. If the clinical value of MRI of the breast can be conclusively demonstrated, then further research can be directed toward the development of a dedicated and less costly system for breast imaging.

REFERENCES

1. Alcorn FS, Turner DA, Clark JW, et al: Magnetic resonance imaging in the study of the breast. RadioGraphics 5:631–652, 1985
2. Bovee WMMJ, Getreuer KW, Smidt J, et al: Nuclear magnetic resonance and detection of human breast tumors. Natl Cancer Inst 61:53–55, 1978
3. Brasch RC: Methods for contrast enhancement for NMR imaging and potential applications: A subject review. Radiology 147:781–788, 1983
4. Carr DH, Brown J, Bydder GM, et al: Gadolinium DTPA as a contrast agent in MRI: Initial clinical experience in 20 patients. AJR 143:215–224, 1984
5. Damadian R: Tumor detection by nuclear magnetic resonance. Science 171:1151–1153, 1971
6. El-Yousef SJ, O'Connell DM, Duchesneau RH, et al: Benign and malignant breast disease: Magnetic resonance and radiofrequency pulse sequences. AJR 145:1–8, 1985
7. Hegwant SSH: Presentation during "Contrast Agents in Magnetic Resonance Imaging." An International Workshop sponsored by the Berlex Corporation, January 17–18, 1986, San Diego, CA
8. Hollis PH, Economou JS, Pavlos LC, et al: Nuclear magnetic resonance studies of several experimental and human malignant tumors. Cancer Res 33:2156–2160, 1973
9. McSweeney MB, Small WC, Cerny V, et al: Magnetic resonance imaging in the diagnosis of breast disease: Use of transverse relaxation times. Radiology 153:741–744, 1984
10. Murphy WA: Magnetic Resonance Imaging of the Breast. A Syllabus for the Categorical Course on Magnetic Resonance. Am Coll Radiol, 1985, pp 274–286
11. NMR—A Perspective on Imaging. Milwaukee, General Electric Company, 1982
12. Partain CL, James AE, Rollo FD, et al. (eds): Nuclear Magnetic Resonance Imaging. Philadelphia, WB Saunders, 1983
13. Pavlicek W, Modic M, Weinstein M: Pulse sequences and significance. RadioGraphics 4:49–65, 1984
14. Ross RJ, Thompson JS, Kyung K, et al: Nuclear magnetic resonance imaging and evaluation of human breast tissue: Preliminary clinical trials. Radiology 143:195–205, 1982
15. Runge V, Clanton JA, Hehyer MS: Intravascular contrast agents suitable for magnetic resonance imaging. Radiology 153:171–176, 1984
16. Wolf GC, Popp C: NMR—A Primer for Medical Imaging. Thorofare, NY, Slack, Inc., 1984
17. Wolfman NT, Moran R, Moran PR, et al: Simultaenous MR imaging of both breasts using a dedicated receiver coil. Radiology 155:241–243, 1985

Index